Engineering the Human Germline

Engineering the Human Germline

An Exploration of the Science and
Ethics of Altering the Genes
We Pass to Our Children

EDITED BY
GREGORY STOCK AND
JOHN CAMPBELL

New York   Oxford
Oxford University Press
2000

Oxford University Press

Oxford   New York

Athens   Auckland   Bangkok   Bogotá   Buenos Aires   Calcutta
Cape Town   Chennai   Dar es Salaam   Delhi   Florence   Hong Kong   Istanbul
Karachi   Kuala Lumpur   Madrid   Melbourne   Mexico City   Mumbai
Nairobi   Paris   São Paulo   Singapore   Taipei   Tokyo   Toronto   Warsaw

and associated companies in
Berlin   Ibadan

Copyright © 2000 by Gregory Stock and John Campbell

Published by Oxford University Press, Inc.
198 Madison Avenue, New York, New York 10016

Oxford is a registered trademark of Oxford University Press.

Library of Congress Cataloging-in-Publication Data
Engineering the Human Germline : an exploration of the science and
ethics of altering the genes we pass to our children / edited by
Gregory Stock and John Campbell.
    p.   cm.
Includes bibliographical references and index.
ISBN 0-19-513302-1
1. Medical genetics.   2. Medical genetics—Moral and ethical
aspects.   3. Genetic engineering.   4. Genetic engineering—Moral and
ethical aspects.   5. Human cloning.   6. Human cloning—Moral and
ethical aspects.   I. Stock, Gregory.   II. Campbell, John H. (John
Howland), 1938–   .
RB155.E56   1999
174'.25—dc21   99-15224

9 8 7 6 5 4 3 2 1

Printed in the United States of America
on acid-free paper

Preface

Germline genetic manipulations are those made to "germinal" or reproductive cells—the egg or sperm—and they can alter both the immediate patient and his or her descendants. This is a major extension of today's genetic therapies and, until recently, most ethicists and scientists have found the idea of allowing such interventions in humans virtually unthinkable. But technology has now advanced to the point where the unthinkable needs to be carefully examined.

This book explores both the prospects for, and the larger implications of, human germline engineering. The book's three sections come at these issues in very different ways. In part I, seven leading scientists lay a solid groundwork by assessing the realistic possibilities and problems of this technology. Too often when genetic engineering is portrayed in the popular media, no distinction is made between fantasy and reality, but the issues surrounding human germline engineering cannot be intelligently debated without a solid grasp of the scientific realities of the technology. These seven essays—each prepared for an audience of nonspecialists—offer us that grasp. Gregory Stock and John Campbell, coeditors of this volume, begin with a vision for practical germline engineering. Leroy Hood, a key figure in the human genome project, describes the relevance of our rapidly expanding understanding of human genetics. Daniel Koshland, editor of *Science* magazine for more than a decade, offers his perspective on issues of safety and ethics. Mario Capecchi, a leading researcher who manipulates the genetics of mice, describes how germline engineering might take place in practice. French Anderson, the father of human gene therapy, lays out his misgivings about near-term use of germline technologies. Michael Rose, an expert in aging research, discusses the feasibility of eventually retarding the aging process. And Lee Silver, an architect of the reprogenetic vision, describes the tight linkages between germline genetic engineering and advanced in vitro fertilization technologies.

Part II is a looser look at the implications of germline engineering, a lively discussion in which the seven scientists from part I are joined by an ethicist, a public policy expert, and Nobel-laureate James Watson, codiscoverer of the structure of DNA and founder of the human genome project. Words are not minced in this extraordinary conversation that opens revealing windows into the issues surrounding the technology of germline engineering as well as the personalities and attitudes of key figures shaping the debate.

Part III—"Other Voices"—takes a broader perspective, through a diverse collection of short essays by scientists, ethicists, lawyers, theologians, and public-policy makers from both the United States and abroad who have thought deeply about these issues and contributed to discussion of them. Together, these essays show the breadth of opinion about the arrival of these genetic technologies looming at our doorstep. Each contributor was asked a specific question, either his or her concerns about widespread use of this technology, or his or her attitude about germline engineering were it ever shown to be safe and reliable. These thought-provoking responses are nuanced by their response to an additional and very personal question that each of us may one day face—"Would you be willing to genetically alter your own child-to-be, given a safe reliable technology offering a tempting possibility?" Their views may help us prepare for that day.

Many people were critical to the creation of this volume. Above all, we would like to thank the speakers at the "Engineering the Human Germline" symposium at UCLA in March 1998. Without the willingness of French Anderson, Andrea Bonnicksen, Mario Capecchi, John Fletcher, Leroy Hood, Daniel Koshland, Michael Rose, Lee Silver, and James Watson to speak publicly and forthrightly about this difficult and challenging topic, our volume could never have been produced. At present, there is considerable discussion of the challenges of human germline engineering in both scientific circles and the popular media. At the time of that conference, however, the climate contained much paranoia about frankly discussing these topics. Indeed, we were even warned that disruptions or demonstrations might well accompany the event. Thus, the speakers' courage in leading the way toward opening up this topic to reasonable discussion can only be applauded.

The book would also not have been possible without the help and support of a number of others. The funders of the symposium—William Stubing from the Greenwall Foundation and Doron Weber from the Alfred P. Sloan

Foundation—were not only generous in their support; they took a personal interest in the project, which was of tremendous value. Their desire to foster increased public dialogue and awareness of the emerging technology of human germline engineering was instrumental in supporting our work. Professor William Schopf provided critical assistance in many ways, but above all we would like to thank him for his faith in the project and his willingness to put the resources of the Center for the Study of Evolution and the Origin of Life at our disposal. The role of Donald Ponturo, the Special Projects Manager of the Program on Medicine, Technology, and Society, cannot be overstated. Not only was he intimately involved in coordinating the symposium and making it a success—he played a major role in editing and organizing this manuscript. Without him, the book could never have happened.

The support of the UCLA administration was also important, and we wish to acknowledge in particular the role of Vice-Chancellor Patel, Provosts Jerry Levey and Brian Copenhaver, and Dean Lenny Rome, who threw the weight of UCLA behind this effort and helped make it a success.

Finally, we wish to thank our agent, Joe Spieler, for his ongoing counsel and support in bringing this book into its current form, and our editor, Kirk Jensen, for his guidance and commitment to making this book all that it could be.

Los Angeles, California   G.S.
March 1989   J.C.

Contents

Contributors

Chapter Authors and Panelists

W. French Anderson is Director of Gene Therapy Laboratories and a professor of biochemistry and pediatrics at the University of Southern California School of Medicine. It was Dr. Anderson's pioneering efforts that led to the first human gene therapy trial in 1990. Dr. Anderson holds an M.D. from Harvard Medical School. He has published extensively, holds many board and editorial positions, and is the editor-in-chief of *Human Gene Therapy.*

Andrea Bonnicksen is a professor in the Political Science Department at Northern Illinois University. Dr. Bonnicksen has written various articles on preimplantation genetic diagnosis of human embryos, germline therapy, and other reproductive issues. She is the author of *In Vitro Fertilization: Building Policy from Laboratories to Legislatures* (New York: Columbia University Press, 1989), coeditor of *Emerging Issues in Biomedical Policy,* and a member of the Ethics Committee of the American Society for Reproductive Medicine.

Mario R. Capecchi received his doctorate from Harvard University and is Distinguished Professor of Human Genetics in the Department of Human Genetics at the University of Utah School of Medicine. His techniques for generating mice with specific targeted genes inactivated ("knock-out" mice) established a new way of exploring how genes work in mammals. He is a member of the National Academy of Science, and his honors include the Bristol-Myers Squibb Award for distinguished achievement in neuroscience as well as the 1996 Kyoto Prize.

John Fletcher received his Ph.D. from the Union Theological Seminary, New York. He researched his dissertation, "A Study of the Ethics of Medical Research," at the Clinical Center of the National Institutes of Health, where he later served as the first chief of its bioethics program. In 1980, French Anderson and he coauthored an influential article on the criteria for any trial of human gene therapy. He was one of the first in bioethics to explore the issues of germline gene therapy. In 1993, he was named Kornfeld Professor of Biomedical Ethics at the University of Virginia.

Leroy Hood received his M.D. from the Johns Hopkins Medical School and his Ph.D. from the California Institute of Technology. He has been a member of the National Academy of Sciences and the American Academy of Arts and Sciences since 1982, and he coedited *The Code of Codes* (Cambridge: Harvard University Press, 1993). Dr. Hood was Bowles Professor of Biology at the California Institute of Technology until he joined the University of Washington in 1992 as William Gates Professor of Biomedical Sciences and the founding chair of the Department of Molecular Biotechnology.

Daniel Koshland, Jr., received his doctorate from the University of Chicago. A professor of molecular and cell biology at U.C.-Berkeley since 1965, Dr. Koshland was the editor of *Proceedings of the National Academy of Sciences* from 1980 to 1985 and of *Science* magazine from 1985 to 1995. He has been a member of the National Academy of Sciences since 1966. Among his many honors are the Waterford Prize from the Scripps Institute and the National Medal of Science.

Michael R. Rose is a professor in the Department of Ecology and Evolutionary Biology at the School of Biological Sciences, U.C.-Irvine, and received his doctorate from the University of Sussex. He is the author of *Evolutionary Biology of Aging* (New York: Oxford University Press 1991) and editor of *Darwin's Spectre.* Dr. Rose's major research focus has been experimental tests of evolutionary theories of aging and fitness. Among other awards, he received the Busse Prize for research on aging from the World Congress of Gerontology.

Lee M. Silver received his doctorate from Harvard University. He is currently a professor at Princeton University in the Department of Molecular Biology, where he conducts research in mammalian genetics, evolution, reproduction, and developmental biology. Dr. Silver is the editor-in-chief of *Mammalian Genome* and the author of *Mouse Genetics: Concepts and Applications* (New York: Oxford University Press, 1995) and *Remaking Eden: Cloning and Beyond in a Brave New World* (New York: Avon, 1997).

James D. Watson, who shared the Nobel Prize with Francis Crick and Maurice Wilkins in 1962 for the discovery of the structure of DNA, received his Ph.D. from Indiana University. He joined the Harvard faculty in 1956 and became Director of Cold Spring Harbor Laboratory in 1976. From 1988 to 1992, Dr. Watson functioned as Director of the National Center for Human Genome Research of the National Institutes of Health, where he helped established the Human Genome Project. Dr. Watson has won numerous honorary degrees and awards and has been the president of the Cold Spring Harbor Laboratory since 1994.

Editors

John Campbell received his Ph.D. from Harvard University and postdoctoral training at the Institut Pasteur, Paris, and the Commonwealth Scientific and Industrial Research Organization (CSIRO) in Canberra, Australia, which runs the main government supported research laboratories in Australia. He is an elected fellow of the American Academy of Sciences, first holder of the Robert Wesson Fellowship on Scientific Philosophy and Public Policy, and the professor of neurobiology at the UCLA School of Medicine. Dr. Campbell's fields of research are genetics and evolutionary theory.

Gregory Stock received a Ph.D. from Johns Hopkins University and an M.B.A. from Harvard. In his 1993 book, *Metaman: The Merging of Humans and Machines into a Global Superorganism* (New York: Simon and Schuster), he examined the evolutionary significance of humanity's rapid technological progress; and at Princeton's Woodrow Wilson School he looked at the implications of recent breakthroughs in molecular genetics. Dr. Stock is now the director of the Program on Medicine, Technology and Society at UCLA's School of Medicine.

Short Essay Contributors

Paul R. Billings, M.D., Ph.D., is Chief Medical Officer and Deputy Network Director of the Heart of Texas Veterans Health Care System. A graduate of Harvard University, he is a clinical specialist in internal medicine and medical genetics. His research has focused on the immune system and, more recently, on the social impacts of biotechnology. He is presently a director of the Council for Responsible Genetics, which opposes germline genetic manipulation.

Lloyd R. Cohen holds a Ph.D. in economics from the State University of New York and a J.D. from Emory University. Dr. Cohen teaches law and economics at George Mason University in Virginia. As an outgrowth of his specialization in the application of economics to law, he has written and spoken extensively on his proposal to create a market in transplant organs as well as on a variety of other health-care issues.

George Ennenga was born in Illinois and was educated in the United States, Canada, and Europe at the Lawrenceville School, Princeton University, the Goethe Institute, the University of Toronto, and New York University. After teaching posts in Canada and the United States, he founded and now directs GXI, a think tank to produce works of art, philosophy, and literature. His works of art are exhibited internationally, and he has written several articles on "artificial evolution."

Kevin T. FitzGerald, S.J., Ph.D., is a research associate in the Departments of Medicine and Medical Humanities at the Loyola University Medical Center in Chicago. He received his Ph.D. in molecular genetics from Georgetown University and a doctorate in bioethics, also at Georgetown. The two principal foci of his research efforts at Loyola are the investigation of abnormal gene regulation in leukemia and the exploration of ethical issues in human genetics.

Rabbi Barry Freundel serves the Kesher Israel Congregation of the Georgetown Synogogue in Washington, D.C. From August 1986 through June 1989, he was Pre-Rabbinics Advisor and Director of Synagogue Services at Yeshiva University. He is an adjunct professor at Baltimore Hebrew University, an adjunct professor at American University, an adjunct instructor at the University of Maryland, and an adjunct professor of law at Georgetown University. In May 1997, he served as a consultant to the United States Presidential Commission on Cloning.

Jan C. Heller, Ph.D., is Director of the Center for Ethics in Health Care. He manages the center's development and its education, research, and consultation services. He is also responsible for ethics-related education and policy review at Saint Joseph's Health System in Atlanta. Dr. Heller is a frequent speaker at conferences, schools, and religious and civic organizations throughout the United States, and he regularly consults on issues in biomedical ethics and health care compliance.

Ruth Hubbard is Professor Emerita of Biology at Harvard University and coauthor, with Elijah Wald, of *Exploding the Gene Myth* (Boston: Beacon Press, 1999). She serves on the boards of the Council for Responsible Genetics and the Boston Women's Health Book Collective.

James Hughes, Ph.D., is a sociologist, bioethics consultant (www.change-surfer.com), and lecturer in ethics and health care administration at the University of Connecticut School of Medicine. From 1991 to 1996, he taught in the University of Chicago's Program in Clinical Medical Ethics. He writes on the topics of genetic engineering and health care policy and produces *Event Horizon,* a syndicated radio show about the future.

Sheldon Krimsky is the professor of urban and environmental policy at Tufts University. Professor Krimsky's research has focused on the linkages between science/technology, ethics/values, and public policy. He is the author of five books and has published over one hundred essays and reviews that have appeared in many books and journals. His latest book is titled *Hormonal Chaos: The Scientific and Social Origins of the Environmental Endocrine Hypothesis* (Baltimore: Johns Hopkins University Press, 1991).

Darryl Macer is an associate professor at the Institute of Biological Sciences of the University of Tsukuba, Tsukuba Science City 305, Japan. He has a Ph.D. in molecular biology, and he teaches and researches bioethics. He is the director of the Eubios Ethics Institute, based in New Zealand and Japan, which includes an international network on bioethics and genetics. He is a member of the HuGo (Human Genome Organization) and UNESCO committees on bioethics and the director of the IUBS (International Union of Biological Sciences) bioethics program. He has authored ten books and over one hundred papers on bioethics.

Alex Mauron initially trained as a molecular biologist and is now an associate professor of bioethics at the University of Geneva Medical School. He has published widely on the ethical issues of genetics and reproduction, as well as on clinical ethics. He is a regular contributor to the daily *Le Temps* and is a member of the Swiss Federal Ethics Commission on Genetic Engineering and of other ethics committees at various research institutions and health-care organizations.

Glenn McGee is an associate director and assistant professor at the University of Pennsylvania Center for Bioethics. The author of more than fifty articles on ethical issues in medicine, his books include *The Perfect Baby* (Lanham, Md.: Rowman and Littlefield, 1997), *The Human Cloning Debate* (Berkeley, Calif.: Berkeley Hills Books, 1998), and *Pragmatic Bioethics* (Nashville, Tenn.: Vanderbilt University Press, 1999). He is an NBC News commentator, director of www.bioethics.net, a 1998 Atlantic Fellow in Public Policy of the British Government and Commonwealth Foundation, and a commissioner on the National Molecular and Clinical Genetics Task Force of the FDA.

Erik Parens is now the associate for philosophical studies at The Hastings Center, a bioethics think tank in Garrison, New York. He has published extensively on the ethical and social questions raised by biotechnological advances; he is also the editor of *Enhancing Human Traits: Ethical and Social Ramifications* (Washington, D.C.: Georgetown University Press, 1998) and coeditor of *Prenatal Genetic Testing and the Disability Rights Critique* (Washington, D.C.: Georgetown University Press, forthcoming).

Gregory E. Pence wrote *Who's Afraid of Human Cloning?* (Lunham, Md.: Rowman and Littlefield, 2000 [3rd ed.]) and has taught for twenty-three years at the University of Alabama at Birmingham, where he is a professor in the Department of Philosophy and the School of Medicine. He wrote *Classic Cases in Medical Ethics: Accounts of the Cases that have Shaped Medical Ethics*, (Boston: McGraw-Hill, 1995) and edited *Classic Works in Medical Ethics* (Boston: McGraw-Hill, 1998).

Sandy Thomas received her Ph.D. from the University of London. She lectured in genetics at London University for several years before moving to the Science Policy Research Unit at the University of Sussex, U.K. Over the next nine years she developed a wide-ranging research program on biotechnology policy and has published several articles on intellectual property issues. In 1997 she became Director of the Nuffield Council on Bioethics.

Stefan F. Winter is the director for science, research, and ethics at the Federal Physician's Chamber in Cologne, Germany. He is a medical doctor and molecular biologist, a former vice-president of the European Committee for Biomedical Ethics, and the present chairman of the European Working Party on Human Genetics. Dr. Winter teaches public health at the Medical Faculty of the University of Bonn and has published in the field of tumor immunology as well as on biomedical ethics and health technology assessment.

Burke K. Zimmerman, whose Ph.D. is in biophysics, is CEO and Chairman of Spectrum Medical Sciences Ltd., a vaccine-discovery company in Helsinki, Finland. He has taught courses in ethics and human values in science, technology, and medicine at George Washington University, U.C.-Berkeley, and Helsinki University. He has held bioethical policy positions with the U.S. Congress and the National Institutes of Health, and he continues to write and lecture on bioethical issues.

Engineering the Human Germline

Introduction

An Evolutionary Perspective

Germline engineering is not a common expression, so it's important to make sure we understand it. Human germline manipulations are those made to the genes of our "germinal," or reproductive, cells—the egg and sperm. In practice, this today means altering the fertilized egg—the first cell of the embryo-to-be—so that the genetic changes will be copied into every cell of the future adult, including his or her reproductive cells. Normally such changes would also be passed forward to future generations; but as we shall see in Mario Capecchi's essay, "Human Germline Gene Therapy: How and Why," this need not always be the case.

Germline technology stands in sharp contrast to the genetic therapy of today, which is "somatic" in that it targets cells of the "soma," or body; for example, genetic insertions to treat cystic fibrosis are directed at cells in the lining of the lung mucosa. Somatic interventions do not reach beyond the patient being treated, so their potential scope is obviously more limited than a germline intervention; but one still might wonder why *germline* therapy is viewed as so consequential a step for humanity. After all, when we use contraceptives, fertility drugs, in vitro fertilization (IVF), or artificial insemination, or even when we choose our mates, the consequences reverberate through future generations.

As manipulations, however, all these actions seem indirect or at least nonspecific when compared to human germline engineering—which, by giving us the capacity to intentionally change the genes of our children-to-be, promises to harness the full power of molecular genetics and turn it back upon our own selves. Germline engineering touches the very core of what it means to be human: It palpably extends human power into a

3

sacred realm, once mysterious and beyond reach. It forces us to look at the degree to which our genetic constitutions shape us. It brings up questions about the adequacy of our collective wisdom. It makes us look at how far we wish to intrude in the genetic flow from one generation to the next.

Even now the evening news routinely features breakthroughs from the Human Genome Project and from work on in vitro fertilization, animal cloning, and artificial chromosomes; human germline engineering will increasingly become a major focus of discussion, soul-searching, and legislation. With human germline engineering, we are beginning to seize control of our own evolution, and yet we have barely begun to grapple with the consequences. Ultimately, we will have to face the question lying at the heart of the emerging international debate about the application of molecular genetics to humans: How far are we willing to go in reshaping the human body and psyche?

By raising the possibility of meaningful human design, germline engineering uniquely captures the challenge of our coming era. Though other technological advances may immerse us in a radically different world, they will by and large leave the essentials of our biology unchanged.

Our lifetimes are so short, our human perspective so narrow, and the changes going on around us so enormous that it is challenging to appreciate just how extraordinary is this moment of time in which we are living. But things are happening today that are absolutely without precedent in the entire history of life on this planet. To see the larger implications of human germline engineering, it helps to step back and consider two other momentous developments underway. The first is space travel: We may be getting blasé about it, but for 3.5 billion years life has been constrained to a thin film on the surface of our planet, and now—through us—it has quite suddenly begun to move out towards the stars. A second is the arrival of the computer chip. It is beginning to seem almost commonplace now, but nonliving material (basically sand) is being imbued with a complexity that rivals that of life itself. These breakthroughs will define our future. And genetic engineering is comparable to them.

As we unravel our own blueprint and begin to tinker with it, we are becoming subject to the same powerful forces of conscious design that have already so completely reshaped the world around us. And as these forces reflect back upon us, life is entering a new phase in its history. Quite literally, we are seizing control of our own evolution, taking the reins, so to speak. How can this not be fraught with controversy? It is mind-boggling to try to imagine the shape of the human enterprise and of our own selves even a millennium from now, much less in the hundreds or thousands of millennia that have been meaningful in traditional evolutionary terms.

To what extent will we transform ourselves? We cannot know, but we can be relatively confident that we will eventually gain the power to do so. Of course, speculation about the shape of the distant future is unprovable, and it is certainly not the subject of this book. We bring it up merely to emphasize the larger implications of the unraveling of our biology. In this text, we will largely direct our attention towards potential human germline interventions that might become feasible in a time frame that is meaningful to us and our children, therapeutic possibilities that may exist or be under serious consideration within a few decades. Trying to look further would almost certainly reveal more about our own hopes and fears than the eventual shape of the future, because critical developments we do not foresee are bound to have major consequences. Even twenty-five years ago, no geneticists imagined that breakthroughs in gene sequencing, molecular genetics, and computers would put us where we are today.

The real question about germline engineering is not whether the technology will become feasible, but when and how it will. The fundamental discoveries that will enable this technology will occur whether or not we actively pursue them, because they will emerge from research deeply imbedded in the mainstream, research directed not towards the goal of achieving human germline engineering, but towards other less controversial goals. Four such arenas of research stand out:

- *Medicine.* The somatic genetic engineering pioneered by French Anderson and others has yet to bring significant new treatments, but it has brought exciting possibilities and is generously supported. Such therapy offers entirely new approaches for treating diseases that have hitherto been untreatable. Society could not easily relinquish such clinical possibilities, and many of the advances developed to achieve them will be readily applicable to germinal cells.
- *Fertility research.* Babies born by in vitro fertilization were once labeled "test-tube" babies and were a subject of serious concern. But now, some twenty years later, IVF has become the obvious choice for tens of thousands of couples who could not otherwise have children.[1] Enormous energies will continue to be devoted to these technologies because they are in serious demand and because society generally approves of giving couples additional reproductive options. When germline engineering appears, it will necessarily be as an adjunct to IVF, so this research effort—driven by its own powerful dynamics—cannot help but lay a foundation for eventual human germline engineering.
- *The Human Genome Project.* Whether the human genome is completely unraveled in the two years now being discussed[2] or in the five years originally projected, it is clear that eventually the information will revolutionize biology and medicine. There will be no turning back from

this grand project, and its fruits cannot help but lay the foundation for both somatic and germline therapies. When coupled with gene-chip technology, which will provide rapid and inexpensive genetic profiling, and genomics, which will elucidate the relationships between our genetics and our physiology, the Human Genome Project will almost certainly yield a host of enticing ways to intervene in our own genetics.

- *Animal research.* Basic research to explore the underlying biology of life is taking place not only in academic institutions all over the world, but also within corporations trying to produce better pharmaceuticals or improve crops and livestock. Cloning was developed for use on animals, not humans, but that will hardly prevent its eventual extension to humans. The same will be true for other breakthroughs in our ability to manipulate the genetics of laboratory organisms, because there is no gulf between human and nonhuman biology.

If it is inevitable that we will gain the capacity to engineer the genetics of our germinal cells, then it is critical to begin to ask who should be allowed to use the technology, when, in what circumstances, and in what ways. In the past, many scientists and ethicists have dismissed serious discussion of this by asserting either that it is not a journey we should begin, or that the technology is so distant that we can let our grandchildren or great-grandchildren grapple with it. But recently we have witnessed the birth of Dolly, the creation of stable artificial human chromosomes, and the culturing of human embryonic stem cells. Molecular biology and genetics are progressing rapidly, and human germline engineering no longer looks so distant. Indeed, rudimentary procedures could be done today— though not with the safety any responsible physician would demand.

The popular media tend to focus on the more lurid and dangerous distant possibilities of human germline engineering, rather than the mundane therapeutic ones that may develop in the immediate years ahead. This is not surprising, for the ghosts associated with the idea of altering the genetics of our children are haunting ones. The pseudoscience of the eugenics movement of the 1920s and Hitler's brutal attempts to create a master race are far too vivid to ignore, but they should not determine our future in a realm where the possibilities and challenges are so enormous. Now, while the technology is still nascent, is the time to examine germline engineering in a frank, intelligent way. The goal of this book is to lay a solid foundation for that examination and move us toward a broad discussion of the technology's implications.

PART I

THE REALITIES OF HUMAN GERMLINE ENGINEERING

JOHN CAMPBELL
GREGORY STOCK

A Vision for Practical Human Germline Engineering

This essay looks as concretely as possible at the practical aspects of engineering genetic changes in the human germline. Engineering our genomes often conjures up science fiction images of turning people into Supermen and Star Trek creatures. In light of the enormous cataclysms of the past century, such vivid pictures cannot help but influence us, but they do not reflect reality. Hollywood scenarios are as irrelevant to evaluating the merits of germline engineering as worries of computers taking over the world are to deciding whether to put computers into the schoolroom. The foreseeable prospects which concern us are for discrete, relatively uncontroversial improvements in our health. For the next decade or two, germline genetic engineering might best be thought of as "germline gene therapy," because most changes that can realistically be expected will be "therapeutic" in one way or another.

Already, genes are being manipulated to fight disease. Somatic gene therapists are currently treating illnesses by putting corrective genes into the body cells of patients. Injecting genes into a fertilized egg will extend gene therapy to the germline. This is an important extension, because it will automatically introduce the genetic changes into every cell of the body without having to intervene in each cell individually. Effects can be limited to the cells that need them by controlling the expression of the altered genes so that they are active only where they should be. This is how the genome operates during normal development. The simplicity of introducing genes through the germline makes it not just another type of gene therapy, but the *ultimate* form of such therapy.

Extending gene therapy to the germline will demand two technical developments: The first is a practical procedure to introduce changes into a human egg. The procedure must be safe, reliable and, above all, practical. Ideally, it should allow us to introduce many improvements into an egg at one time and to do so without interrupting the rest of the genetic program. The second is the creation of genetic improvements with enough promise to inspire us to use them. These two prerequisites are difficult, but geneticists are substantially closer to both of them than is generally appreciated. First, consider how to deliver the genes.

Currently, geneticists manipulate the germline of animals by adding or changing a gene in an existing chromosome of a germline cell. A new approach just becoming feasible is to introduce a new gene on a new additional chromosome. Adding new genes on a newly added chromosome—*double addition*—is the least intrusive strategy, because it leaves the original genome entirely untouched. Furthermore, the technology is rapidly developing. Geneticists already have artificial chromosomes that will persist for repeated divisions when injected into human cells.[1]

A chromosome for double-addition germline engineering (fig. 1) would have no genes of its own but, instead, a series of "docking" sites where designed genes could be inserted using enzymes. It would serve as a universal delivery vehicle for cassettes of genes that medical geneticists fashion for various therapeutic purposes. Initially, only a few safe and effective genetic cassettes will be available, but eventually hundreds might be incorporated into a germline cell, each offering its own particular improvement. The chromosome could be offered to prospective parents in an infertility clinic. These clinics now routinely collect eggs from a woman, fertilize them in vitro, and implant the zygote into her womb. In the future, techicians

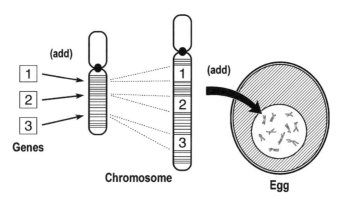

Figure 1. Human germline engineering by double addition. Cassettes of specific genes and their regulatory sequences are loaded at preset docking sites along an artificial chromosome that is then injected into a fertilized egg.

might inject a loaded artificial chromosome into the eggs as an optional extra step.

Chromosomes for human eggs will need other ancillary features. It will be desirable to keep certain gene cassettes inactive until their recipient grows into an informed consenting adult who can decide whether to activate them. It also will be useful to specially design the chromosome to be easy to handle, easy to introduce genes into, and easy to verify that the chromosome and its genes have been properly incorporated into an egg. Most importantly, a mechanism will be needed to prevent the chromosome from being inherited by future generations. Clearly, our earliest genetic modifications should not become permanent parts of the human gene pool. Even were germline engineering perfectly safe, children who received auxiliary chromosomes would one day want to give their own children the most up-to-date set of genetic modifications available, not the outdated ones they themselves had received a generation earlier. It would be difficult to prevent the inheritance of changes scattered throughout the genome, but if changes were confined to an auxiliary chromosome, that chromosome could simply be designed to be nonheritable. Chromosomes could be blocked in a variety of ways from passing through the sexual cycle to the next generation.

Considering the rapid pace of development of artificial chromosomes for the construction of transgenic animals and for human somatic gene therapy, very sophisticated chromosomes will likely be available for human germline engineering within a decade.

A more extensive task than constructing an auxiliary chromosome for human germline engineering will be to design the gene cassettes to place on it. Our understanding of human genetics is still fragmentary; even so, we know enough to begin designing a variety of worthwhile cassettes. Here are two concrete possibilities.

The first protects a person from AIDS. The AIDS virus, HIV, infects only certain cell types made in a person's bone marrow, most notably, T helper cells. AIDS workers are testing a variety of artificial genes which might make engineered T cells resistant to the virus. They include genes for a ribozyme, an antisense RNA, a dominantly defective viral protein, and a truncated anti-HIV immunoglobulin, among others.[2] Gene therapists hope to insert one or another of these genes into bone marrow stem cells of AIDS patients so that they would produce HIV-resistant T cells.[3] Engineering the bone marrow of an adult AIDS patient to produce new T cells is an extraordinarily ambitious goal and might not be possible at all in view of the complex way that mature T cells are formed. It would be far more feasible to introduce the resistance gene into the germline. This would prevent AIDS rather than treat it.

For safety, any resistance gene introduced into the germline should be regulated so that it is expressed only where it is needed, namely, in the T helper cells and their relatives. It seems unlikely that the sorts of molecules used in this case would be harmful to other cells, but the first safety principle for germline genetic engineering should be to express a new or altered gene in the minimum range of cells needed.

Genes are highly amenable to regulation.[4] Chromosomes have two types of genetic elements along their DNA: genes themselves, each of which codes for a unique protein that contributes in some way to the functioning of the organism, and regulatory sequences, which control when and where particular genes are expressed. There are many different classes of regulatory elements. The best understood is the promoter, a short stretch of DNA at the beginning of a gene. Promoters are attachment sites for special proteins that enable the gene to be expressed. These proteins are called transcription factors, because transcription is the first step in gene expression. Every promoter requires one or more particular transcription factor that specifically recognizes that promoter, attaches to it, and initiates the transcription process. If a cell does not make a particular transcription factor, the genes that are dependent on it will not be expressed. Our genome codes for thousands of different transcription factors. Each cell type makes its own unique subset of them for the proteins it needs.

HIV enters only those cells that make a protein called CD4 for their surface.[5] Therefore, an obvious strategy to regulate an introduced HIV-resistance gene is take the promoter (and other regulatory sequences) from the CD4 gene and paste it in front of that gene. That way, the resistance gene will be expressed only in the cells, such as T cells, that the virus can enter.

Actually, the CD4 gene's regulatory sequences are far more complex than just a single promoter. Multiple sites that bind multiple transcription factors are scattered across a long segment of DNA in and around the CD4 gene.[6] Fortunately, vast quantities of DNA shouldn't be a problem for engineering with an auxiliary chromosome, so the inserted HIV-resistance gene could be surrounded by tens of thousands of base pairs of DNA copied from the CD4 region. This would give the inserted gene the expression pattern of the CD4 gene without even identifying the individual controls that were copied.

HIV is a useful example because it is the focus of so much research. The first viral resistance genes developed for antiviral gene therapy may well be for this virus. The general approach we have outlined for HIV could be extended to other intractable viruses as well, admitting, of course, that each will present its own unique challenges. Imagine, for example, a child never getting a cold during his or her entire life. For millions of years, cold viruses have evolved strategies to evade our immune systems, but they will be naive to strategies that genetic engineers can use against them.

Cancer is a second important target for germline engineering. It presents a complex challenge. The key to one strategy for treating cancer is that certain transcription factors activate their promoters only in the presence of a hormone, such as testosterone.[7] Such transcription factors are called hormone receptors because they function only when they bind a hormone molecule. The bound hormone bends the shape of the receptor so that it can attach to its promoter and activate the gene. Without the hormone, the receptor will not even bind to the DNA. The testosterone receptor is, in essence, a switch that testosterone flips on or off. Add the hormone and the gene goes on; remove it and the gene goes silent. Estrogen and other steroid hormones work the same way, each binding its own specific receptor to activate its own hormone-dependent promoters. Even lower animals control gene expression with steroid hormone/receptor systems. For example, ecdysone and ecdysone receptor constitute a system unique to insects.[8]

Figure 2 shows how the ecdysone switch of insects can be fashioned as a cocked gun that could be triggered, when necessary, to surgically excise cancer cells. The gun is the gene that codes for Diphtheria toxin, a lethal cellular poison. The gene is activated by ecdysone, through an ecdysone-dependent promoter. This promoter will be snipped from an insect genome and pasted in front of the toxin gene.

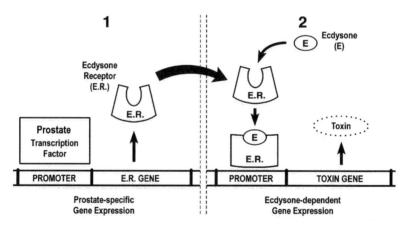

Figure 2. A two-gene cassette to protect against prostate cancer. Gene 1 codes for ecdysone receptor, which is expressed from a prostate-specific transcription factor. Ecdysone receptor functions as an ecdysone-dependent transcription factor to control the expression of gene 2, which codes for diphtheria toxin. When ecdysone is present, the toxin gene is expressed in prostate cells and the cells die. The toxin gene is not expressed in any other cells, because no other cells synthesize the ecdysone-dependent transcription factor.

Humans do not make ecdysone receptor, so its gene must also be taken from an insect genome and supplied in a second module of the cassette. Here, the gene is given a promoter that is active only in the glandular cells of the prostate, which are the ones vulnerable to cancer. This is the same sort of cell type–specific regulation we saw with the CD4 promoter, which was active only in T cells.

This is how the cassette operates: Ecdysone receptor will be synthesized continuously in the glandular cells of the prostate, but nowhere else. It will remain inactive because no ecdysone is present. If prostate cancer were ever diagnosed, or even suspected, a man would get an injection of ecdysone. The hormone would activate the ecdysone receptors in his prostate glandular cells, which would "turn on" the diphtheria gene, resulting in diphtheria toxin that would kill the cells. One shot and the cancer would be gone. Ecdysone would be present throughout the body, but only prostate cells would have the ecdysone receptor to which it would bind, because ecdysone is not a natural hormone of humans.

This strategy is generalizable to other sites. By changing the promoter for the ecdysone receptor gene, this same cocked gun could be aimed at the breast, pancreas, or other vulnerable tissues. These germline engineering approaches for treating AIDS or cancer are not fantasy. They are realistic procedures and strategies that geneticists are already using to create valuable transgenic animals.[9]

The flip side to killing rogue cells is to prevent the death of cells we do not want to lose, for example, neuronal cells in Alzheimer's disease, Lou Gehrig's disease, Parkinsonism, macular degeneration, and stroke. Geneticists are already beginning to test gene insertions in animal models and human cell lines to find ones that might retard these neurodegenerative pathways.[10] When protective genes are finally identified, it will probably be more practical to reach all cells of the nervous system by inserting the genes into an egg than by trying to deliver them to billions of neurons individually.

It is intriguing that neuronal death in patients with neurodegenerative diseases is usually preceded by various combinations of the same common pathologies: oxidative damage, deposition of insoluble proteins, excitotoxicity (excessive stimulation), or induction of programmed cell death.[11] Health providers are especially interested in whether blocking one or more of these pathologies might prevent neurons from dying. If so, it might be that for neurodegeneration, as for cancers and viruses, one basic cassette type could eventually protect against a range of diseases.

Naturally occurring genes in the human gene pool will provide another source for germline improvement. There is enormous genetic variation among humans. Most genes occur in several alternative forms, called alleles, that constitute the genetic differences among people. For example blue and brown eye colors come from alternative alleles of the eye-color gene.

Some mutant alleles are worse than average, as we all know, but some rare gene forms have especially beneficial effects. We suggest the name "superallele" for an uncommon gene allele that notably extends a beneficial trait in the few lucky people who carry it. Geneticists are now developing methods to find superalleles in the chromosomes of particularly favored persons, for example, longevity superalleles in people who are very old and healthy, or protective superalleles in people who have high serum cholesterol levels but little coronary artery disease.

Superalleles are ideal genes for germline engineering. By definition, they have already demonstrated their effectiveness in humans. We can discover if they cause any undesirable side effects simply by examining the people who already have them. Finally, we only need to find superalleles, not understand how they work. Using superalleles for germline engineering holds the promise of enabling any prospective parents to endow their children with selections of the best gene variants our species has evolved.

Of course, we cannot just add a superallele to a fertilized egg, because the egg already has copies of that gene. The introduced superallele must substitute for the copies already present. To do this by double addition, a gene cassette would need a second module to block expression of the existing copies of the gene. Silencing genes is feasible; indeed, this is what the presumptive HIV-resistance genes discussed above would do—silence an essential HIV gene in an infected cell.

How many possibilities are there for germline improvement? No one knows, but when geneticists, pathologists, other biologists, and clinicians— especially experts in aging—put their minds to this problem, they will probably come up with hundreds. Devising these germline improvements on paper is important, both because it could lead to therapeutic interventions and because at this time it is the only way to concretize the immediate possibilities of human germline engineering. The next step is to actually construct DNA cassettes. This would have been a Herculean task fifteen years ago. Now, a good Ph.D. student might handle the challenge. An exciting, if ambitious, thesis project would be to conceive of a germline improvement, make the DNA cassette for it, and insert it into a mouse egg to show that it works. This entire project could be done without in any way using people or human embryos as subjects.

What scientists and the public need to realize is how close human germline engineering may be. The two research efforts needed to bring it into being—one to develop gene therapy strategies, the other to develop a system for their delivery—are rapidly proceeding in parallel. In a decade or two, they will come together, and human germline engineering will suddenly become feasible. Now is the time to begin broad public discussion of what we can, should, and will do with this challenging technology.

The Human Genome Project— Launch Pad for Human Genetic Engineering

Human germline engineering is a discipline of the future. Its objectives will be to reverse genetic defects or to enhance desirable human traits such as emotional stability, intelligence, or longevity. Genetic defects may occasionally be encoded primarily by a single gene and will, accordingly, be simpler to engineer than more complex traits that are encoded by many different genes. It is important to stress that complex traits encompass most of the interesting human features including intelligence, attractiveness, and many other physical and behavioral attributes. Three issues are important with regard to germline genetic engineering. First, what are the technical limitations of germline genetic engineering? Do we have the tools to carry out germline engineering in an effective, safe, and reasonable manner? These questions are covered in other essays. Second, to what extent do we understand the networks of genes that operate in concert to control interesting human traits? We cannot engineer humans without more or less fully understanding the gene systems that control the traits that we would like to engineer. Finally, society must make decisions based on the ethical and social issues surrounding germline engineering. The imperative is to have an informed and thoughtful public that can both understand the issues that germline engineering raises and make rational decisions about the alternatives it presents society. This essay will focus on the Human Genome Project, for this project provides the necessary tools and information for launching attempts to decipher interesting human traits. We will also examine the paradigm changes that the project has catalyzed to lead us to the systems biology that will be the central approach to biology and medicine in the twenty-first century.

Human Genome Project

The Human Genome Project is about deciphering human heredity.[12] Human heredity is encoded by our genomes—the twenty-three pairs of human chromosomes (of twenty-four distinct types, since there are two different sex chromosomes, X and Y) that are present in each and every one of our cells. The fundamental core of each human chromosome is a long string of DNA composed of 50 million to 250 million letters of the DNA language. The DNA language has four different letters, G, C, A, and T, and it is variation in these letters down the long strings of our chromosomes that encode one key type of information: the 100,000 or so human genes necessary for building humans. Indeed, our genome may be viewed as the most incredible software program ever written. It is a program that has been fashioned by 3.7 billion years of evolution, and it dictates the most fascinating of all biological processes, human development—the process whereby we all start as a single cell, the fertilized egg, and after many cell divisions emerge as an adult human organism of 10^{14} cells. There are many different types of human cells—muscle cells, brain cells, and bone cells—each of which carry out distinct functions. These distinct cell types or phenotypes are produced by a chromosomal choreography that specifies the appropriate subset of those 100,000 genes that must be expressed for each cell type to generate its particular functionalities.

The Human Genome Project is about two types of maps—genetic and sequence. To construct a genetic map, chromosomal markers, termed *genetic markers*, are identified across our chromosomes. It is these markers that give us the ability to locate genes which predispose to interesting physiological and/or disease traits. The Human Genome Project has identified 20,000 such genetic markers scattered across the human genome, and this genetic map has been used to identify more than 800 individual genes which predispose to a variety of human diseases, most quite rare.

The second type of map is termed a *sequence map*. It shows the order of each of the letters of the DNA language all the way across each of the twenty-four human chromosomes. It is proposed that the sequence map will be finished by the year 2003.[13] The sequence map is the ultimate map, because it gives us the information necessary to begin deciphering the human book of life, a task which undoubtedly will take one hundred or more years.

If we look back at the Human Genome Project in twenty years, it is apparent that three major benefits will have been achieved. First, we will have determined the periodic table of life. The periodic table of chemical elements, which was established in the ninteenth century, revolutionized our understanding of chemistry by providing insights into the fundamental relationship of the elements to one another. The periodic table of life now being provided by the Human Genome Project will, in the same way, provide the information necessary to gain insights into the fundamental elements of life—the genes and the regulatory machinery that turn genes on at the appropriate time in human development, in the appropriate cells, and express the genes at appropriate concentrations. This periodic table will allow us to take the 100 thousand or so human genes and deconvolute them into their basic building blocks, which are called motifs. These motifs will be important in understanding how the products of the genes, their proteins, actually execute their function. Finally, the periodic table of life will give us the ability to identify and begin to understand the nature of the variation in the DNA letters (polymorphisms) that occur between similar positions on the chromosomes of different individuals. For example, approximately 1 letter in 500 varies between the same chromosomes from two different individuals. Most of this variation has no effect on human traits because genes occupy only about 5 percent of our chromosomes—hence, most mutations lie outside genes. A very few of these polymorphisms modify genes which encode trait variations—for example, some people are tall and others short, some people are fat and others thin. More important, these polymorphisms encode, in part, the entire spectrum of human diversity with regard to interesting physiological and disease-predisposing traits. Therefore, identifying all the human genes, their regulatory machinery and polymorphisms, and their contributions to human traits will be a fundamental aspect of launching the germline engineering of the future.

The second contribution to come from the Human Genome Project will be the development of tools that can decipher biological information at very high rates of speed. Many genes or proteins will be able to be analyzed very rapidly with what are termed *high-throughput analytical* or *global tools*. I'll discuss two of them later.

The third and the most important contribution of the Human Genome Project will be the union of information we obtain from the periodic table of life with very powerful global tools for deciphering biological information; already this union has catalyzed a series of paradigm changes in biology that are leading to what is termed *systems biology*. These paradigm changes provide fundamental insights into how we will go about understanding the complex networks of genes that are engaged in most of the interesting human traits—a fundamental requirement for germline genetic engineering.

Paradigm Changes Arising from
the Human Genome Project

Biology is an informational science. This insight is a fundamental revolution in our view of biology. Biological information is of three different types. The first type is the linear or digital language of our chromosomes. As noted earlier, DNA employs a four-letter alphabet, and it is variation of these letters across the strings of information termed chromosomes that encodes genes, programs the regulatory machinery of genes, and specifies the other types of information necessary for chromosomes to execute their functions as informational organelles. The language of our genes is a code very similar to the digital code of our computers, but it has four rather than two letters. The units of information on our chromosomes, the genes, are expressed in a quantified manner; that is, different genes can be expressed in different cells. For different types of cells, different subsets of genes are expressed, and this leads to the features that distinguish, for example, brain from muscle cells.

The second type of biological information is the final product of the expressed gene information. Proteins are three-dimensional molecular machines that catalyze the chemistry of life and give the body shape and form. In looking at an individual, virtually everything one sees is protein. Proteins are initially synthesized as a linear string with a twenty-letter alphabet. The order of these letters in the string dictates how that string folds into three dimensions to create a molecular machine. Two challenges about proteins are fascinating. First, from the order of letters in the linear protein strings, can we actually predict how the string folds into three dimensions to make a particular molecular machine? The problem is partly experimental and partly computational, and we will have to enlist computer scientists and applied mathematicians to help solve it. Ultimately, however, the solution will rest in our ability to obtain the lexicon of motifs—or building block components—of genes and proteins that will come from the Human Genome Project. The second question about proteins is even more fascinating: Given a particular three-dimensional shape, how do we determine what function that protein executes? Once again, this is partly an experimental and partly a computational problem. Once we have solved these two problems, we will be in a position to carry out protein engineering—that is, the design of diagnostic, therapeutic, and even preventive reagents that may revolutionize medicine in the twenty-first century.

The study of individual genes and individual proteins has been the substrate of biology for the last thirty years or so. It has led to the striking successes of molecular biology. In a sense, the information about both individual genes and proteins is joined to create the third type of biological information—that which arises from complex biological systems and networks. For example, the brain is a complex network of 10^{12} brain cells joined by 10^{15} connections. This network generates fascinating systems or emergent properties such as memory, consciousness, and the ability to learn. In order to understand how these systems properties arise, one can no longer look at single genes, single proteins, or single cells. One has to look at the network of elements as they operate together in the system as a whole. One must be able to take this systems information and create mathematical models that can accurately predict the systems behavior and properties—for it is only through this modeling that we will come to truly understand systems properties. Again, for this, biologists must solicit the help of computer scientists and applied mathematicians. This is the challenge for the future. Global tools will be needed to look at many elements and connections at one time. These global tools will be illustrated shortly.

It is important to understand that there are two meanings to the words "decipher biological information." For example, the Human Genome Project proposes to determine the order of the letters of the DNA alphabet across each of the twenty-four human chromosomes—that is, to sequence the human genome. But determining the order of the DNA letters in human chromosomes is deciphering the DNA language at only one level. Understanding the actual information that 3.7 billion years of evolution has embedded in our chromosomes is another level of deciphering. These efforts will occupy perhaps the next 50–100 years. The following analogy is apt. The human genome contains 3 billion letters of the DNA language. If translated into an encyclopedia of how to construct a human, this text would require 500 volumes, each containing 1,000 pages that each average 1,000 six-letter words of the DNA language. To the biologist, reading this book now would be very much akin to your reading a book of atomic physics. You could understand some words, but most of the meaning would be undecipherable. Thus, biological experiments must be carried out to translate the DNA sequence into knowledge of human biology. In a similar vein, it is one thing to know the three-dimensional structure of a protein and quite another to understand how that three-dimensional structure permits its functions to be executed. Likewise, it is one thing to define the elements and connections of a biological system and quite another to understand how systems properties emerge from this network. Once again, it will be necessary to involve applied mathematicians and computer scientists in creating models to understand how systems properties emerge from the complexity of biological systems. The deciphering (in both senses) of biological information from complex biological systems and networks will constitute the most compelling challenge for biology and medicine as we move into the twenty-first century.

A second paradigm change is the realization that high-throughput analytic or global technologies for studying genes, proteins, and even cells are going to be critical to deciphering biological systems. Let me provide two examples of global tools. In the early 1980s, our group developed an automated machine for sequencing DNA that color codes the four different letters of the DNA language with four different fluorescent dyes.[14] The most advanced form of this machine can sequence almost 40 million letters of the DNA language in a single year.[15] Indeed, within six months, an even more advanced sequencing machine will be able to analyze approximately 150 million letters of the DNA language per year.[16] Large genome centers working on the Human Genome Project may have anywhere between 10 and 100 of these DNA sequencing machines. Thus, one can understand the incredible speed with which DNA sequence analysis can be carried out by this global tool—the automated fluorescent DNA sequencer.

DNA chips provide a second example of a global instrument. Over the past six or so years at the University of Washington, we have developed a technology using commercial ink jet printers whereby we will eventually be able to synthesize up to 100 thousand small fragments of DNA on a glass chip approximately the size of your thumbnail.[17] Other scientists have used the technique of photolithography to create DNA chips.[18] If each of these 100,000 fragments of DNA represents a different human gene, then once the human genome is sequenced, we have the capacity to look quantitatively at all of the genetic information that is expressed in human cells. For example, we will be able to compare the expression patterns of the 100,000 human genes in a normal prostate cell and in a cancer prostate cell to determine how the expression patterns of these genes change when the cell is transformed from its normal to a cancerous state. This global high-throughput analytic technology, accordingly, gives us the capacity to analyze all human genes simultaneously. These chips will also play an important second function by giving us the capacity to look simultaneously at many human genetic markers for polymorphisms.[19] Thus, in a similar manner, 100 thousand fragments of human DNA may let us look simultaneously at 50 thousand different polymorphisms (each genetic marker has two alternative forms). This ability to create very dense genetic maps is going to revolutionize human genetics and give us even more effective means of identifying the genes that control human traits. Obviously, both large-scale DNA sequencing and genetic marker analysis are key technologies for understanding human genes and the roles they play in human traits.

A third paradigm change is the imperative to recruit computer scientists and applied mathematicians into biology. The language barrier between these scientific disciplines presents an enormous challenge in bringing scientists from other disciplines to biology. Curiously, if biology is taught as an informational science, the language barrier can be greatly ameliorated. Computer scientists and applied mathematicians must bring to biology the ability to acquire, store, analyze, model, and ultimately disseminate the enormous amounts of information now being deciphered at all three levels of biological information.

The fourth and final paradigm change relates to the universality of biological information and the unity of life. The Human Genome Project proposes to sequence the genomes of five model organisms: bacteria, yeast, nematode (a simple roundworm), fly, and mouse. The genomes of the first three of these organisms are finished (9, 10, 11).[20] Remarkably, many human genes have identifiable counterparts (homologues) in bacteria, yeast, and the nematode. Therefore, one can study the function of these human homologues in biologically and genetically manipulable organisms to understand how these genes work and to delineate the informational pathways within which they operate. These insights can then be brought to human biology because of the common origin of all living organisms and the universality of their basic biological information pathways. It is proposed that the mouse genome will be finished by the year 2005, at which time we can use the mouse as a model system to understand complex traits shared only by higher organisms (e.g., nervous system, immune system, and so forth). Thus, the model organisms will be Rosetta stones for understanding human biology. Just as knowledge of the Greek language in the original Rosetta stone allowed the Demotic and hieroglyphic languages to be translated, so a knowledge of the bacterial, yeast, nematode, fly, and mouse genomes will allow the human genome to be deciphered.

In summary, four paradigm changes will propel us toward a systems biology that will be the launch pad for germline genetic engineering:

- biology is an informational science;
- global tools are the keys to deciphering biological systems;
- computer science and applied mathematics are critical to deciphering and modeling biological information; and
- model organisms are the Rosetta stones for deciphering human biology.

Germline Genetic Engineering: Simple and Complex Traits

Some human traits may be dominated by a single gene—examples include susceptibility to infectious diseases such as AIDS and certain types of cancer. This does not mean that the corresponding genes are not parts of complex informational pathways, rather that they exhibit a dominant effect in these pathways. In the case of these simple traits, one could think about germline engineering once the technical and ethical issues have been resolved. The interesting question is, how many such simple human traits exist, and which are appropriate for germline engineering?

Complex human traits are encoded in many genes representing complex informational pathways. Thus, complex traits include most interesting human traits—the ability to learn, memory, consciousness, physical attractiveness, and so on. It would be inappropriate to consider engineering these fundamental human traits before we understand the informational pathways and biological networks that encode them. For some of these traits, that may take decades or more.

Germline Genetic Engineering: Ethical Issues

The general public has a general concern, perhaps even distrust, about where human genetics (and the Human Genome Project) is taking us. This distrust arises, in part, from a vague apprehension about where science is taking society (e.g., weapons of mass destruction, the ambiguities of the benefits of atomic power, and so on) and in part from a conviction that genetic engineering of humans is unnatural and therefore wrong. To think rationally about ethical issues in germline engineering requires a basic understanding of inquiry-based analysis and a general scientific (biological) background. Most citizens lack one or both of these educational experiences. My own feeling is that scientists can play a catalytic role in educating society in these regards by making a commitment to helping school grades K–12 science education. Children are excited by hands-on, inquiry-based science experiences, as are their teachers. If all scientists were to make a commitment to improving K–12 science education in their local communities, we might eventually have a society capable of thinking analytically and rationally about the challenges and opportunities of science—including germline engineering.

This education of society is essential, because the Human Genome Project will be a launching pad for understanding systems biology, and once the technical and ethical issues surrounding germline engineering are resolved, humans will be in a position to direct their own evolutionary changes—for better or worse.

Ethics and Safety

From what I read in the press about the state of human germline genetic engineering, there is a large vocal group that says, "Scientists are the heroes of today; they brought us automobiles, pesticides, genetic engineering." And then there is another group, equally vocal, who say, "Scientists are the villains of today; they brought us automobiles, pesticides, and genetic engineering."

Some say that genetic engineering opens an enormous vista for mankind, and others say it's the beginning of a catastrophe, that even a small step such as curing a defective gene is also the first step down a slippery slope to disaster. There is talk of a moratorium before we do any more work on cloning, and there is fear of doing anything to the human genome, even curing a genetic defect.

All agree, however, that no serious catastrophe can result if we start thinking about the subject. Pericles in the glory days of Greece said to his troops, "Let us march." I say, "Let us think."

My aim in this chapter is to tackle the subject of safety and ethics. Unfortunately, there are probably as many ideas about appropriate standards of safety and ethics as there are readers. With so many different moral and safety standards in our population, my job is to try to pave the way to a possible consensus on these subjects. I shall start with safety. There is no such thing as absolute safety in this world, even though some in our legal profession believe that doing anything more dangerous than getting out of bed in the morning must have somebody responsible and financially liable. Yet most of us know that risks are relative and will take them if the potential gains seem to warrant them. So, perhaps a start on the design of safety standards in germline engineering is to ask that the technology be no more risky than the normal process of birth and conception. You might say that this is too tough a standard for a new therapy, because it doesn't allow room for error. But when you think it over, the normal process of conception and birth is really a very risky and dangerous proposition. If our criterion is that the children should turn out to be at least as good as their parents, my guess is that germline engineering will compete very well with those conceived the natural way. And if we make our criterion that the children should be up to their parents' expectations, then I think the engineered child may have a good edge over the child conceived the normal way.

Safety will require, first of all, that there be extensive experiments on animals to be sure that the techniques we would use to correct a defective gene carry only known risks and side effects and do not create any more problems for the mother than would a natural birth. We should expect the treated child to have a better chance of living a longer and more disease-free life than a natural child who has inherited the defective gene.

We must also figure out the dangers to the mother during the implantation, because natural childbirth can bring unforeseen complications, whether or not the child is engineered. Of course, the natural way of conception is going to be more fun, but we will be very solemn and only consider legal and moral risks. The safety issues are not solved yet, but the hurdles are technical and should be solvable in the not-to-distant future.

Now we come to the question of ethics. I looked up the Webster's dictionary definition of ethics. It says, "The study and evaluation of human conduct in the light of moral principles. Moral principles may be viewed either as the standard of conduct which the individual has constructed for himself or the body of obligations and duties which a particular society requires of its members." That struck me as pretty easy. If the standard of moral principles are my own, they are clearly the best. But the definition implies that everyone is entitled to his own set of moral principles. I guess the second part of the definition—that we have to find a set of responsibilities by which society will live—is a better goal. We should start, perhaps, with the question raised by those who say we shouldn't tamper with the germline. I frankly don't understand these people. Where are they living? We are already altering the germline right and left. When we give insulin to a diabetic who then goes on to have children, we are increasing the number of defective genes in the population. No one is seriously suggesting we refuse to give life-saving drugs to genetically disadvantaged people.

We attempt to treat cystic fibrosis, yet we are damaging the germline every day by doing so. Are we doing something terrible by ameliorating the illnesses that our compassionate policies of the present and past have helped create?

I had 20/400 vision when I was a child. If I had been living in the jungle and a saber-tooth tiger had come up fairly close, I would have reached out and said, "Nice kitty," then tried to pet it. I wouldn't have survived for long. But I was nurtured by parents who gave me glasses and kept me in a home free of saber-tooth tigers, so some of my children have inherited my bad vision. If that could be corrected in subsequent generations, should we prevent it?

There are technical difficulties to germline manipulation, and endless problems to be solved, but certainly the emotional statement, "We can't modify the germline," means we must stop all therapies and alter the survival of the less fit as well as block new future germline treatment. As I said at the beginning, "Let us think."

We next come to the question of cloning. There are a number of technical research problems here, too, that must be solved before we can really begin cloning, including, of course, the issue of safety that I mentioned above. But it would be foolish to ignore the high probability that technical problems will be solved. So, we should think about whether we should clone humans if we are able to. If we shouldn't, there's no use even doing the research to make it possible.

My first reaction when I heard the idea of human cloning was: "Oh, that's terrible. This time those scientists have gone too far." Then I started to think a bit, and I thought, "Well, if they had eight people just like me and we were all on the Supreme Court, it would really save the United States." So I thought further.

One of the complaints we hear periodically is that it is the egotists, the megalomaniacs, and the rich who will want to clone themselves, and that isn't fair or good. I am skeptical of this notion. Individuals, and particularly egotists, are usually interested in establishing a life record that is not only considerable but also unique. Some people like to win an Olympic gold medal, be an upstanding leader of the community, be a devoted patriarch of a family, and so forth. Others yearn to be a famous bank robber, or a charming swindler, or a distinguished artist—different goals for different souls, but unique for each. Would they really want to clone themselves? My guess is that people's demands for self-cloning will be very low.

The demand for gene enhancement therapy in order to try to give your children a better chance of success in the world will probably be very large. So outlawing the cloning of one's self seems to me a little like outlawing ballooning around the world. A balloon flying around the world may land in your backyard and do some damage, but the frequency of this really doesn't require that we pass a law against ballooning around the world. And similarly, we should not try to outlaw research on human cloning before any indication of widespread use is apparent.

Cloning, in my opinion, is likely to be most appealing to those who want to emulate someone more clever or more handsome or more athletic than themselves. That will require humility, not egotism. One is saying, "My children will be better with somebody else's genes rather than mine."

Let us imagine an infertile couple faced with the need for artificial insemination. If that's the only way they can get a child, would they be better off taking a natural child with a stranger's genes than a clone from a known person of the family who led a commendable life? As we know, children of even the best parents can turn out to be quite peculiar disappointments. Some just don't care to study and go to college—the same college that Dad and Grandpa or Mom and Grandma went to. Or some child of a long line of clergymen will decide to go into the theater and disgrace the family and run around with loose people. Or others smoke pot and live a wild life and become president of the United States.

It would surely be safer and surer to clone good old Uncle Ebenezer, who paid his bills, went to church, stayed married to the same woman, and voted the straight party line all his life. That would certainly be better than taking part in the gene lottery.

On thinking it over, though, I begin to worry that cloning might be the most conservative thing society could do. We'd all pick successful, humdrum, middle-of-the-road people to ensure that our children turned out all right. We wouldn't take a chance on the new, different, quite strange person that our children might become.

Before we take up the slippery-slope argument, let's think carefully about it, because all human progress can be negated by this argument. I'm sure that in the Middle Ages, if citizens in the time of Henry VIII had been told that serfs would someday ride around in horseless carriages and would someday have enough money to go off on their own and do crazy things like read books and vote, they would have said, "That will be the end of civilization, the family as we know it, and the village as we know it."

There is nothing you can think of that would be worse than having serfs loose all around the world getting educated and voting. It reminds me of the statement made in the early days of aviation by some of its opponents, "If God had wanted us to fly he would never have made railroad tracks."

What strikes me as missing from the doomsday scenarios regarding the ethics and safety of human cloning is the incredibly gradual timetable of events if we allow it. We are not talking about an atomic bomb or a bubonic plague. Procedures for cloning will be expensive and individualized. If we had a few clonings, and people started abusing it, we could always pass a law and stop the procedures.

A few new people can hardly be threatening to society. On average, they would probably be no better or worse than the children who are now produced by statesmen, thieves, scientists, embezzlers, philanthropists, artists, and even politicians—in short, everyone who is now allowed to have children of their own.

If we do go ahead with germline engineering, as I think we should, I can't see any possible reason for not allowing enhancement therapy. We are facing monumental problems with the population explosion, environmental pollution, the shortage of fossil fuels, and the serious lack of leadership. Our science and our compassion prevents us from using survival of the fittest as a process of selection even though it has guided us through evolution up to this point. Should we turn our back on new methodologies that might bring us smarter people and better leaders who are more responsible in their lives? It's going to be tricky, but it seems silly to shut our eyes to a new technology like this.

If, for example, we could clone an Abraham Lincoln or an Einstein or a Beethoven, should we say No? I'm going to use dead people just to illustrate the kind of people to consider, but I'm not hinting we have their DNA. If we could help the common man have children who could more easily get jobs and do better in a computer society, should we say No?

In a democracy, the government of the people must make the final decision on genetic engineering. But we need to discuss how intrusive the government should be in individual matters of genetic engineering and in the cloning of people. If an ordinary person like me wants to clone Franklin D. Roosevelt for one of his children, will he need a license? Will the government say, "No, you really run a terrible household. It's disorganized and you don't take out the garbage on time. Very bad early training for a Franklin Roosevelt."

Or even if they approve it for him, suppose twenty other people want to clone Franklin Roosevelt. Would that be too many in the population? We'd have to make some kind of ruling that if somebody is a Franklin Roosevelt he can't advertise that when he runs for office. If he said, "I have the genes of Franklin Roosevelt," that might get him elected even if he's no good.

If someone wants to clone Jack the Ripper, do we really have anything to say about that? The government is not allowed to say "yes" or "no" on having children now, but cloning presents new problems and, possibly, like driving an automobile, you will need some kind of a license.

So, I think there are major problems, but I think it would be absolutely ridiculous to stop now. It is correct to have a temporary moratorium. We need to think seriously about the consequences from all the angles, assembling people with different thoughts and ideas. We don't need political stump speeches by either scientists or politicians; we need to come together and say, "What are the major problems and how are we going to solve them?"

The easy slogans, such as "It will cure all genetic disease" or "It's a slippery slope to Armageddon" are much too superficial to guide our thinking. These genetic engineering technologies have real benefits and risks, and we'd better think long and hard about them.

I'm reminded of a story about a Maine farmer who'd built a nice-looking farm, in the rather hostile countryside. The farm was in a lovely valley, along a hillside. There were nice furrows plowed in the ground and a stone fence around the property, which clearly showed the generations of toil that had made it a beautiful farm. As the farmer was working, a minister came by and said, "My, that's a beautiful farm you and God have put together." And the farmer scratched his head and wiped the sweat from his brow and said, "You know, that's right, I guess. But you should have seen it when God was handling it alone."

This is an issue that tries men's souls. And all of us are going to have to work together to come to a reasonable solution. Genetic engineering has enormous possibilities for the benefit of mankind, but it also has real dangers of abuse. It is time to take steps, measured steps, to learn the kind of things that are necessary to make it safe and ethical. It is not time to stop even before we start.

Human Germline Gene Therapy

How and Why

In this essay I consider technical issues associated with the implementation of human germline gene therapy, as distinct from human somatic gene therapy. Since, in the latter case, only selected somatic cells are genetically modified, the effects of gene therapy are restricted to the patient. However, in germline gene therapy, all of the cells of the patient, including the patient's germ cells, receive the genetic modification. As a consequence, the newly-introduced genetic change(s) can be transmitted to the patient's progeny. This critical difference between germline and somatic gene therapy makes the issues associated with the merits and justifications for embarking on germline gene therapy much more complex. We need to consider the effects of the therapy upon the health and welfare not only of the individuals directly involved in the procedure, but also of their potential progeny who are not directly involved in the therapeutic protocol. Germline gene therapy is a controversial, complex topic; only through many open discussions of this topic by a broad spectrum of our society will we gain the wisdom needed for proper evaluation of the factors that must be considered before we contemplate initiation of these protocols.

Technical issues directed at evaluating the feasibility, the merits, the ratio of benefits to risks, and the safety of human gene therapy procedures should be part of this discussion. But I want to emphasize that even among the technical issues there is ample room for broad divergence of opinion, because new medical procedures are often introduced without an adequate data base to effectively predict all the consequences, even when there is extensive data from animal models.

Before discussing potential scenarios for human germline gene therapy, it is important to consider the goals of human germline gene therapy and where the pressures for its implementation are likely to arise. In many cases, the justification to use human germline gene therapy is likely to be made in terms of genetic enhancement, rather than in terms of ameliorating a medical problem resulting from a genetic defect. This is because for genetic diseases involving mutations in single genes, there are simpler, cheaper, and more effective means than the use of germline gene therapy to guarantee that a child will not receive a debilitating genetic defect. These methods rely on voluntary abortion of postimplantation mutant embryos or on selection of unaffected preimplantation embryos for implantation. There are rare cases where the above alternatives to human germline gene therapy will not work. Consider, for example, a parent that possesses two defective copies of a gene, such as the dominant mutation associated with Huntington's disease (HD). With dominant mutations, even a single copy of the mutant gene is sufficient to cause the disease. Under these circumstances, all of the embryos produced by that parent will give rise to children with the disease. Although the onset of this disease occurs in adulthood, it is extremely debilitating and leads to early death. Currently there are no known cures for this disease. The only current option for a parent with two copies of the defective HD gene to have healthy children is adoption. However, the drive to have your own biological children can be extremely strong. A small measure of this desire is evident in the extreme monetary costs, as well as physical and mental sacrifices, that parents are willing to tolerate to overcome problems of infertility. In vitro fertilization (IVF) clinics are a booming business. Since approximately 12 percent of couples are infertile, the services provided by IVF clinics will continue to be in strong demand.

It is conceivable that human germline gene therapy could be used to correct the defective Huntington's disease gene, thereby providing the parent who has two defective copies of the HD gene the option of having his or her own healthy biological children. Much of the technology that would be required to perform human germline gene therapy is available in private IVF clinics. Further, should parents desire to implement human gene therapy, and should they find an IVF clinic that is willing to undertake the procedure, there are no laws in place prohibiting it in the United States.

I have brought up this particular example of the use of human germline gene therapy to make two points. The first is that the pressure to initiate germline gene therapy will not likely come from governments or dictators with a desire to make a super race, but rather from parents who desire to improve the chances for their biological children to function effectively within our society. The second point is that, although germline gene therapy is technically demanding, it is not outside the expertise of existing IVF clinics. With a coupling of recombinant DNA technology and the ability to manipulate preimplantation embryos, the core expertise required for doing human germline gene therapy would be at hand.

The example I have chosen—a parent with two copies of the defective HD gene wanting to have his or her own healthy biological child—is obviously a very special, rare case. But it is a plausible case, since over a dozen HD mutant homozygous individuals (i.e., with two defective copies of this gene) have been identified, and many of them have had children.[21] (Surprisingly, the life expectancy of individuals with two defective copies of the HD gene is not measurably different from that of individuals with only one mutant copy of the gene.) Should such a case arise, I believe that few people within our society would question the right of the parents to pursue human germline gene therapy as a means of having their own healthy child. We hold very dear the right of parents to bear their own children. For this reason, we have imposed very few restrictions on IVF clinics. As long as they are run professionally and safely, we allow them to implement new procedures with very few restrictive guidelines. As a result, new innovations are introduced at a remarkable pace by these clinics in efforts to overcome a myriad of infertility problems.

As previously stated, in many cases the proposed goal of human germline gene therapy will be "genetic enhancement." This does not mean that the child will be provided with new human powers, but rather be provided with alleles (i.e., different forms of a given gene) having desirable properties that are not present in either of the parent's genomes. An example would be resistance to HIV infection. Approximately 1 percent of people in our society show remarkable resistance to infection by the AIDS virus. The altered genes (alleles) responsible for conferring resistance to this deadly virus are being identified and characterized. Parents, neither of whom has alleles for such HIV resistance, may nevertheless desire their children to have such alleles. Should the AIDS virus, through recombination with another virus, acquire routes of transmission in addition to those now known, the demand for resistance to HIV would rise dramatically. Although multidrug treatment, particularly involving protease inhibitors, has made significant progress in arresting HIV infection, the ability of these viruses to rapidly generate drug-resistant variants is dramatic. It is still unclear whether the pace of new drug development will outrun the virus's capacity to generate new resistant variants. One can imagine many other examples of alleles present within the human gene pool that, could we choose our parents, we would be happy to have. This would include alleles that reduce rather than increase our risk of acquiring diseases such as diabetes, heart failure, stroke, cancer, neurological pathologies, and so on. We must keep in mind, however, that susceptibility to disease is a complex process usually involving the interactions between several genes. Thus, the beneficial effects of alleles that cosegregate with a lower incidence of a disease, such as atherosclerosis, may depend on the presence of other alleles within the fortunate carrier. As a consequence, the transfer of that allele to a new individual may not confer the same benefit.

Before the cloning of the sheep Dolly by Wilmut and his colleagues[22] and the cloning of mice by Wakayama and his colleagues,[23] human germline gene therapy was a theoretical possibility, but its implementation faced so many technical hurdles that we could safely dismiss its potential use on pragmatic grounds alone. However, the demonstration that a nucleus from a differentiated cell could be completely reprogrammed by immersion into the cytoplasm of an enucleated oocyte and that this hybrid embryo could produce viable offspring has potentially eliminated the pragmatic arguments.

Vast experience with the mouse as subject has demonstrated that the safest, most versatile means of altering the genome in a mammal is to use gene targeting to modify an existing gene.[24] However, the process of gene targeting is not very efficient and must be done on a population of cells in order to allow the investigator to identify the rare cells that carry the planned modification. Because of the need to work with populations of cells, it is not practical to do gene targeting directly on one-cell embryos, because these embryos can be obtained only in relatively small numbers. In mice, we circumvent this problem by using embryonic stem (ES) cells. ES cells, which can be cultured in vitro, are derived from the early mouse embryo and are pluripotent.[25] That is, they are not committed to a particular differentiated cell type such as liver cells, bone cells, nerve cells, and so on. When ES cells are returned to an early embryonic environment, they participate in making all of the tissues of the mouse, including the germ cells. Using this technology, a genomic modification introduced by gene targeting into mouse ES cells can be transmitted to the mouse germline. By breeding, we can then generate as many mice as we want with the desired genetic change which had been originally introduced into the ES cells. Gene targeting in mouse ES cells is now used routinely, in hundreds of laboratories all over the world, to generate mice with designed genetic alterations. All of these mice, in effect, are generated by mouse germline gene therapy.

ES cells, however, are not an attractive option for human germline gene therapy. The reason that ES cells are a good route in mice, but a poor route in humans, is that genetic diversity plays a very different role in these two situations. In our experimental mouse population, we normally try to reduce genetic diversity. Any genetic alteration that we introduce into these mice can then be evaluated on a uniform genetic background. For this purpose, we utilize inbred lines of mice that were generated by brother-sister crosses for over twenty successive generations. In the human population, on the other hand, we treasure genetic diversity. One of the pleasures of having children is that, with the exception of identical twins, each child receives a very different complement of genes from each parent, thus contributing to the child's uniqueness. With one's own children there is a pleasant blend of resemblances and differences.

In our desire to maintain overall genetic uniformity in our mouse experiments, we use the same starting ES cell line to generate many mouse lines, each containing a different genetic alteration. To use the ES cell route for human germline gene therapy, and also maintain the same degree of genetic diversity that is generated during normal human conception, would require preparation of individual ES cell lines from each embryo. This would be prohibitively labor intensive. However, the nuclear transfer technology used to clone Dolly provides an alternative route that could be applied to individual embryos (see fig. 3).

In vitro fertilization using sperm and eggs donated by each set of parents would be used to generate one-cell embryos (fig. 3). In culture, the embryo would be permitted to progress to the four-cell stage. The embryo would then be separated into four cells; three of these cells would be frozen for later use. These are procedures routinely carried out in IVF clinics. Each of these four cells, frozen or unfrozen, would have an identical set of genes and would be capable of generating a normal child. The fourth cell would be allowed to divide in culture until a million cells were generated, taking approximately twenty cell divisions to achieve this number. Different embryonic cell types would be present within this cell population, but this diversity should not affect the procedure. One million cells is an ample population size to permit the use of technologies, such as gene targeting, to introduce the desired genetic alteration into a subset of these cells. The subset of cells containing the desired genetic alteration would be isolated from the remaining cell population and carefully characterized to ensure that the genetic modification was accurate. At this point, the nucleus of one of the mother's oocytes would be removed and replaced with a nucleus from the expanded pool of cells containing the prescribed genetic modification. In this cytoplasmic environment, the modified nucleus would receive instructions to commence making an embryo. The cells would be allowed to divide in culture once or twice, and then the embryo would be surgically transferred to the mother's womb to allow pregnancy to continue. A child produced in this way would contain the genetic modification, introduced in cell culture, in all of his or her cells, including the germ cells.

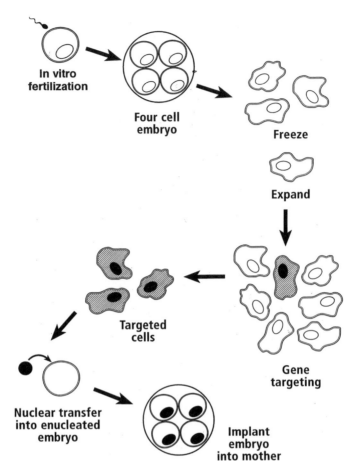

Figure 3. A scheme for human germline gene therapy using nuclear transfer. The first step is to generate the one-cell embryo by in vitro fertilization. Next, the embryo is incubated for two cell divisions to generate the four-cell embryo. The zona pellucida is removed and the four cells are dispersed. Three of these cells are frozen for later use; the fourth is expanded in culture to produce a population of cells to be used for gene targeting. A clone of cells, containing the desired genetic modification, is isolated and synchronized in culture to arrest them at Go. A nucleus from a cell containing the desired genetic modification is then transferred into an enucleated embryonic cell, this being any of the three original embryonic cells frozen in step 3. In the new cytoplasmic environment, the nucleus is reprogrammed to initiate embryogenesis (I. Wilmut, A.E. Schnieke, J. McWhir, A.J. Kind, and K.H.S. Campbell, "Viable Offspring Derived from Fetal and Adult Mammalian Cells," Nature 385[1997]:810–13.). The embryo is cultured in vitro to form a four-cell embryo and then transferred into the mother's fallopian tube to allow development to progress from implantation, to formation of the fetus, and finally to the newborn child. Every cell in the newborn child, including the germ cells, will have the genetic modifications introduced in culture by gene targeting.

In the above scenario, I suggested using gene targeting to introduce the desired genetic modification. There are alternative procedures for introducing genetic modifications, which I will discuss shortly, but gene targeting has a number of clear advantages over other approaches. Modifications introduced by gene targeting take place at the gene's normal chromosomal location. The activity of a gene is normally controlled by the interactions of regulatory transcription factors with DNA sequences surrounding the gene. The pertinent DNA sequences can be located hundreds of thousands of DNA nucleotide base pairs away from the gene. Placing a gene in an inappropriate chromosomal environment can result in perturbation of the gene's activity or in no gene activity at all. Modification of a gene in its normal environment, on the other hand, allows the gene to be properly regulated so that it functions in the right cells, at the right time, and at the right level.

A problem with the use of gene targeting to introduce genetic modifications is that it is normally employed for only one modification at a time. With the view of being able to introduce many concurrent modifications, investigators are developing artificial chromosomes that could simultaneously carry many modified genes with their appropriate regulatory sequences to ensure proper gene expression. This technology is currently in its early infancy but has a potentially promising future.

A potential problem with the use of artificial chromosomes as a route for human germline gene therapy may occur in the second generation. Pairing of chromosomes is an important step during meiosis (i.e., during the formation of germ cells). To ensure proper chromosome pairing, two artificial chromosomes can be introduced during the human germline gene therapy procedure. This will also ensure that each germ cell will receive one artificial chromosome. However, in the second generation, the only way to ensure proper chromosomal pairing is for both parents to contribute related artificial chromosomes (i.e., capable of pairing) to the embryo. The inability of chromosomes to pair may lead to sterility. Should this be the case, the problem may be solvable in an IVF clinic by introducing the artificial chromosome into the oocyte (female egg) or spermatocyte (precursor to the sperm) of the parent that does not harbor the artificial chromosome.

Whereas the ethical issues associated with human germline gene therapy are more complex than those of somatic gene therapy, some of the technical hurdles are actually less complex. Though considerable effort has gone into somatic gene therapy, the success has been meager. Three major obstacles have been encountered: gene delivery, gene expression, and immunological nontolerance. For example, if the genetic defect results in the absence of a particular enzyme normally produced in the pancreas, then the ideal somatic gene therapy protocol would be to deliver a nondefective gene encoding the enzyme to a majority of the pancreatic cells. Further, gene activity in the pancreas would be modulated in a normal manner in response to metabolic need. Instead, what is often observed is that a minority of cells of the appropriate tissue receive the gene and further, that the transgene (gene of exogenous origin) is expressed at suboptimal levels because it is located in a foreign chromosomal environment. However, this small amount of gene product is still sufficient to elicit an immune response, so even what little that has been produced is cleared from the body. These difficult technical hurdles would not be encountered in germline gene therapy since the altered gene would automatically be delivered to all cells in the body. If, as already discussed, gene targeting were used to introduce the genetic alteration, then the altered gene would also be in the proper chromosomal environment to ensure proper expression. Finally, since the gene is likely to be expressed during fetal development prior to the establishment of the host immune system, the altered gene product will be recognized as self and not elicit an immune response.

A major consideration with human germline gene therapy is that the genetic alterations would be transmitted from generation to generation. It would become a permanent record within the family. Because human germline gene therapy would be mediated by human beings, and we are far from perfect, there is a potential for error. In addition, no matter how much thought went into the process, twenty or thirty years henceforth the procedure may appear naive in the context of the technology available at that time. Furthermore, whatever improvements could be made at that future date, they too would be subject to being outmoded. For these reasons, it is important that whatever procedures we might adopt for human germline gene therapy, they should, at the very least, be reversible. Fortunately, this can be accomplished.

An example of how genetic information added to the patient's genome could subsequently be deleted is illustrated in figure 4(A). This selective deletion takes advantage of a site-specific recombinase known as CRE.[26] This enzyme performs recombination (i.e., exchanges) between specific thirty-four-base-pair sequences known as *loxP* sites. The consequences of activating CRE-mediated recombination between two *loxP* sites oriented in the same direction (i.e., head to tail) is deletion of all intervening DNA sequences (fig. 4[A]). Note that, in this approach, at the same time as new information is introduced into the germline, the *loxP* sites and CRE recombinase gene needed to reverse the change would also be introduced. This would, at the patient's discretion, allow subsequent deletion of all information introduced into his or her germline, leaving only one *loxP* site behind. This single *loxP* site does not have a coding or regulatory potential on its own and therefore could be placed within the genome so that its presence remains neutral. The CRE recombinase could be accompanied by control elements to allow it to be activated in response to a drug taken by the patient, which would result in deletion of essentially all of the added the information from his or her germ cells. Thus, the added information would not be transmitted to subsequent offspring.

For other experimental objectives, we have tested this procedure in mice under conditions designed so that the exogenous information flanked by the loxP sites was automatically deleted from the germ cells in the first generation of mice.[27] Under these circumstances, the genetic alteration was restricted to the somatic cells of the first generation mouse and not transmitted to any progeny. We tested over 100 second-generation offspring and none received the exogenous information, which was, by design, intended to be deleted. As planned, however, the CRE recombinase was not activated in any of the mouse's somatic cells.

The procedure described above works to delete added information. Germline gene therapy may, however, require replacement of one piece of information with another. For example, we could replace the HD mutation with the normal sequence, or replace a more common allele with the allele that confers HIV resistance. Could replacement processes also be done so as to be reversible (i.e., permitting restoration of the original replaced sequences)? The answer is yes, one approach to this end being outlined in figure 4(B). The open arrow in that figure represents an exon (coding sequence) of a gene containing the sequences that we want to replace (the HD mutation). It is drawn as an arrow because exons have a functional direction. In the opposite orientation, an exon loses its function, that is, it is not seen by the cellular processing machinery as an exon. The introduced targeted sequence (second line) contains the replacement exon (arrow with cross hatch) plus the original exon, with the latter in the opposite orientation, so that it is not functional. In addition, the gene targeting event introduces three loxP sites, two in the same orientation, the third in the opposite orientation, as well as the coding sequences for the CRE recombinase. In the absence of activation of the CRE recombinase, the only functional unit within this construct is the new exon (cross-hatch) that replaces the old. On activation of CRE, the new exon would be deleted and the orientation of the old exon would be reversed and therefore become functional again. The reason that the orientation of the old exon would be reversed is that CRE-mediated recombination between loxP sites in the opposite orientation (head to head) results in inverting the intervening DNA sequences, rather than deleting them. It may be asked how the CRE recombinase knows which pair of loxP sites should be recombined, but, in fact, the order of these events does not matter. In either case, the final

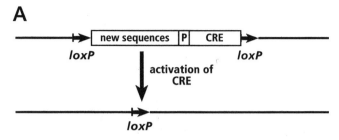

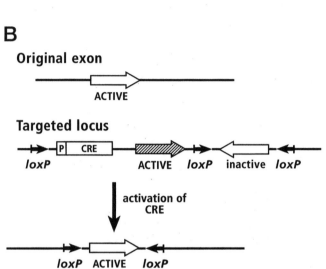

Figure 4. Human gene therapy can be designed so as to be reversible. A: An approach permitting deletion of added information from the germline. The new sequences added by the germline gene therapy procedure could encode a single gene or multiple genes present on an artificial chromosome. These new sequences would also include the gene encoding the CRE recombinase. All of the sequences would be flanked with *loxP* sites oriented in the same direction. On activation of CRE, recombination would take place between the flanking *loxP* sequences resulting in the deletion of all of the intervening DNA. Activation of the CRE recombinase gene could be made dependent on a drug taken by the patient in order to delete the exogenous information from his or her germ cells. B: A procedure for reversing the consequences of a replacement re-action. In this sceme, rather than deleting newly added information, the objective is to revert to the original information which was replaced by the gene-therapy procedure. For simplicity, the scheme illustrates the replacement of one exon (gene coding sequence) with another. The top line represents the exon to be replaced. It is drawn as an arrow because exons have a functional direction. In the opposite orientation, an exon loses its function—that is, it is not seen by the cellular processing machinery as an exon. The second line represents the targeted locus generated by the gene therapy protocol. It contains the new exon (arrow with cross-hatch) which will replace the old exon, plus

(continued)

result of these two reactions is the same. It may be noted that continued inversion reactions can yield half of the cells with the old exon in the correct orientation and the other half with that exon in the opposite orientation. In further refinements of this scheme, the sequences of the *loxP* sites can be designed so that they allow the initial recombination reactions to occur, but discourage further reaction. With such refinements, the recombination reactions can be directed so that restoration of the original exon in the correct orientation is greatly favored.

Unless an error were made, it is difficult to envision a situation in which once a defective gene, like the one for Huntington's disease, had been corrected, it would be in the patient's interest to reverse the procedure. However, procedures involving the incorporation of alleles conferring HIV resistance may be more complex. Although such alleles do provide resistance to HIV, they might also compromise the immune system such that carriers of these alleles may be more sensitive to other, as yet undefined, pathogens. This latter case points out the importance of having a full understanding of the biology of a system before attempting to change it.

In summary, I have tried to underscore the fact that plausible scenarios can already be envisioned for methodologies by which human germline gene therapy could now be accomplished. I have also outlined examples of problems that could be approached by this technology. The contemplated procedures are not overly complex and are within the expertise of existing IVF clinics. Ironically, many of the technical hurdles encountered in human somatic gene therapy are obviated in the apparently more radical human germline gene therapy. I have also argued that any procedure utilizing human germline gene therapy need not be, and should not be, regarded as an inevitably permanent alteration but can, and should be, designed from the outset to be reversible.

The pressures to undertake human germline gene therapy are likely to come from the desire of parents to provide their children with improved opportunities to function more effectively within our society. While there remain many technical issues to be explored before germline gene therapy

Figure 4. *(continued)* the original exon in the opposite orientation so that it is now nonfunctional. The targeted locus also contains three *loxP* sites, two oriented in the same direction, and the third in the opposite direction, as well as the coding sequences for the CRE recombinase. In the absence of activation of the CRE recombinase, the only functional unit within this construct is the new exon (cross-hatch) that replaces the old. On activation of CRE, the new exon would be deleted, the orientation of the old exon would be reversed, and therefore the old exon would become functional. The orientation of the old exon would be reversed because CRE-mediated recombination between *loxP* sites in the opposite orientation results in inversion of the intervening DNA sequences.

is actually implemented in humans, it seems likely that most of these can readily be approached with animal models. Eventually, the difficult questions will not involve the methodology by which human gene therapy can be accomplished, but whether to initiate the procedures and, if so, for what purposes. The technology, though now relatively straightforward, is extremely powerful. With recognition of this power comes a responsibility for social deliberation to seek ways to ensure that human germline gene therapy can be used in productive ways that keep the interests of individuals and of society in balance.

W. FRENCH ANDERSON

A New Front in the
Battle against Disease

At the center of this discussion of the potential for genetic engineering of human beings over the next twenty years is the question of germline gene therapy. Let me present my position at the beginning. I believe that it would be unethical to attempt germline gene transfer at this point in time. We have neither the scientific ability to do so safely, the medical knowledge to do so effectively, nor the ethical competence to do so wisely. However, we do now have the expertise to attempt in utero gene therapy of somatic cells and this new approach does offer a new front in the battle against disease.

Genetic engineering of human beings can be classified into four categories:[28] somatic cell gene therapy, germline gene therapy, enhancement genetic engineering, and eugenic genetic engineering.

Somatic cell gene therapy is a treatment procedure whereby a therapeutic gene is inserted into a patient's somatic (body) cells in an attempt to treat a disease. In contrast to somatic cell therapy is germline gene therapy, whereby the gene is inserted into the germline cells, the egg or sperm. Inserting a gene into somatic cells affects only the patient being treated, similar to when a patient undergoes surgery, takes a medication, or receives a limb prosthesis. However, with germline gene therapy, a gene is inserted into the DNA of an egg or sperm so that children of the patient will have the inserted gene. There are two proposed ways to attempt germline gene transfer. One is to insert the gene into the pre-embryo, perhaps even at the four-to-eight cell zygote stage. The other is to target germline cells in the fetus, child, or young adult. The technology to carry out either procedure in a safe manner does not now exist.

The third category, enhancement genetic engineering, would involve an attempt to "improve" or "enhance" a normal individual, for example by inserting extra copies of a growth hormone gene to try to make him or her taller. A line can be drawn between therapy and enhancement. Therapy occurs in response to illness, when a person is below what is considered a healthy state, and the attempt is to bring the patient up to normal. Enhancement is the idea of trying to go from "normal" to above normal. As I have discussed elsewhere,[29] I am strongly opposed to attempts at enhancement genetic engineering for a number of reasons: scientific, philosophical, and societal.

The final category, eugenic genetic engineering, is defined as the ability to modify complex human traits such as body structure, personality, intelligence, and so on. In 1982, when I put this classification scheme together,[30] I thought that eugenic genetic engineering was so difficult that modification of complex traits would not be possible for many decades. And yet, only seventeen years later, the incredible pace of gene discovery and genetic research is such that attempts to "redesign human beings" have become a distinct possibility in the next twenty years.

Ethical Considerations Involved in Human Genetic Engineering

What are the ethical considerations that should be taken into account before attempting a new therapeutic procedure with a human being? In 1980, John Fletcher and I attempted to answer this question with regards to somatic cell gene therapy.[31]

The medical abuses that occurred in Germany during World War II led to an in-depth analysis of what ethical rules should be followed before initiating experimental therapy with human beings. Beginning with the Nuremberg Code, a body of ethical guidelines has accumulated. Central to these ethical guidelines is Rule 3 of the Code:[32]

> The experiment should be so designed, and based on the results of animal experimentation and a knowledge of the natural history of the disease or other problem under study, that the anticipated results will justify the performance of the experiment.

Henry Beecher summarized the ethical considerations governing the initiation of a new experimental treatment with a patient by stating: "A study is ethical or not at its inception; it does not become ethical because it succeeds in producing valuable data. . . ."[33]

The report of the Belmont Commission[34] is the most definitive statement of the ethical guidelines that govern experimental clinical research. The Belmont report stressed that the paramount question to ask is: Is the risk/benefit ratio acceptable for the patient? To assist in assuring that this question is appropriately answered, the Belmont report recommended two new procedures which, although controversial at the time, are now considered mainstays of clinical research: the establishment of local review committees called "institutional review boards" that must approve any experimental procedure before it is carried out with a human being, and the requirement for a written informed-consent document.

For any new procedure to be carried out with a human being, whether it is a new surgical operation, a new drug, a new medical procedure, or gene therapy, the issues are the same. What are the potential risks for the patient? What are the potential benefits for the patient? Is the ratio of risks to benefits appropriate for the patient? These questions can best be answered, in most cases, by carefully-conducted studies in animals. Two categories of data need to be obtained: One, efficacy—will the new procedure be effective in treating the disease? And, two, safety—how significant are the risks of harm from the procedure itself? Whether the new procedure is medical, surgical, pharmaceutical, or genetic, these requirements need to be met. Thus, there are no unusual or new criteria for genetic engineering that are different from any other new experimental procedure.[35] The issue is to evaluate, on a patient by patient basis, the risk/benefit ratio.

The determination was made in 1990 by the appropriate government regulatory groups (the National Institutes of Health Recombinant DNA Advisory Committee [NIH-RAC] and the Food and Drug Administration [FDA]) that the animal and other data justified an attempt at human somatic cell gene therapy.[36] If we replace the phrase "somatic cell gene therapy" with "germline gene therapy," we can use the somatic cell gene therapy review process as a means to determine what needs to be done before an attempt at germline gene therapy should be approved.

Ethical Considerations Involved in Germline Gene Transfer

We do not have the expertise to attempt germline gene therapy.[37] There are three criteria that need to be satisfied prior to any attempt at modifying the germline of human patients.

First, there needs to be long-term experience with somatic cell gene therapy. Before attempting to manipulate the germline of human beings by genetic engineering, we need to know what are the long-term consequences of carrying out somatic cell gene therapy in patients. At present, we have only limited experience with somatic cell gene therapy: nine years of experience with the first two girls that were treated in 1990 and early 1991, a number of cancer patients who have survived, and a few other surviving patients. But this represents only several dozen patients over a short number of years. We need to have experience for ten or fifteen years, with hundreds if not thousands of patients who have undergone somatic cell gene transfer, to be certain there will not be serious long-term negative effects. It is possible, though highly unlikely, that patients who have exogenous genes placed into their cells might have a very high risk for cancer ten years later. Lack of data does not constitute negative data. We simply do not know what the long-term risks may be from genetically engineering human cells. Consequently, it would be ethically inappropriate to attempt an irreversible and multigeneration procedure such as germline gene transfer without initially having long-term experience indicating that there is a low risk with somatic cell gene transfer.

Second, there needs to be a reliable, reproducible, safe procedure.

We read about new transgenic mice that have been developed, new "knock-out" mice that mimic human disease, and about Dolly, Polly, and other cloned and transgenic livestock. The impression is that it may be a simple step to go from germline genetic engineering in mice and livestock to germline genetic engineering in humans. This impression is incorrect. Ninety-five to 99.9 percent of all "engineered" embryos are damaged; most are lethally damaged and do not lead to live births, but even those that do are frequently deformed and later die. Even in mice, where separate inbred strains of animals can be optimized for each step of the procedure, the success rate has not improved that much over the past fifteen years. Only a few percent of animals are born as "healthy" transgenics, and these are the ones we read about in the press; the failures are often reported only in the scientific literature. In livestock, which are partially inbred, the success rate is down to less than 1 percent. In humans, who are totally outbred, the success rate with the present procedures would be expected to be extremely low. What this means in practical terms is that the vast majority of attempts at germline gene transfer would result in deformed or dead embryos. It would be unethical, I believe, to attempt such a procedure in humans until the success rate in animals is significantly improved.

Successes in the field of in vitro fertilization and reproductive biology are indeed impressive. It is becoming possible to take one cell from a eight-cell zygote and analyze it for a range of genetic defects. Perhaps, over the next twenty years, it will become possible to safely insert a functional gene into one of the cells in a mammalian zygote and, thereby, carry out germline gene transfer efficiently. The technique would then need to be shown to be reproducible, reliable, and safe in nonhuman primates, since these animals are the closest to humans. If healthy baby monkeys carrying a functional gene can be born, then, I believe, it would be ethical to transfer the procedure to human beings for the treatment of serious disease.

It could be argued that injection of a therapeutic gene into a human zygote may be possible without any apparent ill effect, so why not try it? Unfortunately, one can only know that there is a problem when one knows how to look for it. But we do not know what to look for. The only way to measure an effect now, with our present state of ignorance, is either to have a gross defect or death. We simply cannot know what the effect is in the zygote when an exogenous gene is injected, whether we "see" any problems or not.

Third, there needs to be societal approval prior to the first attempt at germline gene transfer. Almost all medical decisions are made between the patient and his or her physician, whether it is with regard to tranquilizers for nerves or cosmetic surgery for personal pride. Our rationalization for this freedom is that "my body belongs to me." But our genes do not belong to just ourselves. The gene pool belongs to all of society. No individual has a right to intentionally change the gene pool without the consent of society. Thus, the final criterion is that there should be societal awareness and approval before germline gene transfer is initially attempted.

In Utero Gene Therapy

Expertise in the area of gene transfer has now attained a sufficient level to consider an attempt at in utero gene therapy.[38] A gene transfer procedure into the mid-trimester fetus would be into somatic cells, although there is a potential for a low level of inadvertent gene transfer into the germline cells. Therefore, the criteria outlined above concerning societal approval may also apply to fetal gene transfer. The purpose of developing in utero gene therapy is to attempt to treat those genetic diseases that cause irreversible damage before birth and for which there is no other therapy available.

My colleague, Esmail Zanjani, and I, together with our collaborators, have developed two different procedures as possible techniques for carrying out in utero gene transfer. After twelve years of study in sheep and monkeys,[39] we believe that there are sufficient animal data to consider developing clinical protocols.[40] To this end, we submitted two "preprotocols" to the NIH-RAC for discussion at their September 24–25, 1998, meeting. The committee agreed that the time was appropriate to begin the discussion and that animal work should proceed with regular public review. We anticipate that it will be at least three years before sufficient data will be available to justify the submission of clinical protocols.

The two pre-protocols we submitted to the NIH-RAC can be summarized as follows. The first is in-utero gene therapy for the treatment of adenosine deaminase (ADA) deficiency. We propose a direct injection into the 13–15-week fetus of a retroviral vector carrying a normal copy of the human ADA gene controlled by human genomic ADA regulatory sequences. Because it is a direct in vivo injection, an occasional vector particle may enter an egg or sperm, thereby resulting in germline gene transfer. The magnitude of this risk will be determined by animal studies over the next two to three years.

The second is in-utero gene therapy for homozygous alpha-thalassemia. Homozygous alpha-thalassemia is a particularly tragic disease, because the fetus dies in utero and produces toxic symptoms in the mother. The standard therapy is an abortion at 24 weeks to protect the mother. We propose to remove blood cells from the fetus at 17–20 weeks, insert ex vivo a copy of a normal human alpha-globin gene controlled by human genomic alpha-globin regulatory sequences, and then transplant the gene-engineered cells back into the fetus. Because the gene transfer would occur outside the fetus in this procedure, there would be less danger of germline gene transfer, but the cell transfer approach is not as efficient as direct vector injection.

Because of the concern relating to inadvertent germline gene transfer in these in utero procedures, the ethical issues surrounding germline genetic engineering are now under active public discussion.

Conclusion

We know so little about the human body and so little about living processes, we would be unwise to attempt genetic engineering to try to treat, much less "improve," the human zygote or embryo. What our society may want to do 100 years from now is its business. It will not care what we think any more than we care what people 100 years ago thought we should do. However, it is our duty to go into the era of genetic engineering in as responsible a way as possible. This obligation means that we should utilize this powerful new technology cautiously until we learn its problems, and even then, use it only for the treatment of disease and not for any other purpose.

MICHAEL R. ROSE

Aging as a Target
for Genetic Engineering

This essay is divided into three parts. I begin by discussing the interesting nature of the problem of aging, continue by looking at the new promise of aging research, and conclude by considering whether at this point aging is an appropriate target for genetic engineering.

The Problem of Aging

One perspective on aging is that it concerns death and when you get to die. Right now, in the United States, life expectancy averages about seventy-five years. If your're male, it's about four years earlier than that; if you're female four years later, which some might take as yet another indication of which sex is superior.

By contrast, we can look at the demographic pattern of a nonaging human population. Such populations don't actually exist, but we can estimate their properties using the low mortality rates of humans between the ages of ten and fifteen in the United States and other OECD (Organization for Economic Cooperation and Development) countries. The survival of this age group is better than that of any other, and if every American, irrespective of age, could have and maintain these optimal survival statistics, a cohort of such Americans would have a life expectancy of 1,200 years,[41] and a few people would live some 2,000 years. These are just numbers, since no one is now in a position to make people nonaging, but this simple calculation reveals that, if we didn't age, we'd have an order of magnitude greater life span. Yet it might be said, "Well, who needs more than that? Seventy-five years is plenty."

So, what is enough of a lifespan? There is a spectacular pediatric disorder known as Hutchinson-Guilford's progeria, which is thought to be a genetic disease. Sometimes this disorder is called "accelerated aging," though this label is controversial. Afflicted children live about ten to twelve years, with a variety of symptoms that become progressively more severe. They "look old," and come to lack the physical abilities even of children, but they remain cognitively normal. Could it be said that their lifespan is perfectly acceptable? Most dogs live about that long. Most rodents don't even approach such an age. Nonetheless, most people regard progeria as a tragically curtailed lifespan.

But why is the lifespan of a progeric tragically short, while that of the present average American is not? Do contemporary citizens of OECD countries live a perfectly appropriate life span? Do they enjoy their "God-given life span"? Would it be appropriate to extend present-day lives, or is this something too Promethean to contemplate?

Even if you aren't interested in when you die, you may still have some interest in how you die. It's one thing to imagine dying climbing Mount Everest or sky diving. It's another thing to die of cardiovascular disease, stroke, or cancer, which is how most of the elderly die. As time goes on, the health of the elderly deteriorates until, by eighty-five years of age, only 30 percent are ostensibly free of a major disease. And the elderly have any number of aggravating diseases like gout, diabetes, and impotence. As time goes by, it's not true that you're getting older but getting better. You are deteriorating.

There is much you can do to change when you will die. You can die sooner by a variety of pretty reliable methods: acute physical stress, hypoxia while climbing Mount Everest, hypothermia. Those are fast ways to die sooner. Almost as reliable, but somewhat slower, is smoking, but it has the fringe benefit of addiction to make you less likely to change your mind. Exposure to contagious disease is making a comeback thanks to HIV, though there are also resurgent disorders from the nineteenth century, such as tuberculosis and influenza. Still common are various sources of fatal injury, from driving without a seat belt to drunken navigation of watercraft. As long as we are willing to truncate our lives, we can certainly control when we die.

What is unclear is what we can do to die later. Many people suppose that, if they exercise fanatically for ten or twenty years, they're adding years to their life span. But there's very little evidence for that. Exercise does improve your short-term morbidity, your short-term likelihood of developing a variety of diseases, but it does not appear to radically transform your life expectancy. The nostrums and prescriptions gleaned from health magazines are not likely to change the essential numbers. As we get older, after forty or so years of age, we are more and more likely to die, to contract a disabling disease, and to look bad in bright light. For the fatalist, this is as it should be, and everyone is entitled to this point of view. But for those who are interested in amelioration or extension of their lives, this prospect must seem pretty grim.

New Hope for Aging

Despite the scenario just sketched, there are reasons for thinking that there may be some new hope coming from basic biological research. In fact, it might be argued that aging is now a solved biological problem. We know why aging occurs, and from that we know how to shape it, at least on the level of basic science.

The solution to the scientific problem of aging is that aging is caused solely by a decline in the force of natural selection with increased age, in adult organisms that reproduce using eggs or seeds, which is what most organisms do. This seemingly enigmatic statement deserves some explanation.

Consider an organism that reproduces strictly by splitting in two as, for example, bacteria do. This organism practices binary fission, in the terminology of science. If, through successive divisions, the descendant cell lineages deteriorate, you have a process that's somewhat like aging, but the lineage eventually will terminate. For these organisms, aging and extinction are the same, so the process of natural selection is going to strongly select against aging. And it doesn't matter whether an organism is unicellular or multicellular. It's all the same. Sea anemones provide examples of multicellular organisms like this; quite a few anemones reproduce by strictly splitting in two, and they can live forever, with no signs of aging.

Humans, on the other hand, are organisms that grow from an egg or a seed into a mature organism that, in turn, reproduces using eggs or seeds. When this situation is considered formally, using mathematics, one can calculate the force of natural selection acting, for example, on American males at any particular age.[42] This calculation shows that the force of natural selection is very powerful at early ages. Evolutionary biologists know that this has produced a wonderful adaptation at these early ages, something we might call "health." But once reproductive age is reached, the force of natural selection progressively weakens, hitting zero around age forty, using the simplest assumptions. After this point, metaphorically speaking, natural selection does not care whether you live or die. This causes many males to panic and buy a sports car.

The only upside of this grim conclusion is that it can bring an understanding of the genetic fabric of aging. One possibility is that because the force of natural selection collapses later in life, mutations that affect us only then are unshaped by natural selection. Basically, any genetic garbage can accumulate as long as it doesn't alter our reproductive success. The other possibility—and this is an important issue for genetic engineering—is that of genetic trade-offs. It's also called "you can't get something for nothing." This possibility would come about by natural selection enhancing early fitness through genetic effects that are deleterious later in life. Something may be good when you're young, but bad later. Either or both of these possibilities can lead to aging and all it entails.

But this is just verbal gloss on mathematical theory. Let us consider the data. Most of the data on the evolution of aging are collected on fruit flies, partly because they're easy to study. The bottom line is that we test the validity of the evolutionary analysis of aging by manipulating the force of natural selection so that it postpones aging. If the theory were incorrect, we couldn't do this. But we can. The most elementary experiment is one where you discard the eggs of younger flies and thereby increase the age at which you first allow female fruit flies to reproduce successfully. When this procedure is sustained for many generations, the results are very consistent, as long as there is genetic variation to begin with. Postponing reproduction maintains the force of natural selection at high levels in middle age. Theory predicts that this should eventually cause the evolution of increased longevity. And it does. This has been the result in one experiment after another since I began them in the 1970s.[43]

For example, in an experiment that has been ongoing for about eighteen years, the average life expectancy has doubled, and the maximum life expectancy has slightly more than doubled. We are not just compressing morbidity by getting the flies to die closer to some natural limit. We are, instead, shifting the pattern of aging. Otherwise we wouldn't have doubled the maximum life expectancy.

We know many things about the physiology of the longer-living flies. They are much more robust than their controls. They can survive extremes of starvation and desiccation that kill normal flies. Both males and females can reproduce vastly more when they're older. They have much better endurance at the athletic level. These are not flies that do as little as possible for a very long time; their metabolic and sexual activity is considerably in excess of the meager lives of normal fruit flies.

These points undergird the contention that aging is a solved problem. We not only have essential theory; it has been validated by tests of its predictions. So, the problem of aging is something we can address in theory and resolve—at least in fruit flies.

How to Postpone Human Aging

But what can we do about human aging? How can we engineer postponed aging in humans? There are all kinds of possibilities that would be bad ideas to carry out. One is breeding humans for postponed aging. That would require the forced use of contraception by everyone under age thirty-five, if not forty. This is a *Nineteen Eighty-four* or *Brave New World* fantasy. Not enough people would cooperate, and the coercive system necessary would be worse than aging itself. Like Soviet socialism, it would mainly serve to make the alternative look attractive.

Another idea, which the French are fond of, is to use only human genetic data to unravel human aging. The basic problem with this is that you don't get enough information fast enough. Human genetics, on its own, will never advance as quickly as genetics that uses "model systems" such as fruit flies, nematodes, yeast, and bacteria. Among other difficulties, it is hard to arrange the human matings that are the most interesting scientifically.

Another procedure that would be inappropriate would be the untested injection of fly genes directly into humans. However well we know how the fly works, particularly its genes, we can't assume that all that knowledge will apply to humans. Tests with other mammals will be needed first.

And there is a final, more controversial point: Genetic manipulations that make the cells of our body capable of unlimited division are now becoming available. But what works for cells won't necessarily be beneficial for whole organisms, so I do not support this approach. Unlimited cell division, for example, raises the risk of cancer, even if cell-division controls are added.

Instead of these approaches, I propose the following scenario. Start work with simple animal experiments. We can identify more genes for postponed aging faster using invertebrate "models" such as the fruit fly and the nematode. Then, from those model systems, work must progress first to mice and then to humans. This is a multistage, multimodel approach to postponing aging in humans.

We have just mentioned fruit fly selection experiments that produced postponed aging. They are only the beginning. There are other manipulations one can use to postpone aging in fruit flies and nematodes. It is possible, for example, to manipulate diet and thereby change their aging patterns. In fruit flies, genetic engineering has been going on for almost two decades. In the nematode, one can use wholesale mutation as well as genetic engineering to postpone aging. With mice, we can select for postponed aging. Once you have mouse lines that have been selected for postponed aging, you can identify the specific genes involved and, very importantly, you can start to work on physiology. It is not enough just to think genes; you must to think of inparting meaningful physiology to the organism, particularly if you are to avoid problems with side effects.

Once we learn enough about aging in the mouse, we will be able to genetically engineer postponed mouse aging. We are not at this point yet, but we could easily get there someday, and then some will undoubtedly say we should proceed to genetically engineer postponed aging in humans.

But there's another alternative. We might also figure out how to emulate the effects of genetic interventions using more conventional therapies such as oral provision of hormones or protein injections. This would be the more cautious strategy, and I think that at this stage there's a lot to recommend caution. For example, once we have shown that tweaking a particular hormone in a mouse gave postponed aging, we could try tweaking that hormone nongenetically in humans. Indeed, at present, there are a number of physicians having their patients try out hormone antiaging interventions before there are proper results in well-understood laboratory experiments or appropriate clinical trials. The fact that these people are operating more on hope than knowledge doesn't mean that someday we won't have useful hormone interventions for aging. The present approach suggests the need for more research at the preclinical level, but there are, in fact, very good reasons for thinking that conventional medicine may fail to address the problem of aging correctly. The conventional medical model is about the alleviation or amelioration of specific conditions, effects of specific pathogens, and specific genetic defects. That's the way medicine works. It cures disease.

But aging has no such disease status. We are all going to age. Approximately 70 percent of the United States population will die of an aging-related disorder such as cardiovascular disease, cancer, or stroke. Aging is not something weird. It's something that's predictably going to happen to us unless we get hit by HIV or a big RV on the freeway. So aging is not a disease in the traditional sense.

Aging is a failure of adaptation. In aging, you are seeing the effects of natural selection abandoning you. In aging, you are seeing the power of evolution by natural selection in reverse, namely, when it stops working. When you look at what an eighteen-year-old can do, you are seeing the power of what natural selection can accomplish. When you look at yourself in the mirror and you're sixty-eight years old, you're seeing what happens when natural selection just doesn't bother.

To address this kind of problem, you need different approaches. Serious antiaging medicine, if it can be called medicine, depends on addressing problems that involve many genes, some of only minor effect. These problems will require powerful, complex, and well-balanced interventions. But that's not how medicine works; medicine is specifically targeted. One possible technological need created by the polygenic nature of aging is for artificial chromosomes, so that numerous genetic alterations can be brought together in one physical structure. Artificial chromosomes will allow the assembly of many genetic loci to do a variety of things that our aging bodies fail to do. What may be required is "genomic" engineering, well beyond genetic engineering.

The timing of intervention is an important issue when considering the genomic engineering of aging. One approach would be to wait until the last minute. So you are sixty-seven years old and you say, "Okay, Doc. Shoot me up with all the latest artificial chromosomes." A good thing about that is that you wouldn't pay any earlier physiological price for the treatment. All of the physiological costs would be paid at that time. On the other hand, there may be a lot of medical problems you can't solve at that point. At least with this last-minute, desperate approach you wouldn't have any effect on future generations.

Then there is the hard-core germline approach. Let's say you went after the gametes because you wanted your descendants to have the best possible genes. So right from the start—right from the zygote or close to it—you intervene. The advantage is that the benefits will go to all your descendants, but there's a disadvantage in that early problems associated with your artificial chromosome would be expressed through growth and development. It is very fashionable for genetic engineers to say, "Ah, yes, but we will only turn on those genes later." Well, indeed, they may be able to turn on transcription at high levels later, but there will still likely be some genetic side effects at early ages even though they tried to shut everything down until later years. There is also the problem of evolutionary instability, of permanently having in your germline an artificial chromosome that is simply not going to be as stable as a regular chromosome. And then, finally, you have the problem of possible homogenization, which is like all of us driving Toyota Camrys. If we all have exactly the same anti-aging chromosome and, as it turns out, that makes us prone to infection by a virus we've not yet seen epidemiologically, then we could all be stricken and the consequences might be dire.

So it seems reasonable to conclude that hard-core genetic engineering presents us with some very substantial problems. A compromise might be appropriate. One such compromise might be to supply any artificial chromosomes to the adult body before aging really begins, in the hope of alleviating much of the damage of the aging process, so that when you do hit age sixty-seven or sixty-eight you're in relatively decent shape. Not all disorders associated with aging will be preventable using this kind of intervention, because some later medical problems may arise from growth patterns established in the fetus, such as patterns of vascularization. However, this does leave the germline free, and it avoids deleterious effects during childhood. Therefore, early adulthood intervention is the most reasonable choice for prudent genetic engineering to postpone aging. Now, if only we could get people to quit smoking.

Reprogenetics

*How Reproductive and Genetic Technologies
Will Be Combined to Provide New Opportunities
for People to Reach Their Reproductive Goals*

The Impact of In Vitro Fertilization

A singular moment in human evolution occurred on July 25, 1978, with the birth of Louise Joy Brown to Lesley and John Brown in the Oldham and General District Hospital in Oldham, England. Nine months earlier, a single egg had been removed from Lesley's ovary and placed into a small plastic dish by Patrick Steptoe. Sperm obtained from John Brown were added to the same droplet of culture fluid, and the dish was placed under the microscope where Steptoe's colleague, Robert Edwards, watched as fertilization took place. The fertilized egg was allowed to divide three times and was then placed into Mrs. Brown's uterus. At the end of July 1978, Louise Brown was born.[44] Why did I call the birth of Louise Brown a "singular moment in human evolution"? Medical science in the twentieth century has had enormous success developing cures for many once-fatal illnesses. Why should a cure for infertility—and an imperfect one at that—be singled out as more important than all of the hundreds of other medical advances that have occurred during our lives? Aren't cures for diseases that used to kill or lame children, in particular, more significant to our society?

I don't think a cure for infertility should be placed on a higher pedestal than the development of a polio vaccine or cures for childhood cancers. But this isn't what I had in mind when I used the phrase *singular moment*. Rather, it was the conviction that although in vitro fertilization, or IVF, was developed as a means for treating infertility, it will now serve as a stepping stone to many reprogenetic possibilities that go far beyond its original purpose. By bringing the embryo out of the darkness of the womb and into the light of day, IVF provides access to the genetic material within. And it is through the ability to read and alter genetic material inside the embryo that the full force of IVF will be felt.

Most people are aware of the impact that reproductive technology has had in the area of fertility treatment. Louise Brown is already nineteen years old, and the acronym IVF is in common use. The cloning of human beings has become a real possibility as well, although many are still confused as to what the technology can and cannot do.[45] Advances in genetic research are in the limelight, with almost weekly identifications of new genes implicated in diseases such as cystic fibrosis and breast cancer, or personality traits such as novelty seeking and anxiety.

But what has yet to catch the attention of the public-at-large is the incredible power that emerges when current technologies in reproductive biology and genetics are brought together in the form of reprogenetics. With reprogenetics, parents can gain complete control over their genetic destiny, with the ability to guide and enhance the characteristics of their children, and their children's children as well. As the editors of *Nature* put it in 1996, "That the growing power of molecular genetics confronts us with future prospects of being able to change the nature of our species is a fact that seldom appears to be addressed in depth."[46]

The development of IVF marks the point in history when human beings gained the power to seize control of their own reproductive and evolutionary destiny. In a very literal sense, IVF allows us to hold the future of our species in our own hands. The possibilities that open up with the use of IVF as a foundational technology can be grouped into two broad categories. The first is the enhancement of reproductive choice. In addition to providing a means for infertile heterosexual couples to overcome their infertility, extensions of the IVF technology will soon allow single adults to reproduce completely alone (through the procedure commonly referred to as cloning) and homosexual couples to reproduce children that share their genetic inputs. Although these alternative methods of reproduction will never be used by more than a fraction of the population, they will provide a benefit to society as a whole by allowing this group to reach their reproductive goals and achieve happiness through the birth of children who will be loved and cared for.

The second category is based on the fact that IVF and its associated protocols will provide access to the genetic material within the embryo. And it is through the ability to read and alter genetic material inside the embryo that the full force of IVF will be felt ultimately.

Will the Technology Be Used?

Before I describe the reproductive and reprogenetic possibilities made possible by IVF, it is important to consider whether people would actually be willing to sever the link between sexual intercourse and babies in an attempt to achieve some sort of reproductive goal, also whether they would be able to find professionals willing to work with them on the task. It depends, of course, on what the goal is. There's a big difference between curing infertility, on one hand, and trying to make sure your child inherits your curly hair, on the other. More than 75 percent of Americans now feel that IVF is an acceptable solution to infertility, while many fewer accept its use for purely cosmetic reasons.[47] But there are many reprogenetic goals that lie between these two extremes. Where will people draw the line?

No matter where it is drawn today, it will almost certainly be drawn to include more reprogenetic possibilities in the coming years, and more still in later years. This is because breakthrough technologies are always viewed as alien when they first appear—many people are instinctively opposed to things they are not accustomed to. But as the physicians Kleegman and Kaufman observed in 1966:

> Any change in custom or practice in this emotionally charged area [of assisted reproduction] has always elicited a response from established custom and law of horrified negation at first; then negation without horror; then slow and gradual curiosity, study, evaluation, and finally a very slow but steady acceptance.[48]

The public's opinion of IVF has evolved in this very way. When news of its development by Steptoe and Edwards reached the media during the 1970s, there were editorials calling for the abandonment of all further research on "test tube babies." And when the first IVF baby was born, most Americans found the notion so bizarre that they couldn't think about using it themselves. Over the period of a decade, however, IVF has been transformed from an alien concept to a broadly accepted medical approach for treating infertility.

Let's consider the arguments that can be made against the possibility that IVF will be used for purposes other than the alleviation of infertility. One argument is that people will not be willing to subject themselves to an alien technology that separates sex from reproduction just for the purpose of providing their children with some advantage that they might not otherwise have. Either ethical or emotional concerns, or both, could be at the root of this unwillingness.

A second argument concerns cost. Even if people had no objections to using the technology per se, they might not be willing to spend $30,000 or more for this purpose. A third argument is that even if people were willing to pay, they wouldn't be able to find clinics that were willing to provide the nonessential reprogenetic services that they desired. This could be because the technical expertise itself might not be available, or because those with the technical expertise have ethical objections to using it in this manner.

There is no doubt that in Western societies today, many people have a strong "gut reaction" against the use of reprogenetic technologies for nonmedical purposes. I observed this "gut reaction" when I asked a class of about 100 senior college students in a 1996 "Biotechnology and Society" course at Princeton whether they would ever consider the use of genetic engineering on their own children-to-be for any reason. More than 90 percent said no. But when I presented a hypothetical scenario in which genetic engineering might be used to provide absolute protection against AIDS, and posed the question again, half changed their minds. In a matter of minutes, they switched from rejecting a reprogenetic technology to accepting it.

What about the cost? Would $30,000 be too much to pay to ensure that a child would be born healthier or wiser in some way and better able to compete in the world? In fact, it is not uncommon for American parents to spend more than five times $30,000 to provide a child with four years of college education. And what is the point of this expenditure? It's to increase the chances that their child will become wiser, in some way, and better able to achieve success and happiness. If parents are willing to spend this money after birth—with no guarantee of a return on their investment—why not before? Parents might be willing to spend this money, you might say, but only the wealthy will be able to afford it. This notion is belied by the entry of so many middle-class couples into current IVF programs. In one well-known case, a Tennessee couple with a joint annual income of just $37,000 was able to come up with the money required for seven separate IVF attempts at pregnancy over a four-year period.[49]

Finally, there's the question of whether there will be clinics that are willing to provide these nonessential services. In this regard, there can be no doubt of the answer. IVF practitioners are expanding so rapidly that they are bound to reach a point where the pent-up demand from infertile couples is satisfied. When this point is reached, if not sooner, some will go looking for new customers.

Many practitioners, including those associated with major medical centers, may worry about political backlash from conservative political groups before proceeding. But consider the countries where IVF is being practiced successfully today; consider as well the hundreds of private clinics that operate in the United States; consider the amount of money to be made; and consider the fact that as of January 1999 there are no federal laws that regulate the services that private IVF practitioners can offer to their clients. If there are people who desire reprogenetic services, there will be others willing to provide them.

"Cloning"

The first method of alternative reproduction that I will discuss is cloning, which became a real possibility with the announcement in February 1997 that a healthy sheep named Dolly had been cloned from an adult cell.[50]

On January 6, 1998, less than a year after this announcement, an unemployed physicist named Richard Seed told a radio interviewer in the United States that he planned to set up a private clinic for cloning human beings. The media response to Dr. Seed, with television coverage and front page newspaper articles, was as immediate and nearly as explosive as the response to Ian Wilmut's announcement of Dolly. And yet, the actual accomplishments of Dr. Wilmut and Dr. Seed are as far apart as can be.

Dr. Seed did once dabble in fertility work, but that was over a decade ago. At present, he has no laboratory facilities at his disposal, no private or public funding, and no demonstrable commitment from actual physicians or reproductive biologists to perform the work. Indeed, there is no evidence whatsoever—and much to the contrary—that he can set up a clinic, let alone carry out the cloning protocol on human cells. Indeed, Dr. Seed does not even seem to appreciate the overwhelming technical obstacles that currently lie in the way of human cloning.

So why has a man on the street who says he plans to clone human beings garnered so much attention, including a direct response from the President of the United States? I believe the answer lies not in what Dr. Seed himself can, or cannot, do, but rather in the startling realization by the American public, in particular, that human cloning may be pursued in private clinics, no matter how many government officials, scientists, and bioethicists argue against it in public.

Although human cloning is not feasible today, I have no doubt that it will become so one day. Dr. Wilmut and his group proved that the clonal production of a healthy mammal was scientifically possible. The transformation of this scientific result into a usable technology will almost certainly follow the same path as other science-to-technology conversions in the field of biotechnology. In the wake of Dr. Ian Wilmut's announcement, numerous researchers have jumped into the cloning fray, working on a variety of different animals. Already, a more efficient method for producing cloned animals by somatic cell nuclear transfer (cows, in this case) has been published by an independent group,[51] and live-born monkeys have also been born by a separate cloning technique.[52] Over the next several years, it is very likely that the biotechnical community, as a whole, will resolve the technical problems associated with cloning, increase its efficiency, ultimately demonstrate its safety on a monkey species closely related to humans, and optimize the protocol to the point that it could be used to create human embryos for development into children. The question, in my mind, is not whether this will happen, but when.

The initial reaction to the announcement of Dolly's birth—from the public around the world—was one of hysteria. In retrospect, it's not hard to understand why the public reacted this way. In the absence of scientific understanding of what actually took place in Scotland, people had no choice but to visualize human clones through the images fed to them by popular culture—as full-grown replicate, but perhaps inferior, copies of human beings that already exist. Not surprisingly, these ghoulish images led to a sense of revulsion.

Even with an accurate scientific understanding of what cloning can and cannot accomplish, there are still many who adamantly oppose its human application. First, they worry about safety and efficiency—perfectly legitimate concerns, but ones that will surely be made moot, sooner rather than later, if we use past history of technological advances as our guide. Then they worry about the psychological well-being of the child. They fear that a cloned child will have a reduced sense of individuality, will not be treated with dignity and respect, and will be ostracized by society. To my mind, these fears are mainly based on an exaggerated expectation of what cloning can accomplish as well as an exaggerated notion of genetic determinism.

Right now, there are children being born somewhere in the world who will mature into a "spitting image" of one parent or the other, just by chance. Other children will express a personality and behavior that is a replica of one parent, just by chance. And for a small number of children born every day, it will be both: a "chip off the old block," as the old saying goes. Indeed, there are surely people alive today, around the world, who are actually more similar in both looks and personality to a parent than might be expected, on average, with a child who is a genetic clone! For this reason, observers will never know for sure (in the absence of DNA testing) whether a child is really a clone or just a parental look-alike.

As is so often the case with new reproductive technologies, the real reason that people condemn cloning has nothing to do with technical feasibility, child psychology, societal well-being, or the preservation of the human species.[53] The real reason derives from religious beliefs. It is the sense that cloning leaves God out of the process of human creation and that man is venturing into places he does not belong. Of course, the "playing God" objection makes sense only in the context of one definition of God, as a supernatural being who plays a role in the birth of each new member of our species. And even if one holds this particular view of God, it does not necessarily follow that cloning is equivalent to playing God. Some who consider themselves to be religious have argued that if God didn't want man to clone, "he" wouldn't have made it possible. Should public policy in a pluralistic society be based on a narrow religious point of view? Most people would say No, which is why those who hold this point of view are grasping for secular reasons to support their call for an unconditional ban on the cloning of human beings. When the dust clears from the cloning debate, however, the secular reasons will almost certainly have disappeared. Then, only religious objections will remain.

But just because something can be done does not mean that it should be done. Will the cloning of human beings provide any benefit to society? The answer is Yes. It will provide a means for a small fraction of the population to achieve their reproductive goals, and by increasing happiness in these people, it will benefit society as a whole.

The desire to have biological children is a deeply ingrained instinct, second only to self-preservation. In the United States, couples unable to have children because of fertility problems can spend $30,000 or more to obtain treatments that can include in vitro fertilization, sperm donation, egg donation, or the services of a surrogate mother. Cloning, better labeled somatic cell nuclear transfer (SCNT), is one more tool that could be used by fertility clinics to help clients achieve their reproductive goals. As one example, SCNT may provide the only means by which a couple that is unable to produce either sperm or eggs could still have a biological child (or two, with one related to each parent). In such a case, the U.S. Constitution might legitimize this couple's right to nuclear transfer as a matter of procreative liberty.

As another example of who might want to use the "nuclear transfer" technology and why, I want to present a fantasy story that takes place fifty years in the future. It is the story of an American woman named Jennifer.[54] Jennifer is single, forty years old, financially secure, and the happy mother of a seven-year-old daughter from an earlier marriage. Even though she doesn't have a man in her life, Jennifer wants to have a second child. She knows that menopause is on the horizon, and she must act quickly. Many other women in her situation have used anonymous sperm donors to achieve pregnancy, but for Jennifer, a new option has become available. A reproductive clinic in Indonesia has recently begun to offer "nuclear transfer" as one of its many services. Although the price is steep at

$100,000, Jennifer knows she can afford it. And so Jennifer compares her options. She could use a sperm donor to fertilize her eggs, or she could initiate a pregnancy with one of her own cells. Which method should she choose? An anonymous sperm donor could bring all sorts of unknown genes and undesirable traits into her child so what would she gain? On the other hand, what would be so terrible about having a child who carried 100 percent of her mother's genetic material, if no one knew?

Jennifer makes up her mind to go abroad for a two-week holiday by herself. One month after she returns, her gynecologist confirms her pregnancy. He knows that she is a single woman, but he doesn't ask—and she doesn't tell—how her pregnancy began. Eight months later a newborn baby is delivered. Jennifer names her Eve. To the nurses and doctors on the maternity ward, Eve is just one more baby, just like all the other babies they've seen in their lives.

Eve will grow up in a loving household like many other children her age. Occasionally, people will comment on the striking similarity that exists between Eve and her mother. Jennifer will smile at them and say, "Yes. She does have my facial features." And she'll leave it at that. And then one day, when Eve is well into her teens, Jennifer will explain to her how her development began. And like other children conceived with special reproductive technologies, Eve will feel . . . special.

No matter what the laws are in Jennifer's home country, they will have no impact on her ability to use the "nuclear transfer" process at a clinic somewhere in the world where it is not illegal (it is illegal in most of the United States at the present time). But in the final analysis, SCNT won't make a bit of difference to society at large. No heads will turn when an SCNT child walks down the street, just as no heads now turn at the sight of a child born through IVF, egg donation, or artificial insemination. And as times passes, in the decades ahead, more and more individuals and couples who must now seek out sperm (or egg) donors to achieve pregnancy, will ask themselves, "Why not just use one of my own cells?"

Shared Genetic Motherhood through Embryo Fusion

Cloning is just one new way in which some people of the future will choose to reproduce. Many happily bonded couples view the birth of a child who brings together their genetic material as the ultimate consummation of their love for each other. And when barriers lie in the way of achieving this goal, many couples will do anything within their power to overcome them. A certain type of happily bonded couple, however, has never even considered the possibility of joining their genes together in a child. I am speaking, of course, of same-sex couples.[55]

Most people think it is biologically impossible for two unrelated women (or men) to both pass on their genetic material to a single child. But twenty years ago, a Polish embryologist demonstrated the feasibility of a protocol for accomplishing just this result in mice. Tarkowski reasoned that if very young embryos could be separated into individual cells which could then go on to develop independently as identical twins, triplets, or quadruplets, it should be possible to reverse the process and combine multiple embryonic cells to form a single animal. Tarkowski reasoned further that if cells originating from the same embryo could be brought together, it should also be possible to bring together cells from different embryos or even cells produced by different mouse parents.

Tarkowski's simple method worked like a charm, and since his original publication in 1961, the method has been repeated in hundreds of laboratories.[56] When embryos produced by pairs of mice from two strains with different fur colors are merged together, the success of the protocol is clearly visible in the offspring born. If an albino-strain embryo is mixed with a dark-colored one, the resulting offspring exhibit a patchwork coat with alternating areas of dark and white fur.

It is important to understand what is and is not happening inside a merged embryo from two sets of parents. At the cellular level, nothing happens. Each individual cell retains its identity; no fusion between cells takes place. But, as the embryo develops, the cells derived from different parents mix together and communicate with each other as if they are all members of the same team. And when the animal is born, every tissue within it—including the brain and gonads—is a mixture of cells from the original two embryos. Now creating chimeric mice is all well and good, but how do we know that we could actually accomplish the same thing with human embryos? I could remind you that mouse, human, and all other early mammalian embryos are virtually indistinguishable from each other and will almost certainly respond to manipulations in the same way. This is the logic that Steptoe and Edwards followed in their decade-long quest to perfect conditions for in vitro fertilization in humans.

But I don't need to rely on this logic at all, because mother nature has already done the experiment for us. Since the 1950s, more than 100 natural-born chimeric human beings have been identified by medical geneticists. Each of these people emerged from the fusion of two embryos that resulted from the fertilization of two eggs that the mother had simultaneously ovulated. We should not be surprised by this rare, but natural, process because we already know that embryos can spontaneously fall apart to form identical twins. If scientists can get two mouse embryos to stick together on contact in the lab, then the same thing should occasionally happen spontaneously in a woman's reproductive tract.

In almost all respects, a chimeric person—like a chimeric mouse—is indistinguishable from other human beings. But, like mice, there are two ways to recognize some chimeric humans. If the two embryos that merged together had genetic makeups programmed toward very different skin or hair colorations, then the chimeric person could have a patchy complexion or hair color. Among naturally-born chimeric humans, this type of abnormality is rarely observed.

The second distinction occurs when an embryo with an XX genetic constitution merges with an embryo having an XY genetic constitution. During fetal development, the tissues that differentiate into the sex organs will be bombarded by conflicting signals. More often than not, signals from the Y chromosome predominate, and the individual develops normal, or nearly normal, male genitalia. But the gonads themselves will often develop as mixtures of ovarian and testicular tissues. In some cases, the combination of male and female signals can cause the external genitalia to develop into an intermediate configuration with an enlarged clitoris (or reduced penis) and other tissue intermediate between a scrotum and a vulva, with perhaps a shallow vagina or none at all.[57] In fact, intersex chimeras can have genitalia ranging anywhere from normal female to normal male. And perhaps surprisingly, intersex chimeras can be fertile and have children, sometimes as a father, sometimes as a mother.

It is only when their genitalia are what physicians call "ambiguous" that chimeric human beings usually are detected. However, for every chimeric person identified through ambiguous genitalia, there are likely to be four or more other chimeric individuals who have gone through life unnoticed. These include essentially all of the chimeric people formed by the merger of two same-sex embryos as well as many intersex chimeras who have developed as normal men or women.

With intentional embryo fusion, the possibility of intersex formation can be eliminated by pre-sexing the embryos and choosing two of the same gender. Thus, embryo fusion technology could provide a means for same-sex couples to combine their "bloodlines" in a single child, just as heterosexual couples do all the time.

Reprogenetics

Amazingly, as the world's attention has been focused on the prospect of so-called human cloning, other powerful technologies with a much greater potential for altering the nature of the human race have been developed without much fanfare over the last twenty years. This enormous potential will emerge when current technologies in reproductive biology and genetics are brought together in the form of "reprogenetics." With reprogenetics, prospective parents will gain the power to select which of their genes to pass down to their children and whether to add in other genes to protect their children from diseases, both inherited and infectious.

Already, embryos produced in the laboratory can be genetically screened so that parents can begin their pregnancy with one free of a particular disease—such as cystic fibrosis or Tay-Sachs disease. And, in fact, children have been born disease-free this way.[58] But this technology can just as easily be used to select for the presence or absence of any known gene. And within twenty years, we will know every one of the 100 thousand human genes. The implication of this knowledge is profound. It means that parents will be able to select genes that provide their children with resistance to what many consider to be less-serious diseases such as obesity, alcoholism, or clinical depression. Ultimately, it means that parents might be able to select for positive traits like height, happiness, or inborn talents in one realm or another.[59]

Some scientists don't believe that the technology of embryo screening will ever become this powerful. These scientists claim that the genetic component of these positive and negative traits is too complex and that the technology of embryo screening is not powerful enough to do such complex screening.

But these same scientists would have told you just twelve years ago that DNA screening of embryos would forever be impossible. Indeed, every scientist thought it was impossible, and now there are children alive today based on the use of this so-called impossible technology. Thirty years ago, scientists thought we might never be able to characterize all 100 thousand human genes, and now we are only a few years away from accomplishing the feat. Just five years ago, most scientists still thought it would be impossible to rapidly screen all those genes in any individual, and now the technology to accomplish this very task—based on DNA chips—is already in use. As the physicist and visionary, Freeman Dyson, says in this regard: "The human species has a deeply ingrained tendency to prove the experts wrong."[60]

But there is an inherent limit to what embryo selection can accomplish by itself. All it can ever do is allow a couple to choose from among their own genes to give, or not give, to their children.

Germline Genetic Engineering

A reprogenetic technology that will allow prospective parents to go beyond their own genes is called germline genetic engineering. It could allow parents to enhance their embryos with genes that they themselves do not carry. Genetic engineering is already routine in laboratory animals such as the mouse.[61] and it has been performed with success in pigs, sheep, cows, and goats as well.[62] There is no limit to the kind of genes that can be added to the embryo. Genes from one species can be manipulated before they are placed into another to carry out their designated task. So a cow, for example, can be engineered with a manipulated human insulin gene to produce human insulin in its milk.

This ultimate reprogenetic technology has not yet been applied to human embryos for two reasons. First, it has not been very efficient. Second, apart from issues of efficiency or safety, the idea of manipulating human genes is deeply troubling to many people.

Once again, problems of safety and efficiency may soon be resolved. Indeed, probably the most important implication of the nuclear transfer technology is that it provides a means for solving the efficiency problem.[63] Thus, there is every reason to believe that genetic engineering could become feasible on human embryos in the near future.

What reason might people have for wanting to use this technology? One answer is to provide protection against disease. In fact, we can already imagine a way to use genetic engineering to provide absolute genetic protection against infection with HIV, which causes AIDS.[64] And as we learn more and more about our own genetics, it will become possible to develop more and more sophisticated genetic enhancements for parents to use to give their children other health advantages.

The Final Chapter:
Extending the Human Mind

"Have you ever imagined what might become of our race in the future?," asked the bright young man. "Do you think future people could have intellectual powers far, far beyond our own?" The village elders shook their heads as they smiled in unison, seeming to say, "Been there, thought that." "No," they explained, "it is not possible. The problem, my bright young man, is that our brains are so unbelievably complex that any tinkering meant to improve one aspect of mental processing would surely diminish another. *We are the final chapter.* We are exactly what God intended us to be."

Beginning almost two centuries ago with Mary Shelley's *Frankenstein,* countless works of fiction have focused on the theme of humans who succeed in creating human life or enhancing known human life beyond its "natural" form. While the stories differ in detail, the moral is always the same: Anyone who tries to play God is not only doomed to fail but to cause ghastly pain and destruction. We humans are the final chapter, these stories assert. We are exactly what God intended us to be. Given the complexity of our bodies and brains, not to mention our *souls*, there is not merely a possibility of unintended consequences for attempting to usurp God's power—there is a natural *law* to prevent it.

Although the creation of humanoids has a long history in literature, it was impossible for anyone—scientist or nonscientist—even to imagine the genetic enhancement of natural-born human beings before the discovery of the molecular structure of the gene by Watson and Crick in 1952. Since the 1970s, there has been a rapid increase in the number of science fiction writers who have taken a stab at this idea, often in ways much less fantastical and more realistic than previous portrayals of humanoids.

Nevertheless, the moral remains the same. In two excellent examples from this genre—*Brain Child* by George Turner[65] and *Beggars in Spain* by Nancy Kress[66]—genetic engineering is used to provide children with superior abilities. But—and there's always a but—these "superior" children are deficient in some way. In both novels, as in Philip K. Dick's *Do Androids Dream of Electric Sheep?*,[67] which gave rise to the film *Blade Runner,* genetically enhanced children lack empathy, and their "race" is doomed. In the 1997 movie *Gattaca,* the most fully developed, genetically enhanced characters are actually weaker in body and mind than the unenhanced protagonist and hero. Indeed, there is a common, if unspoken, implication in all these works that genetic engineering for the purpose of enhancement is, and always will be, morally wrong. And it's not just the fiction writers who moralize. Dean Hamer, one of the top scientists studying genetic links to such human behaviors as homosexuality, curiosity, and anxiety, agrees with this point of view in his recent book, *Living with Our Genes.*

What exactly is the moral objection to genetic enhancement? Well, that's not always clear. Writers' and scientists' views on this subject are laden with emotion; when all else fails, they fall back on the assertion that it shouldn't be done because *it won't work.* As Hamer says, "Using genes to select elaborate traits in children before they are born will *always* be an exercise in frustration because of the *inevitable* trade-offs that parents will have to accept."[68] The words *always* and *inevitable* leave little room for maneuvering, yet this respected scientist fails to shore them up with any logical argument.

The *law* of unintended consequences. Yin-yang. What goes up, must come down. The light that burns twice as bright burns half as long. And so on, and so on. These are the clichés that writers, social commentators, and some scientists have long used to pooh-pooh the idea that humans might someday succeed at creating or enhancing human life beyond its "natural" form. As the village elders said, "We are the final chapter."

Old clichés die hard. What goes up need *not* come down—anymore. The so-called law of inevitable trade-offs is based on religion or ideology, not science. This is not to say that there aren't sometimes unintended negative consequences of attempts to improve the human condition. Of course there are, and there always will be. But the twentieth century has witnessed a series of medical and technological advances that have greatly improved human health and increased longevity. We have gone higher and higher without stumbling.

But our minds are different, you might say. They represent the essence of humanity, and it's pure hubris to imagine that we could improve upon them. Really? What if the exchange between the bright young man and the village elders had taken place among early *Homo erectus* individuals, 1.5 million years ago rather than today? Since that time, a doubling in brain size has led to a massive increase in intellectual capacity, which has brought about civilizations in which most people are protected from the cruel hand of nature. The *Homo erectus* elders would have been proven wrong.

So why couldn't we evolve even further in the direction of increased intellectual capacity? Well, for one thing, it won't happen "naturally." The most important evolutionary consequence of civilization is that greater intelligence—no matter what its root basis—does not lead a person to have more children. And only genes that increase reproductive output are "naturally" selected. Thus, the natural evolution of intelligence has come to a grinding halt.

Nevertheless, I am convinced that further evolution of our minds will occur. It's just the driving force that will be different. Instead of evolving naturally, the present-day human species is on the verge of self-evolving. If our civilization doesn't self-destruct, and if our world is not destroyed by an asteroid, the human race has five *billion* years left on the planet earth before the sun burns out. That's a very long time. Can you really believe that we will never figure out how to enhance intellectual capacity *without* any trade-offs, when the technology is practically at our doorsteps today? If not in the next decade, what about the next century, millennium, or million years?

Of course, just because something *can* be done does not mean that it *will* be done. But the driving force behind self-evolution is as transparent as can be. Parents have always wanted to give their children all possible advantages in life, and what could be more advantageous than increased intelligence? And where there's a demand, there will be a market.

Not so, some say. The government will control the use of genetic technology. Look at the massive governmental effort to identify all 70 thousand human genes, an effort molded by public debate on the uses and abuses of the information obtained.

Incredibly, in May 1998, while no one was looking, the Human Genome Project was snatched up by a private biotechnical company that will do it faster, cheaper, and without any oversight whatsoever. How long will it be before clever scientists use the information generated in this project to develop reprogenetic technologies that meet the market demand, which is sure to expand along with the power of the technology itself, for genetic enhancement? Those who condemn any talk of cognitive enhancement as an act of hubris have it backwards. The real hubris is displayed by those who claim confidently that we are the final chapter.

PART II

THE ROAD AHEAD

A Panel Discussion

This part offers a unique view of the feasibility and significance of germline engineering and a look at where the technology lies within our present medical, scientific, and societal landscape.
In addition to the authors of the book's essays, the discussants included
John Fletcher, a distinguished ethicist; Andrea Bonnicksen, a public policy
expert; and Nobel laureate James D. Watson, codiscoverer of the structure
of DNA and founder of the Human Genome Project. Gregory Stock, director of UCLA's Program on Medicine, Technology, and Society, moderated.
Though this remarkable discussion took place before a large audience, pre-
sentations and questions from onlookers were avoided. The discussion's
course went wherever the panel's exchanges led it. The spontaneity of the
participants and their candor in addressing even the most controversial
issues surrounding human germline engineering make this exchange as
provocative and stimulating today as it was in 1998, when it took place at
the UCLA symposium, "Engineering the Human Germline," the first major public forum where key scientists and educators openly explored the
topic before the public.

———————

GREGORY STOCK: Dr. Fletcher, you have a doctor of divinity degree, so I'd
like to ask what role you feel religion plays in our evaluation of the pro-
priety of germline engineering and other sorts of genetic technologies?

JOHN FLETCHER: Actually, I don't have a doctor of divinity degree. I received my doctorate at Union Theological Seminary in 1969, and in
those days you studied ethics and received a doctor of theology degree

with a specialty in ethics. But so many of my colleagues who received the degree couldn't get employed that they petitioned Union, which then petitioned the Board of Regents of the State of New York to change the nomenclature, and by action of the Board of Regents we all became Ph.D.s. Also, in the interests of full disclosure, inthe late eighties, after thirty-five years of trying to hold together the beliefs of Christian theology and modern biology, I gave up the struggle and resigned from the Episcopal ministry and became a friendly critic of religion.

I am not an enemy of religion. I recognize its power for good and for evil. My view of religion is that it is an evolutionary program fulfilling a very important function: to make you aware that you're part of the whole. Human beings are the only species who are aware they are part of a whole, and that is an awesome insight that binds us all together. I think the concept of God blurs that insight for the most part, rather than magnifies it. Religion plays a powerful part in the development of peoples all over the world, especially in our culture, where religion is so vibrant and alive and where there are so many types of religious movements.

On the whole, religion plays a very conservative role in response to genetics. And it actually, in its worst features, makes people afraid and passive in the face of terrible things that nature and genetic roulette can do to children.

I think one of the greatest harms of some religions in the world today is the doctrine that unprotected sex is sanctified. The idea behind the doctrine is to promote unity between sexual love and reproduction, but unprotected sex is the greatest threat to women in the world. It's also a threat to men, but it's certainly a threat to women.

In my experience, very few deeply religious people are open to understanding biological evolution. It is not hard to understand why. Evolution by natural selection powerfully answers how we and all living things descended from one source, a tree of life that slowly evolved over billions of years. This answer offends many deeply religious people who attribute all power to a God who, they believe, created them and everything else as Genesis described it. The biblically literalistic churches wage "culture wars" against this answer and misinform children about the development of life on the planet. However, evolution need not offend an inquiring religious mind. It is a very large step from the question, "Why and how did living things come to be?" to "What is the meaning of life?" The second question involves choices between world views and ultimate loyalties, and Darwin's answer to the first question implies but does not dictate a particular philosophy of life. Noting these differences, moderate and liberal religious traditions make room for evolutionary science in the anterooms of their theodicies and theologies. So, religious views of science and evolution create a spectrum of responses to human genetics and genetic technologies. Although conservatives lack the social power to block advances in human genetics, they have blocked federal funding of genetic research involving living human fetuses or embryos.

Public life in a democracy is like a large table to which parties willingly and openly come for discussion. There is a minority of the religious who shun this table. Among them an even smaller minority dangerously acts out their hatred of science. A so-called Army of God bombs abortion clinics. I know of a scientist in a well-known university who works with stem cells derived from electively aborted fetal tissue. He takes a different way to work every day because he is afraid that somebody with this mindset may harm him.

So, you have posed a complex question about the role that religion plays in evaluating germline engineering and genetic technologies. The answer is complex, but in the public affairs of science, religion is a force with which to reckon. Anyone who underestimates the power of religious groups in this nation is politically naive. If one is involved in the public process, the table had best be set so that all can come, express their views, and have a role in settling questions like germline genetic modifications. Neglect of religion will mean that before the end of the process, hostility will prevail, which comes back to harm you.

GREGORY STOCK: Thank you. I think it's going to be very difficult to come to a consensus on these issues, because they affect us so deeply and fundamentally. Dr. Bonnicksen, you've written about international perspectives on genetics. There are such different attitudes about germline engineering and genetic engineering in general; could you say a few words about the key differences that exist globally?

ANDREA BONNICKSEN: I can best answer this by looking at a few national perspectives, a regional perspective, and an international perspective, because many different voices around the world have been heard about germline manipulations. These voices have come to the forefront of national and transnational governments more vocally than they have in the United States, where the federal government has not created the opportunity to discuss the issues.

One example in Europe of what I would call a permissive climate is the United Kingdom, which has a licensing system for embryo research and in vitro fertilization. The law setting up this system has been in effect since 1990, and it leaves the door open for germline manipulations and other medical innovations. It states that there will not be germline interventions unless they meet regulations, but this leaves the door open, so I would consider it permissive.

Other nations are permissive by default, not having a national law on embryo research.

And some are restrictive. There are two kinds of restrictive voices: one includes countries that have restrictive embryo research laws that are so broad they would, in effect, prohibit germline manipulations. This leaves the door open, because if embryo research were to reach the point where germline interventions were safe, then perhaps their application would be appropriate.

Another restrictive type has an embryo research law that specifically mentions germline interventions. Germany would be an example of a highly restrictive law. Its Embryo Protection Act has been in effect since 1990. Here there is concern for individual rights. but there is more distrust of the ability to draw lines against technological change. There is also a concern for the human genome as a common heritage of humanity.

On the regional level, the Parliamentary Assembly of the Council of Europe in 1982 issued a recommendation stating that there is a right to inherit a genetic pattern that has not been interfered with, except according to certain principles. What might those principles be? The Council of Europe produced in 1997 a bioethics convention now out for the signatures of the Council's member states. Twenty-two nations have already signed it. This convention looks for principles that would guide such things as the deliberate intervention in the human genome. A key phrase states: "An intervention seeking to modify the human genome may only be undertaken for preventive, diagnostic, or therapeutic purposes and only if its aim is not to introduce any modification in the genome of any descendants." This indicates a more or less closed door, but still only half of the member states have signed the convention.

Another international body is the United Nations Educational, Scientific, and Cultural Organization [UNESCO], which has a global rather than regional orientation. One-hundred-eighty-six nations signed the Universal Declaration on the Human Genome and Human Rights in 1997. This declaration was four years and nine drafts in the making. It was designed to balance individual rights with the promise of genetic inquiry for all people. It did not forbid germline interventions, so it left the door open. It did, however, call for further discussion about practices that "could be contrary to human dignity, such as germline interventions."

There are other organizations as well, but in the interest of time let me make a couple of summary points. First, national laws on germline gene therapy are caught up in broader laws on embryo research and assisted reproductive technologies. We cannot talk about germline therapy without considering the policies on embryo research. And much of the concern relates to the sanctity or the non-sancitity of the embryo. What the embryo is will determine what people believe about what should be done with it.

Second, there is no single approach to germline manipulations. There are polar worldviews, illustrated by differing policies in the United Kingdom and Germany, so this is not a simple matter to discuss. International documents have attempted to bridge these polar views, and the UNESCO declaration is an effective example of that.

Third, germline policies are efforts to protect human rights before the techniques have even been developed, and the result is an odd mixture of definitions and notions. If you look at the different documents and the national laws, you have to scratch your head a bit and say, "What exactly is being forbidden here? And when we hear about all of the things that were discussed today, are they or are they not forbidden?" This is one of the perils of advance regulation.

And a final point, these regulations do not deal explicitly with enhancement. They all deal with germline gene therapy.

GREGORY STOCK: Thank you. You mention how restrictive the laws are in Germany and in a couple of the other countries in Europe. Dr. Watson, you've spoken very eloquently about the legacy of eugenics and the abuses of Hitler. What are your thoughts about the impact that legacy has had on our perception of genetic engineering and germline engineering?

JAMES D. WATSON: I think people are frightened by the term *gene*, frightened that genes are powerful and can be used against people. The main message we need to draw is to keep, insofar as possible, the state out of any form of genetic decision. Consider what happened in Russia, where they essentially banned genetics because the concept of genetic inequality didn't appeal to them. Since there is genetic inequality of all sorts, it's denying reality.

In the case of the eugenics movement, genes are often used to justify racial, class, and religious prejudice, and in a very awful way. This left a legacy, particularly in Germany, which I think still hasn't really faced up to what they did.

When Benno Muller published his very popular book, *Murderous Science* [Cold Spring Harbor, N.Y.: Cold Spring Harbor Press, 1997], he only received one review in all of Germany, and he hasn't been elected to any German academy, despite the fact that his work with Wally Gilbert on the lactose repressor was very major science. So Benno has simply been penalized for drawing attention to what happened in Germany.

I think the complexity of genetics makes regulation very difficult. For instance, the term *enhancement*. Should you restrict abortions only to serious genetic diseases? What may be serious to one family isn't serious to another. What's frivolous to some people isn't frivolous to others. Very few cultures are monolithic; and particularly in the United States it's hard to form a consensus for letting people go their own way.

I'm very afraid of the middle class deciding what's best for poor and unfortunate people. I think they're patronizing, and they distrust the notion of trying to improve human beings, because they think they're pretty well off. In reality, they're not really worrying about the people who suffer from what I call "genetic injustice."

Evolution can be very cruel. There's an enormous amount of variation that is there to create the variations that have been necessary in the past for survival in changing environments. We have quite a high mutation rate, so many people are born with very obvious defects where their genes don't let them function as well as other people.

I certainly was very conscious of eugenics and, particularly, the role of my own institution, Cold Spring Harbor Laboratories, in the eugenics movement in the United States. When we started the Human Genome Project, we decided to spend 3 percent of our money for the discussion of ethics, and I think that's been among the wisest money we've spent. We simply tried to co-opt as many people as possible into discussing genetics. I think, as you discuss it, you realize how difficult it is.

My principle here is pretty simple: Just have most of the decisions made by women as opposed to men. They're the ones who bear children, and men, as you know, often sneak away from children that aren't healthy. We're going to have to feel more responsible for the next generation. I think women should be allowed to make the decisions, and as far as I'm concerned, keep these male doctor committees out of action. The French are the perfect example of that. Their policies are a mistake. . . . Keep them away. . . .

W. FRENCH ANDERSON (interrupting): Am I a good example or a bad example?

JAMES D. WATSON: You're a terrible example of trying to tell other people what to do. We will not know whether things work perfectly. You sounded so conservative I just couldn't believe it. We are going to make mistakes in this world. Mistakes are made all the time. Someone gets a bad surgeon and they die. If the surgeon continues to make mistakes, he loses his license, and at least you know where he is. Some people are going to have to have some guts and try germline therapy without completely knowing that it's going to work.

It seems obvious that germline therapy will be much more successful than somatic. If we wait for the success of somatic therapy, we'll wait until the sun burns out. We might as well do what we finally can to take the threat of Alzheimer's away from a family or breast cancer away from a family. The biggest ethical problem we have is not using our knowledge, . . . people not having the guts to go ahead and try and help someone. We're always going to have to take chances.

It seems to me the question we're going to have to face is, what is going to be the least unpleasant? Using abortion to get rid of nasty genes from families? Or developing germline procedures with which, using Mario Capecchi's techniques, you can go in and get rid of a bad gene.

Right now, abortion, unpleasant as it is, sounds to me a lot easier and more predictable. But assuming that research goes forward, you may reach a situation where people will say that germline modification is safer and causes less stress to the people involved. One doesn't want to justify a procedure on something you can't predict, but having good germline therapy to protect us if a terrible virus suddenly occurred on the face of the Earth might be a very good thing.

We could have these techniques on hand so that we could at least see that the children who are going to be born won't die of a new plague. It's common sense to try and develop it. I think the slippery slope argument is just crap. If you get a Hitler, nothing's going to protect us. Societies thrive when they're optimistic, not pessimistic, and the slippery slope argument sounds like one from a worn-out person who's angry at himself.

And the other thing, because no one has the guts to say it, if we could make better human beings by knowing how to add genes, why shouldn't we do it? What's wrong with it? Who is telling us not to do it? I mean, it just seems obvious now. I think, and Mario Capecchi knows all too well, that these procedures are difficult. But if you could cure what I feel is a very serious disease—that is, stupidity—it would be a great thing for people who are otherwise going to be born seriously disadvantaged. We should be honest and say that we shouldn't just accept things that are incurable. I just think, "What would make someone else's life better?" And if we can help without too much risk, we've got to go ahead and not worry whether we're going to offend some fundamentalist from Tulsa, Oklahoma.

GREGORY STOCK: Well, I hope Dr. Watson's frankness and openness is a model for everyone on the panel. Let's try and get at the core of these issues in a very concrete way. Safety and reliability have come up a number of times, and Dr. Anderson has stated very stringent requirements—including primate testing—as to what would be safe. I'm not sure all his requirements have been met even for somatic testing, certainly not for some fetal therapies. Does anyone else have some thoughts about the levels of safety that are required and when we might achieve those? Lee?

LEROY HOOD: Mario would be more qualified. I have opinions but not facts.

GREGORY STOCK: Well, why don't you give an opinion then, and afterwards Mario can give us the facts.

LEROY HOOD: I agree with Jim [Watson]. I think science proceeds and succeeds by doing. And I think what we're talking about here are incremental advances with enormous implications. If we're shackled by "You can't do fetal research. You can't do this; you can't do that. . . ." Some of the laws that have come up to ban cloning would ban everything that has anything to do with the word *clone.* That includes DNA as well as cells. I think that's something we can't afford to have in our society. You need to be reasonable and rational. Yes, you should do animal testing, but how far you have to carry it I'm not certain.

Some of the well-known model systems will give us much of the information we need, but it would be a shame if we were really inhibited by society. Again, I agree with Jim [Watson]. The great thing about American society is its enormous diversity. It's the equivalent of what Mario [Capecchi] was talking about regarding genes. An implication of that is that people have to have the right to make decisions based on what their diversity is all about. If we follow that to its logical conclusion, I would say that we have unique opportunities to bring together the kind of things we've talked about today, and we can make enormous changes. In twenty-five years we'll be, as Mario [Capecchi] said, ahead of anything that we can conceivably imagine now.

I think the specific details of what we can do may be answered when we get to the point where we know exactly what tools are available. At that point we can formulate theories on how to proceed, rather than talking well before the fact and trying to set up abstract rules and regulations. So, how about some facts, Mario?

GREGORY STOCK: Mario, do you have any comments?

MARIO R. CAPECCHI: First, in terms of safety, the issues can actually be addressed in fairly simple organisms—for example, mice. How much damage do you do if you micro-inject? Those issues haven't been examined in detail because nobody has had reasons to address such questions. But if we have the impetus, such issues can be addressed. One thing I am afraid of is to set stringent guidelines saying you have to go through animal A, B, C, D, and E. Certain questions can be addressed in certain organisms, and other questions will have to be addressed in other organisms. For example, when you make transgenic animals of domestic quality, you find mosaics much more frequently than when you do it in a mouse. So, doing experiments in different species is of value. But that doesn't mean every time you want to do a protocol you should go through animals A, B, C, and D. What it means is that certain safety tests are done in different species but that most could be done in species such as mice. It saves money, it saves time, and, I think, limits the need for regulation. The criterion should be that you have demonstrated that the procedure is not doing harm. A remarkable fact is that we've been using recombinant DNA technology for twenty-five years, and there's very little evidence any harm has ever been done. That's quite remarkable compared to any other industry. So I think we should be proud that there have not been the catastrophes that people envisioned, and just march forward—but at the research level.

GREGORY STOCK: Thank you. Dr. Koshland, you had a response?

DANIEL KOSHLAND, JR.: I want to come in on the side of more hope and optimism. I was listening to French [Anderson] and it sounded to me that, based on the hazards and the problems, we should give up sexual intercourse for about ten years until we really understand what's going on. To be serious, when you look at something new, the benchmark for safety must be how hazardous the present process is. When you think of childbirth and conception, it really is a hazardous undertaking—let alone how the children grow up.

Absolute safety is never going to be possible. At a certain point, the advantages are going to be clear for an individual. What is good about cloning is that we're not doing it to everybody all at once; we're doing it incrementally. In the case of a childless couple, using a process that will give them a child means an enormous amount; it is very different from a couple with several children interested in a slight enhancement. Individuals are going to have to decide how much risk they'll take to try to get an optimal result. I think we need to be careful about flat prohibitions.

GREGORY STOCK: Dr. Anderson, you wanted a chance to respond?

W. FRENCH ANDERSON: Yes. I'm having a wonderful time, because having endured a considerable number of death threats when we pioneered somatic-cell gene therapy, and now facing another onslaught of these when we announce fetal gene therapy, to be attacked because I'm a fundamentalist from Tulsa, Oklahoma, is extraordinary.

It might sound funny, but I agree with what everybody says. I think the difference is that perhaps my perspective is slightly different in the sense, at least for somatic-cell, and it appears, for fetal gene therapy, I'm the guy behind the eight ball. If we produce a defective fetus, I'm the guy who's going to get sued, and I'm the guy who will have to face the parents and the press. So, yes, I'm a little more conservative than others.

GREGORY STOCK: Another aspect of this is that you had to go through some fifteen committees and present all sorts of evidence to Congress. It must be very difficult to convince officials to allow you to do what you're doing.

W. FRENCH ANDERSON: It does warp the mind a bit, yes.

GREGORY STOCK: Thank you. Now, John Campbell, I've noticed there has been a little sniping at you today. You've proposed a double-addition approach to germline engineering. What are your thoughts about the safety of such procedures?

JOHN CAMPBELL: It's clear that this engineering must be done in the safest way possible. Some of the safety issues are real, but I think some can be looked at as problems to be solved. The crucial factor is to understand the expression of our genes. If genes are expressed only in a very specific cell type, then some of the problems dissolve, especially where you're trying to eradicate a disease. If that construct can be kept silent beforehand, then you need only worry about what it will do when it is expressed in the cells you're trying to eliminate.

As far as keeping the addition silent, we have to study that, but it's the sort of thing that can be assessed. There are special reporter genes we can put in to make sure these constructs are not expressed in cells we don't want. We'll need empirical evidence of that. If they are expressed, you go back and redesign your control systems to add another lock or another safety feature If you can't do that, you say, "Well, that won't work. We've got other opportunities, and we'll just have to put that one back on the drawing board until we can make it safe."

JOHN FLETCHER: This is a question for Mario. I gather you don't agree with French that you would need to do germline gene experiments in higher primates; you think you could stop with the mouse.

MARIO R. CAPECCHI: No. I'm not saying that. I'm saying you don't need to do *all* experiments in primates. It would be good to do a certain number of experiments in nonhuman primates, which then establishes the protocol. Once you've learned what you can from that particular process, you move on. You have to be selective. The problem with bureaucracy is that you set a train of events in motion, saying you must go through these particular hurdles over and over, and it may be a waste of time and resources. So, I'm saying you must do some experiments in nonhuman primates, because otherwise you won't know. The biology may be different in a mouse and a primate, but it should not become a part of the bureaucratic protocol.

GREGORY STOCK: A key aspect of John Campbell's notion of double addition was the ability to turn the added genes on and off. Does anyone have a thought about whether that is really practical or could be practical within a decade or so?

DANIEL KOSHLAND, JR.: It seems to me that when you're repairing a defective gene such as a defective insulin gene, in the long run the more economical and safe method is going to be homologous recombination, which is where we excise the bad gene and put a good gene in its place.

I think there are a lot of clever ideas about the addition of an extra chromosome, and turning it off with a hormone and so forth, but by removing a bad gene and replacing it with a normal gene, you're really bringing back the normal person. Controls in the interactions and the secondary interactions with other systems are minimized. If you had a gene on an extra chromosome, you'd have to turn something off in the bad gene's transcription to be sure the good gene took over. That seems a lot more complicated than homologous recombination.

LEROY HOOD: Yes, I would concur. Further, I think an amazing thing is that the manipulations to do those kinds of experiments are actually much simpler in germline than in somatic therapy. If I had to project, I think fifty years from now we will be doing everything through the germline rather than in somatic tissues.

JOHN FLETCHER: I want to go back to Dr. Watson's appeal for gutsy investigators to go out and just do it. Jim, there's a distinction between being a fool for genetic science and a damn fool for genetic science. I would like to see the best investigators turn their attention to therapy. There's a huge discrepancy between what we can diagnose and what we can treat. The more excellent investigators we have involved in therapy the better. But there is a system out there that has evolved in clinical investigation and human experimentation that you need to respect.

And, although you didn't say it explicitly, the vision I got was that you wish that somebody would just go on and try it and be successful. And that's been tried, Jim, right here in this town, and it didn't work.[1]

JAMES D. WATSON: You know that was premature. It was twenty years ago. I'm just afraid of demanding a consensus of committees of elders to decide whether we should use a new technique. They are always going to say No. So you're going to be as dull as Germans who want the State to make all the decisions. I think the healthiness of America is keeping the State out of it, educating your people well, and not having cowboys doing things they shouldn't. One's not for that. If Edwards and Steptoe had needed to get the consensus of the American public to go ahead with their work, it would not have happened. That's what I'm trying to say. So we've got to be careful about demanding consensus. We should say that it's none of their business.

If there's a terrible misuse and people are dying, then you can pass regulations. That's how society goes. We're in the position of passing regulations without anything bad happening. That's a very different situation, and a very dangerous one, because you don't know your enemies and yet you're passing laws against them. Biology is so complicated that this is a very misguided way to go. I'm afraid of asking people what they think. Don't ask Congress to approve it. Just ask them for money to help their constituents. That's what they want—money to help their constituents. They don't want to deal with diabetes. They don't want Parkinson's. Frankly, they would care much more about having their relatives not sick than they do about ethics and principles. We can talk principles forever, but what the public actually wants is not to be sick. And if we help them not be sick, they'll be on our side.

GREGORY STOCK: There's certainly an extraordinary hesitance to regulate areas that are considered natural, even if they are known to be extremely dangerous. You had a comment, Lee?

LEE M. SILVER: There's an interesting analogy from the fertility field. Until 1992, men who could not produce motile sperm were completely infertile, and nothing could be done for them. But, in 1992, they tried a completely untested technique, which was to inject sperm directly into the oocyte, and it worked. It had never been tested on other animals but it worked. You got babies out. And within three years, not knowing anything about long-term effects, 80 percent of the fertility clinics in the United States were using this technique.

It's important to understand the driving force here. There was a demand from infertile individuals whose only way to have a child was to use this technique, and fertility clinics met their demand using an untested technique, and children were born from this technique—the oldest ones are not more than five years old. That gives you a sense of what's going to drive this technology. There was a sense that this technique would work, that it shouldn't be bad. But they weren't sure.

GREGORY STOCK: Let's shift gears a bit and discuss genetic patrimony and the sanctity of the human germline. It has been said that our germline is something owned by all of us and that it shouldn't be tinkered with. This was brought up earlier by Dr. Anderson. Do you have some thoughts about this issue, Dr. Watson?

JAMES D. WATSON: I think it's complete nonsense. I mean, what or who sanctifies? I can't indicate how silly I think it is. I mean, we have great respect for the human species. We like each other. We'd like to be better, and we take great pleasure in great achievements by other people. But, saying we're sacred and should not be changed? Evolution can be just damn cruel, and to say that we've got a perfect genome and there's some sanctity? I'd like to know where that idea comes from, because it's utter silliness. We should treat other people in a way that maximizes the common good of the human species. That's about all we can do.

Terms like *sanctity* remind me of animal rights. Who gave a dog a right? This word *right* gets very dangerous. We have women's rights, children's rights; it goes on forever. And then there's the right of a salamander and a frog's rights. It's carried to the absurd.

I'd like to give up saying *rights* or *sanctity*. Instead, say that humans have needs, and we should try, as a social species, to respond to human needs—like food or education or health—and that's the way we should work. To try and give it more meaning than it deserves in some quasi-mystical way is for Steven Spielberg or somebody like that. It's just plain aura, up in the sky—I mean, it's crap.

GREGORY STOCK: Does anyone else have anything they'd like to add to the notion of the germline having some sort of a sanctity that shouldn't be tampered with?

JOHN FLETCHER: The concept of genetic patrimony, or the way that it's put in Europe, is that every individual has a right to an untampered genetic patrimony. If you study the origins of this concept, it's really a way to smuggle natural law into the debate. Its roots lie in theological sources. This is a very powerful motif in the Council of Europe's deliberations. I neglected to say earlier, when I was talking about religion, that traditions of religion supply strong resources and inspiration for morality. They supply stories, parables, myths, and symbols that are tremendously important for civilization.

But the idea of natural law is one that I think is not a viable concept when it comes to the gene pool. One of the first thought experiments I did when I began thinking about this was: Suppose we really knew how to treat cystic fibrosis or some other very burdensome disease and didn't do it because of the belief that people had a right to an untampered genetic patrimony. Then, you met a person twenty-five years later and you did the Golden Rule thing and said, "Well, you know, we could have treated you for this, but we wanted to respect your right to your untampered genetic patrimony. Sorry."

It doesn't take a high-falutin' ethicist to realize that's just plain wrong. You violate one of the basic principles of morality, namely that you want to treat a person as you would want to be treated. And what person who is sick and suffering wouldn't want to avoid it, if it could have been done safely and effectively?

I have lived long enough in this country to know, and Dr. Anderson, who is also coming from experience, knows that, for the well-being of a germline therapy movement, you have to do it as well as you can the first time it is tried. If you get concrete results, you'll see considerable backing and filling in Congress. And those early results are going to come from privately-funded research efforts.

We live in two worlds now. There's a publicly funded world that Congress has got by the throat, and there is a privately funded world that comes through university funds, clinical earnings, foundations, private donors, and pharmaceutical and biotechnical firms. It is that world that is going to supply the money in order to get this done.

W. FRENCH ANDERSON: John [Fletcher] has presented, very eloquently, my exact feeling. Of course, the two of us have been working hand in hand for thirty years, so that's not too surprising.

The fact is that I'm the one who has been in a position to pioneer procedures. Because of the concern that if it's done wrong, the field will be set back, the criteria I've set for myself and the field are conservative. But, as I pointed out in an editorial in the Journal when we did the first somatic-cell gene therapy, if it was successful it would open the door for a vast number of protocols. We are now seven years later, and there are over 300 approved clinical protocols.

The same thing will happen, I hope, if we do the first fetal gene therapy correctly, which I am now proposing. If we are successful, it will open the door, and if nobody else does it, I'll be the first one that does germline gene therapy. But we're going to do it in a safe way, when the time is right, and not when it's premature.

GREGORY STOCK: I think that gets at the issue of how these things should be regulated, if at all. In vitro fertilization presents an interesting model where there are local regulations, sometimes very restrictive, sometimes very loose. There has been tremendously rapid progress in that field, and there are probably some risks as well. Do any of you have thoughts on this? Because there have been strong efforts to try and gain international consensus on a uniform approach of some sort.

JAMES D. WATSON: I think it would be complete disaster to try and get an international agreement. I just can't imagine anything more stifling. You end up with the lowest possible denominator. Agreement among all the different religious groups would be impossible. About all they'd agree upon is that they should allow us to breathe air. But even regarding food, their opinions are not in common. I think our hope is to stay away from regulations and laws whenever possible.

There were all these efforts to get laws about recombinant DNA in about 1977. We fought it, and thank God we did. Efforts like the Council of Europe are dull and ineffective, and all it will do is put Europe more in the backwater.

DANIEL KOSHLAND JR.: I agree with Jim [Watson] in the following sense: When you're dealing with something like global warming, that's a case where you want all nations to come together. In that case an international agreement is important.

With something like genetic engineering, it seems to me there isn't any great potential catastrophe. And I agree with French completely, that what we need to do is have some cases that are really good examples for the public, and then you may have to take some chances. Maybe it won't turn out perfectly, but I have a great deal of confidence in the people who are doing it, and in French's work, and I'm confident they will pick a specific case and do a good job. It seems to me the United States will be in the forefront of this research. We're more likely to carry it out successfully than almost any nation in the world. To try and get all the nations of Europe to agree with us, let alone all Africa and Asia, will significantly hinder us.

If we go ahead and set a successful example, most people will want to follow that example. We also have to set some priorities. For instance, I really loved Dr. Rose's talk, but I was really against putting any priority on lengthening our life span.

The one way I personally don't want to go is by dying of natural causes. I mean, who needs to be eating oat bran and sitting away from a draft? I want to die in an open roadster going eighty miles an hour and getting hit by a truck. That's the way to go.

We're living long enough, and the bad thing at the moment is that some of us are not living so well in our current lifespan. We have bad diseases: arthritis, which is painful; Alzheimer's, which is emotionally awful. Anybody who has a good idea should be considered, and I thought John Campbell's ecdysone suggestion was just terrific in terms of getting at prostate cancer and breast cancer. One of the things scientists can do is to make priorities of the conditions that are going to be most important and most efficacious. And, of course, in a democracy, the people as a whole have to decide whether we're going to go ahead.

MICHAEL R. ROSE: Can I respond to that?

GREGORY STOCK: Yes.

MICHAEL R. ROSE: Some of your own [Dr. Koshland's] remarks contradict themselves in that . . .

DAN KOSHLAND, JR.: I never wanted to be consistent.

MICHAEL R. ROSE: You and Winston Churchill. Why not give people the choice? It's certainly not my argument that everyone should postpone their aging. But if, with this technology, we could actually do it for some people, that would be very attractive. And if you want to die next week in that roadster, going down Highway 405, that's great. As long as no one else dies.

GREGORY STOCK: You wanted to make a comment, Andrea?

ANDREA BONNICKSEN: Yes. I don't want to defend genetic heritage and genetic patrimony, so much as to comment that it suggests an alternative to the autonomy model that is prevalent in the United States by suggesting there's a collective model too, representing a more collectivist world view. The United States is part of a number of nations. As it develops its regulations and its models, it should keep in mind that there are alternative positions throughout the world.

Because we lack a regulatory model in this country, the more we can develop incremental policy from the clinics on up, from the scientists on up—to be able to work on these questions of when it's ethical to begin, at what stage safety is assured, at what stage the effectiveness is appropriate—the more that can substitute for governmental interventions.

Those in the scientific and medical community have a responsibility to try to develop their own working rules of thumb, and that's why this conference is so important, because you are suggesting that germline interventions might be coming about. Let us begin to think about this in concrete ways, in ways that can be publicized and published, and we will be able to develop our own regulatory models that might preempt governmental regulation or serve as a model for it, if it comes to be.

LEE M. SILVER: If we look at the fertility reproductive technologies, this country is unique in that there are no federal regulations of IVF clinics. There are hundreds of private clinics that carry out IVF and, for the most part, there have not been catastrophes because the situation is self-controlling. If you had a clinic producing deformed children, it would very quickly be run out of business, and the doctors would go to jail.

I don't see why you need extra regulations for germline engineering. The IVF-clinic model in America seems to be working quite well for the most part. You can extend this, hopefully, to the further examples we've been discussing.

GREGORY STOCK: Well, litigation and liability is certainly a strong force.

LEE M. SILVER: Yes, exactly.

GREGORY STOCK: Dr. Watson?

JAMES D. WATSON: It was correctly said that this is the first gathering where people have talked openly about germline engineering. Partly, it was in order to get somatic therapy going that it was said, "Well, we're not doing germline. That is bad. But somatic is not bad morally." It virtually implied there was a moral decision to make about germline, as if it was some great Rubicon and involved going against natural law. I've indicated, I think, that there is no basis for this view.

So, we are fighting the statement that somatic is safe, therefore, germline is unsafe; whereas, in fact, if anything is going to save us, if we need to be saved someday, it's going to be germline engineering.

GREGORY STOCK: Dr. Watson, you had a large part in creating or making successful the Human Genome Project. . . .

JAMES D. WATSON: No. No. Lee Hood. He got the machine. Without him the sequence of the human genome would be just hot air.

GREGORY STOCK: Well, Lee Hood may have made it work, . . . but you were certainly involved in some *small* way. What I wanted to ask is this: If there is no Rubicon to cross with germline engineering, and some approaches have a greater possibility of success than others, is human germline work something we then need to be thinking about trying—at least at a research level—to see whether there are possibilities worth realizing? Should there be some sort of a project toward this goal?

JAMES D. WATSON: Well, I wouldn't make it difficult to do the experiments, which is what the proposed laws against human cloning would have done. [Those laws] could make it very difficult to do the sort of experiments Mario [Capecchi] would like to do on homologous recombination, which is simply "correcting" a gene. We've got to be very careful not to admit at the outset that we're three-quarters evil and a quarter good. I just don't see the evil nature of what we're trying to do.

Genetics, in many people's eyes, has a bad connotation of the State or others determining people's lives. Which is why, again, the State should stay out of it. My feeling is, the State shouldn't tell a person either to have it or not to have it. If the procedures work people will use them, and if they don't work or if it's dangerous, it will stop.

The real enemy is a preexisting genetic inequality which makes some people unable to function well in the world. Terrible diseases— that's the enemy. Whereas some people are convinced the enemy is the people who study the genes, that we are evil people. I don't think we're any more evil than the people who run this Music Department. You know? I don't know if we're better or worse. And I suspect we're deep down trying to respond to a long-term need, and the music people are making us happy by singing hymns, which cheers us up. We should be proud of what we're doing and not worry about whether we're destroying the genetic patrimony of the world, which is awfully cruel to too many people. And I think that that's what we're all trying to fight. French, I think you know we basically agree, but it's the image. I'm sure I will be misquoted by someone who's says I'm gung ho to go ahead and do it [human germline engineering]. I would do it if it made someone's life better. We get a lot of pleasure from helping other people. That's what we're trying to do.

GREGORY STOCK: Thank you.

JOHN FLETCHER: Since we are talking about regulation, I'd like briefly to review what university-based or industry-based scientists need to know.

Somatic-cell transfer research in humans is now regulated, in all of its phases, by the Food and Drug Administration [FDA]. What about crossing the line to human germline gene transfer experiments? The NIH's Recombinant Advisory Committee's [NIH-RAC] policy on intentional germline transfer is that it "will not now entertain" protocols with this aim. Obviously, much more research in animals must occur, as well as public discussion, to cross this line. Since germline gene transfer experiments will occur in gametes or embryos, the one area to watch carefully is research with embryonically derived stem cells. In 1994 Congress prohibited federal funding of any research that would harm human embryos. But this ban does not apply to privately funded research.

If your research is privately funded, there are no federal legal barriers to deriving stem cells from embryos. One needs to know if state law permits this research, before submitting a protocol for the research to the Institutional Review Board [IRB]. If your institution has signed a Multiple Project Assurance with the Office of Protection from Research Risks at the NIH, you promise to abide by the regulations to protect human subjects, no matter the source of funding. The "protection of human subjects" issues do not apply to embryos, but to the persons who are sources of embryos to be used experimentally. The privacy of couples in infertility treatment or donors of gametes needs to be protected. A process of informed consent for donating embryos or gametes for research needs review and approval. Finally, there are some ethical considerations about the outer limits (14 days) of permissible embryo research and prohibiting any future uses of research embryos for implantation. The report of the NIH Human Embryo Research Panel and the British guidelines for embryo research provide guidance on these points. The important message for local IRBs is that it is not illegal to do privately funded embryo research, as long as the personnel, facilities, and equipment to be involved in this research are not substantially subsidized by federal funding. Research that involves putting genes into human cells or embryos requires the approval of the NIH-RAC and would also be regulated by the FDA.

JOHN CAMPBELL: Most of the research I envisage being done in the next five or ten years would be animal work. So, even if there was a prohibition on actually putting genes in human cells, it would not be decisive in inhibiting the research that needs to be done.

GREGORY STOCK: Dr. Watson dismissed the slippery-slope argument earlier, the argument some people make that, if we once start to do these things, then gradually we will go down to who knows where. It has always seemed to me that either we're already on that slippery slope, and so might as well forget about it, or that it doesn't exist. Does anybody have any thoughts about the nature of the sort of reinforcement and self-reinforcement that occurs with these kinds of developments?

ANDREA BONNICKSEN: I would like to suggest a couple of other metaphors for the slippery slope that I've seen in the literature. One is to talk about us rapelling down the slope—that is, rather than just slipping on down without any stopping point, we can repel from the building back and forth with stopping points. Another metaphor is that of the ramshackle staircase: instead of sliding down the slope, we instead are going down a rickety kind of staircase, and at points we stop and look back and fix it, and then we keep going. These metaphors suggest that—with these new techniques—we face not a slope but a course of action with stopping points and places to draw lines.

GREGORY STOCK: Lee, did you have a comment to make?

LEROY HOOD: I related to this idea of the sanctity of the human germline. Remember, each of our chromosomes differs by 1 letter of the DNA language in every 500. And each of our chromosomes, when it goes through the necessary manipulations to make sperm, actually undergoes recombinational events where the information is scrambled. Indeed, there are an enormous number of other events where information is altered, is rearranged, and is changed.

I would reject, utterly, the idea of a slippery slope, because it seems to be arguing that we're doing something unnatural. In fact, it is quite the contrary. We're using exactly the same kinds of techniques used by evolution, but what we're attempting to do, in a thoughtful and rational way, is to facilitate evolution, so it doesn't operate in a blind fashion—most of the changes being neutral or deleterious—but in an optimizing fashion. It's exactly the same as the analogy for antibiotics. You could argue that maybe some human would someday run into the fungus that made penicillin, but on the other hand is it unnatural? Is it a slippery slope to manipulate molecules that could kill bacteria?

The other point I would make is that there should be a fundamental distinction between basic research—learning how to do this in animal models and so forth—and the application of that research, which is where we obviously have to show a great deal more caution. What is absolutely fearful about a lot of the laws that came up in response to cloning is that they made no distinction. They went all the way back to the very core of this kind of research. Meetings like this are important because they help people gain an understanding about these distinctions and respond when laws are absolutely inappropriate.

One of the things that terrifies me about how laws get written is the realization that they're written by twenty-three-year-old staffers who are out to make a name, who studied this subject for three or four weeks. In general, those in Congress have even less idea of what this is all about, so it is a process that is not conducive to writing laws. But in spite of that, it ends up working surprisingly well.

GREGORY STOCK: Does anyone else have a comment to make about this subject? Lee?

LEE M. SILVER: There is this false notion that species try to preserve their gene pools to try to preserve themselves. That is completely false.

Species are always changing, and they even transform from one species to another. And as they change, their gene pools change naturally. This notion of a species trying to preserve itself is a false one right from the start.

GREGORY STOCK: Michael?

MICHAEL R. ROSE: I would like to address the evolutionary issue. Lee Hood has presented the technological case, and I'm very sympathetic to it. Evolution is an incredibly complex process which is not suited to platitudes. Evolution can be spectacularly creative, so much so that many of the problems in artificial intelligence are now being solved using evolutionary algorithms. When design and optimality approaches fail now, artificial intelligence designers are using evolutionary techniques—basically, natural selection and genetic recombination—on computer programs. But just as you have to acknowledge the power and creativity of evolution, you also have to acknowledge its complete indifference to us as individuals. That's not what evolution is about at all. Evolution is about the transmission of DNA sequences down through time. We're just incidental things that get in the way. We're like the foot soldier in World War I, and we're sent out of the trenches into the enemy machine guns, and we die in our millions. And that's fine with evolution as long as our DNA gets into the next generation. This is, perhaps, part of my rebelliousness to the notion of "normal." I think what is normal is a catastrophic waste, and if one were simply to accept what evolution does as normal then, hell, you can give up on most everything that medicine does. You have to reject this concept of normal. You have to take what evolution does and look at it askance, exploit what it does well, and provide what it does not provide. And, of course, for those poor individuals who are afflicted by genetic diseases—which are the products of an evolutionary process in which mutation and selection together do not guarantee that everyone of us is genetically perfect, but only that most of us are genetically pretty good—their afflictions are a concrete example of where evolution has to be firmly rejected. The fact that, to evolution, we are disposable past a certain age is another candidate for rejecting what evolution normally does and doing something completely different. I think we need to seek an appropriate balance between respect for and use of what evolution does and rejection of what evolution does.

GREGORY STOCK: Along those same lines, I would like to express the notion that evolution, as it has operated in the past, has essentially stopped for the human species. Our future evolution will be intimately connected with the technologies that are being developed today.

When you look forward, even a few centuries, it is difficult to imagine how you could separate any changes that occur to the human species from the technology that is evolving now and is now reflecting back upon ourselves. Does anyone have a comment to make about that general notion? John?

JOHN CAMPBELL: I suspect that the idea of us grabbing the reins of our own evolution is not new. Students of human evolution recognize that the major factor in the past history of humans—the past several million years in the development of humans—has been the tampering by humans with their own reproductive system, through sexual selection. Indeed, Darwin believed that sexual selection was the main factor that caused humans to evolve. He did not talk about the evolution of humans in his *Origin of the Species by Natural Selection.* He put it in a separate volume on natural selection in relation to sex and the origin of man. So, he put the origin of humans right in with sexual selection. Leakey thought the way to think about how we originated was that we autodomesticated ourselves. Other people have thought that the most important factor was the parent-offspring relationship, that the real selection pressure was the degree to which a mother protected her offspring. Undoubtedly, humans have been the main instruments in their evolution, the process which brought them to the status of being human. If we now start to tamper with our evolution, we are not doing something that is unique or unnatural or something that hasn't happened before. What I see as unique is that now we can bring our rationality to it, instead of having it based on sexual preference.

GREGORY STOCK: Dr. Koshland?

DANIEL KOSHLAND, JR.: We're doing evolution in test tubes now. In my laboratory we're using what's called combinatorial chemistry, which is what happens in evolution. You combine chemistry with the idea of selection in biology, and you make billions of mutants, of, say, little peptides. Then they are selected in your laboratory. Basically, that's what happens over evolutionary time in millions of years. This is now spreading throughout industry; the biotech industry, for instance, is using it to develop new drugs.

In some ways this comes back to germline engineering, because we've decided as a society that it's too cruel to get rid of less-effective or defective people, like those, for example, who have glasses. It really is crazy to discard a rational approach to helping our species, since we really have rejected the system that, as Dr. Campbell pointed out, has in a cruel way, over years and years, discarded the less fit. Now say we don't want to improve the species, because that would be too mean and inappropriate to the less able.

GREGORY STOCK: Dr. Hood, you would like to make a closing comment?

LEROY HOOD: There is another way we can use evolution in absolutely incredible ways to help us decipher some of the most complicated of these "complex traits." One of the speakers mentioned—I think it was Lee Silver—that chimps and humans are 99 percent identical in their sequences. One incredibly fascinating project would be to have a Chimp Genome Project and to compare the results with those from the Human Genome Project. The genes that would be enormously fascinating to compare are those that regulate the nervous system, for therein would be a great deal of the information that separates what we can do with our minds and learning and thinking from what a chimp can do. Also, you can use evolution in a lot of ways to gain fundamental insights into the kind of things we need to be able to manipulate in the future, if we want to fundamentally change schizophrenia, manic depression, and a lot of these very, very complex multifactorial diseases.

GREGORY STOCK: Does anyone else have a closing comment they feel burning within them?

LEE M. SILVER: This is not something that is going to happen overnight or even within the next thirty or fifty or a hundred years. But for the first time we understand that as a species we have the ability to self-evolve. That's what the difference is with this new technology versus the sexual selection which occurred subconsciously in previous years. I mean, this is an incredible concept: that our species has the ability to self-evolve. I wanted to make that point.

GREGORY STOCK: This has been an incredibly rich day, and a long one. I would like to thank our speakers. It's wonderful to have a discussion that is as open and frank as the one that occurred today, and I hope it moves out beyond this room.

DANIEL KOSHLAND, JR.: And I'd really like to thank you [Gregory Stock] and Dr. Campbell, because I think you stuck your necks out and did a great job.

GREGORY STOCK: Thank you. And with that, the "Engineering the Human Germline" symposium is closed.

PART III

OTHER VOICES

This final part offers additional perspectives on human germline engineering through short essays from ethicists, lawyers, theologians, public-policy makers, and scientists from both the United States and abroad who have thought deeply about the issue. To emphasize the breadth of opinion about this genetic technology, each contributor has written an essay based on one of only three question sets about key issues concerning human germline engineering. Each question has thus been answered by several contributors. But their answers are neither commentary on previous portions of the book nor on each other's essays. Rather, this is a collection of independent snapshots of opinion.

The first set of questions confronts the issue of human germline engineering head-on by circumventing the matter of safety, which has often muddied discussions about the technology. Safety is a distinct issue of its own. Opinions differ about what level of safety would be adequate, but no one argues that we should apply the technology to humans before it is medically "safe." To imagine how we would view the technology if it were truly safe brings our different attitudes about human germline engineering into sharp relief.

If germline engineering procedures were demonstrated to be no more risky in humans than natural conception, what limits would you place on the types of interventions allowed? Would your opinion be altered if the technology allowed the blockage of transmission of these alterations to future generations?

The second set of questions seeks commentary about some of the more commonly expressed worries about germline engineering and attempts to gauge concern about the technology.

Some have asserted that altering the genetics of human germinal cells would be an assault to human dignity, others that it would lead down a slippery slope with dire consequences. What is your assessment of the eventual possibilities and dangers of human germline engineering, and what are your biggest fears about its implementation? Would humanity be better off in a distant future where no direct modification of the genetics of human germline cells were allowed, or in one where significant modification were available?

The third set of questions is straightforward. Given the powerful dynamics bringing technologies like germline engineering into the realm of possibility, should we try to erect international measures to control them?

Some have advocated the development of an international policy on germline engineering and cloning. Do you think this would be preferable to a patchwork of national policies and, thus, worth pursuing?

Each contributor has been identified by a short biographical blurb, but to give readers a context in which to read the essays, we've also included his or her answer to a hypothetical personal question that may offer readers even better insights into the thinking of these individuals. Perhaps their views on this will help us prepare for that day when we or our children are confronted with a similar question.

Imagine you were conceiving a child by in vitro fertilization, and your obstetrician convinced you that the embryo of your child-to-be could, without additional risk or cost, be given an artificial chromosome to increase his or her life expectancy by a decade. Would you use the procedure?

Beyond the Issue of Safety

If germline engineering procedures were demonstrated to be no more risky in humans than natural conception, what limits would you place on the types of interventions allowed? Would your opinion be altered if the technology allowed the blockage of transmission of these alterations to future generations?

Glenn McGee: "Parental Choices"

The human germline is not sacrosanct. For the sake of argument, we will assume that alteration of the genes of the yet-to-be born, yet-to-be conceived, or their progeny poses no special health risks to anyone involved or yet to be involved. Why ought we be fearful, then, of altering our inheritance through direct physical changes to germline cells? The principal objection to germline alteration has been that it crosses a bright line between the bucolic operations of nature and the engineering of humans by humans. It is supposed to be dangerous to cross this line—dangerous to the children involved and dangerous for our species.

If we eliminate the danger of overt physical toxicity for the offspring involved, what dangers remain for these individuals? I would argue that human germline modifications are, under these assumptions, no more dangerous than other kinds of parental choices. More specifically, I would argue that the means we use to secure our desired procreative outcome are strictly linked to the ends in view. The means alone are not the issue. The question is how well the means suit our ends, and how well our ends square with what is ethically acceptable for parents to desire. If germline alterations can be used responsibly, within the context of parental common sense and as part of institutions designed to carefully monitor the outcomes of those alterations, then it is hard to see how they will harm children or future generations. There is no reason to be opposed in principle, either, to the improvement of human beings or to the direct actions aimed at that goal. Of course, the devil is in the details. Which human parental goals are intelligent, and which pose profound dangers? In an article in *Hastings Center Report*, "Parenting in an Era of Genetics [March 1997]," I argue that there are several clear "sins" that we encounter in parenthood, whether our means of "engineering" is high- or low-tech. These dangers of parenthood, and the ethnographic means of assessing them, should be the focus of bioethics in an era of germline therapy. We have to distinguish between the uses of parental wisdom that are to be allowed, and those that should be disallowed by the institutions involved: medicine, family courts, churches. Beyond the obvious question of which uses of genetic technology should be banned or regulated, moreover, is the issue of the rhetorical role for bioethics: should bioethics be in the business of recommending to parents that they choose or forego particular kinds of germline modifications? Arguably, bioethics in this area has focused too much on what should be allowed and too little on what should be recommended.

Dangers to the human species are more intractable. Virtually every author of a recent tome on genetics has suggested that we are moving into a new evolutionary period, in which human beings describe and promulgate the kinds of creatures that will be born. The observation is profound, and it points to a fundamental truth. People can observe, classify, and control more of human embodiment than ever before in recorded history. The development of molecular biology and biophysics, as well as their clinical corollaries, portends more such control. But, again, where is the bright line that divides nature's machination from human engineering? Elsewhere I argue[1] that theories of "genetic progress" and dystopian analyses of genetic downfall are almost always predicated on a Luddite refusal to analyze the distinctions between technology and nature with rigor and care. Technological innovations aimed at improving human health are age-old, and, indeed, we have taken many steps toward improving our ability to conceive children whose lives will be improved by virtue of our actions. Fears of eugenics are not without meaning. We could, indeed, make mistakes with our species that would cost the lives of many, and genetic policy could indeed cheapen the lives of those yet to be born or yet to procreate. But the lesson of eugenics is a special and historically-situated one. Today, our fears about germline genetic engineering should center on the danger to our species of thoughtless, libertine progress into the breach. We proceed headlong into genetic engineering without even a casual glance in the direction of reforming family law, research restrictions, or our educational institutions. Families taken off guard by genetic technology thus rebuke it as "playing God." The greatest threat to our species is the ignorance within our social institutions whose role it is to provide support for good decision making. Genetic counselors cannot replace town hall meetings, church discussion, and good educational institutions.

> If you could do so safely, would you use an artificial
> chromosome to extend the lifespan of your child?

I would probably be among the thoughtless, casting my own love of life into a bid for my child's immortality. When I was a boy, I wondered about when and how my parents would die. I hoped that I would never see that day, and that I would somehow be forever young. Deep in us is a fear of death, a fear of loss of meaning. The danger of technologies that promise a longer life is that they commodify what should be a spiritual conversation about what it means to want to live, and what it means to want to live longer. In principle, I see no reason to object to having a longer life. I'd like to see people in space. I would like my child to have more time to grow and love and learn. But the plain question is, at what cost?

The danger of genetic choices such as this is that they cast parents in a more perilous role. How will I relate to my child? Parents already come to resent their children as they age. My child's promise—which liberates me at one level by relieving my burden and offering solace in my aging—is also a yoke I must bear. I feel myself dying, even as my child grows and grows out of the society and needs that, for me, are most important. Will my choice to give a child more years come to haunt me and our relationship? Moreover, what will I have wrought on the world? Would a collective choice to live longer in the American style cost so much money for so many as to implicate my child in the exploitation of the poor? I'm not sure. Finally, I would be among those paying for extra years. But I am not so sure that such a choice should be mine in the first place.

Sandy Thomas: "Thoughts on the Ethics of Germline Engineering"

A major objection to germline engineering is the notion that a person's genetic makeup should not be directly determined by the deliberate choice of another. It can be argued that preimplantation screening, prenatal screening, and even abortion allow manipulation of an individual's genome. However, the potential impact of germline gene therapy on the next and future generations raises additional concerns. Here, the parents are not merely considering the best interests of their unborn child, but those of their child's unborn descendents. Concern has focused largely on the irreversibility of genetic changes effected by germline gene therapy and the denial of decision making by future generations. There is anxiety that if therapeutic interventions were permissible, genetic enhancement would soon follow.

We are currently at an interesting stage of knowledge in the field of human genetics. Our understanding of diseases caused by single genes has grown rapidly, and nearly all diagnostic genetic tests are for these diseases. At the same time, we are beginning to see that the role of susceptibility genes in many common diseases is complex, that such genes may have multiple effects, and that interaction between genetic and environmental influences may be difficult to unravel. Our knowledge about genes for personality traits, for intelligence and behavior, is by contrast very limited.

If germline gene therapy were no more risky for humans than natural conception, would there be ethical objections to eliminating disease genes? For example, the replacement of recessive cystic fibrosis alleles by dominant normal genes through homologous recombination in fertilized eggs could be viewed as a positive intervention which justified the deliberate determination of the genetic makeup of future generations.

In reality, few situations are likely to be as straightforward. Where a disease gene is dominant, as in the case of Huntington's disease, homologous recombination at both gene loci would require very high levels of efficiency. If a couple at risk of carrying a single-gene disease had gone to the trouble and expense of in vitro fertilization, preimplantation screening of embryos would provide a much simpler way of offering the family reproductive choice. Moreover, engineering for complex diseases is unlikely to be viable, and "success" will be impossible to measure. Even if germline gene therapy allowed for blockage of transmission of these alterations to future generations, the same limitations would apply. Under what kind of circumstances should we be considering germline gene therapy for a single generation? Would we be doing so for that small group of patients who object to abortion following an adverse result from prenatal testing? I would argue that this is an unrealistic scenario except, perhaps, for the most serious genetic diseases. In any event, unless gene transfer in embryos was 100 percent efficient, the procedure of selecting some embryos and rejecting others might be unacceptable to these patients

The costs of allowing clearly defined medical interventions, as in the case of cystic fibrosis, might be the opening of the door to enhancement.

The idea of "designer babies" raises a whole range of serious ethical questions. The view of some scientists that because something is technically possible, it will invariably be done, is misplaced. Scientific possibilities should not, in and of themselves, determine policies that need to reflect ethical, legal, social, and economic considerations. The application of germline gene therapy to effect novel and beneficial therapies is one thing. It is quite another to think in terms of use of the technology to allow parents to improve their chances of having an above-average child.

Even with our limited knowledge about the heritability of, for example, intelligence, musical ability, and sporting prowess, it is clear that we are not simply the "sum of our genes." For many traits (and most common diseases), both genetic and environmental factors are likely to be important. Even if the genetic influences affecting a trait are well understood, there is likely to be variation in the symptoms and outcomes observed. To encourage the idea that we should manipulate the genome to "make better human beings" raises major ethical and scientific problems. From the viewpoint of ethics, the notion of enhancement ignores the fundamental principle of respect for persons which is expressed in action and procedures that give due weight to personal autonomy and integrity. By introducing selected specific traits of this kind into an embryo, a parent imposes his values of what is "better." How could the teenager or young adult rebel against his or her selected genes? Parental choice would extend into the child's life in a way that could compromise his rights as an individual to pursue his *own* path.

Raising potentially unrealized expectations of parents in the abilities of their unborn child is unlikely to be in the child's best interests. Ambitious parents who have invested in gene therapy to secure a bright future for their child may not be well placed to cope with failure. The child who has been unsuccessfully enhanced for intelligence may suffer low self-esteem and be denied the right of being valued for himself, regardless of his abilities. If enhanced intelligence is seen as a means of "bettering" one's children, there is a real danger of an increased stigma being attached to people who are less intelligent. The stigma associated with mental disorders should serve as a warning to us.

In conclusion, advances in human genetics will bring benefits to a wide range of people through the development of more effective drugs and prenatal genetic testing for a wide range of common diseases. In contrast, germline gene therapy is unlikely to make a significant contribution to public health within the next thirty years. Our limited understanding of how human genes behave and interact should restrict, delay, and, if appropriate, prevent some applications, including those in germline engineering.

> If you could do so safely, would you use an artificial
> chromosome to extend the lifespan of your child?

I would not use the procedure involving the addition of an artificial chromosome to increase the life expectancy of a child. The development of new medicines and medical procedures should be focused on improving the *quality* of people's lives. As new therapies are developed to treat common and debilitating diseases of old age, longevity will be enhanced. The notion that medical research might be directed at increasing life expectancy per se is, in my view, misguided and ignores the right of *future* generations to their own autonomy. Germline gene therapy to eliminate heart disease or cancer would be less controversial, in that they could be seen as being in the child's best interest. There is doubt, moreover, that the introduction of artificial chromosomes into the germline could be designated as risk free, since the effects in future generations could not be thoroughly evaluated.

Sheldon Krimsky:
"The Psychosocial Limits
on Human Germline Modification"

Our thought exercise assumes that the health risks of human germline genetic alteration have been reduced to rates that fall below genetic abnormalities of natural reproduction. This means that the genetic modification of germ cells (GMGC), including deletion, addition, duplication, rearrangement, immobilization, or expression of gene sequences, coding or noncoding, would produce only the desired ("positive") outcome. Or, in the case that a genetic modification produces multiple genomic or phenotypic effects, it also assumes that those effects would not add any risks to the health and well-being of the individual (over his or her lifetime) beyond the background risks we attribute to natural conception. It shall also be assumed that any decision to undertake GMGC in procreation is strictly voluntary, has an economic cost, and has perceived benefits to the parents.

The most serious moral problem that I see in permitting the voluntary use of GMGC in human reproduction for any purpose whatsoever is that it will establish a role for genetic technology in raising aspirations of prospective parents for attaining a culturally defined but morally impoverished ideal of the genotype/phenotype of their progeny.

Among the most problematic cases are those involving the uses of GMGC for procreating children of a particular sex, body size, shape, or skin color. Offering people the opportunity to choose the phenotype of a child will result in psychosocial pathologies, including deeper class and racial divisions within society.

The use of GMGC or other techniques to determine the sex of a child can, in a patriarchal society, lead to the superabundance of males with unanticipated consequences to traditional courtship patterns and gender equity. In many parts of the world where racial prejudice based on skin color is pervasive, some blacks may feel pressured to avail themselves of GMGC to insure light-skinned offspring. If this genetic modification were possible, it would reinforce social prejudices by connecting "medical procedures" with racist stereotypes that imply "whiter is better."

The same may be said of body types. Young adolescent girls, responding to media messages of "perfect body image," are prone to anorexia nervosa. Abnormal dieting and obsession with caloric intake are pervasive among normal preteens and adolescents. Women who recall their own pained adolescent years struggling with body image might be inclined, if offered, to choose a body type for their offspring that more closely resembles contemporary media images. While people may aspire to have children resembling our contemporary media "gods" and "goddesses," it would be a grave human error to use GMGC to narrow the genotype/phenotype of the population. The public identification of genetics for this purpose reinforces the dangerous notion that there are universal standards of beauty and that science supports such standards. Even if there were but a few wealthy individuals who could afford to use such methods (assuming they were effective and safe), the symbolism that science has developed a reproductive technology that offers parents choices of body types for their offspring has profound psychosocial implications. And while cosmetic surgery responds to similar social cues and prejudices, it cannot affect the genotype and therefore will not narrow genetic diversity and serve a eugenics purpose. The psychosocial arguments against modifying germ cells for "enhancement" apply whether or not the alterations are transmitted to future generations. The availability of eugenic techniques in reproduction to a minority of affluent people will support the "geneticization" of a society, enabling an aristocracy with so-called proper genes to use it to their class advantage.

What about the selective use of GMGC for deleting or repairing life-depriving genetic defects? Can we establish a reasonable and sustainable moral boundary that prohibits modifying clinically normal germ cells yet accepts the repair of abnormal ones? Theoretically, we might be able to justify a boundary that permits the use of GMGC in conjunction with in vitro fertilization exclusively for extreme genomic abnormalities. Realistically, our decentralized institutions providing reproductive services, including infertility clinics, sperm banks, and prenatal care, would make it virtually impossible to maintain a boundary between the use of GMGC for life-threatening genetic diseases, "enhancements," and the vast grey area in the middle. Just as surgeons have great latitude in the use of cosmetic surgery, and physicians can prescribe drugs for uses other than those approved in drug trials, if GMGC were approved for some uses of human reproduction, there would be no centralized system of control to prevent slippage.

Assume a best-case scenario: two heterozygotes, carrying single copies of a gene that is life-threatening for homozygotes, who do not wish to pass the gene to their offspring, seek relief through GMGC. We must ask if there are reasonable alternatives to germline modification, such as egg selection or sperm donation. If germline modification is the procedure of last resort for producing a healthy offspring, then we must balance the interests of parents with the broader social concerns that this first step will be the starting point for less agreeable (more morally ambiguous) forms of germline changes. With no assurance that our institutions and laws can prevent slippage in applying GMGC, any decision should weigh heavily on the side of "no first use." An international convention on proscribing the use of GMGC can set the framework for civil laws against eugenics on the part of signatory nations.

> If you could do so safely, would you use an artificial
> chromosome to extend the lifespan of your child?

If I am given a hypothetical choice that allows me to endow my offspring with excellent health and longevity without compromising the child's personhood in any way, which does not compromise the health of my wife, which does not have any adverse implications on race, class, gender oppression, which is universally available, and for which there are no trade: offs (the procedure is just an add on), I would accept it. Of course, in vitro fertilization implies extracting eggs from a woman, which can have adverse effects. Perhaps we can add the proviso that the method adds no risk to the egg donor. I would do lots of things I don't ordinarily do (such as pray or live on a macrobiotic diet) if I had certainty it would create a better world or healthier children. Of course, I have to assume that if this were such a perfect and cost-free method to insure the health and longevity of my progeny, one that is universally available, many others would avail themselves of it and there would be no stigma associated with its use. It would be like a smallpox vaccination. Some people may be opposed on some principled grounds to vaccinations, but by and large having the availability to vaccinate against diseases has been a positive contribution to human civilization.

Perhaps some day there may be "genetic vaccinations" for men and women. The purpose of these "vaccinations" would be to repair mutations of germ cells in vivo before conception. If that ever were possible, it would make me rethink the "no germ line intervention" stand. Presumably, if the State were responsible for such "vaccinations," then a centralized guidance system could prevent its use for "enhancement" purposes that tend toward the medicalization of social or cultural ideals.

Kevin T. FitzGerald: "Do We Know Ourselves Well Enough To Be Engineering Humans?"[2]

Germline genetic technology could significantly change our understanding of human nature as well as radically alter procedures for treating human disease. Since ethical decisions concerning the proper uses of new medical technologies are grounded in concepts about human nature, it follows that we need to scrutinize these concepts as to their completeness in describing and explaining what it means to be human.

Presently several concepts of human nature can be found within the ethical frameworks used to address the issues raised by germline interventions. Most of these concepts have a particular field of academic inquiry (e.g., science, philosophy, or theology) as their primary source, though that source may not be explicit.

Some concepts commonly employed are based on philosophical and/or theological tenets about human characteristics. Since these tenets generally were formulated hundreds or thousands of years ago, the science which informed them is quite dated and results in somewhat rigid or "static" concepts of human nature. Overreliance on these concepts creates heuristic frameworks often at odds with contemporary scientific knowledge. Hence, even though those who apply this type of ethical framework may intend to protect and to value human nature, the discontinuity of their concepts of human nature with contemporary science weakens their arguments.

In what may be an overreaction to static concepts of human nature, other concepts are used which too readily embrace contemporary scientific knowledge. These concepts are bereft of religious, moral, and other humanistic knowledge about human nature and rely solely or predominantly on scientific information. This lack of nonscientific sources of knowledge leaves these concepts of human nature with an impoverished description of humanity by reducing the human to the merely biological or physicochemical. How can such concepts be employed in a heuristic framework to assess the total impact that genetic research and its applications will have on human nature and society?

Still another option often suggested is to focus almost exclusively on individual choice and allow the marketplace to decide the issue. For example, let parents decide how to apply germline genetic interventions for their own children. This option has two major problems. First, the vast majority of those who promote such an approach also want to prevent blatant misuse by limiting interventions to "responsible" ones made by "responsible" parents, so it still must be determined who and what is "responsible."

The second problem arises from the first. If the marketplace is to be the arena wherein the choices of what constitutes good germline intervention are to be decided, then what about those "responsible" parents who cannot afford any of the selections? The bottom line for this approach isn't morality or science, but economics. By default, those who are considered "responsible" parents will be determined by their financial status. Hence, this option faces the same difficulty as those previously mentioned—an incomplete consideration of the total human situation.

Is there a better alternative to the three approaches mentioned above? In my judgment, such an alternative would include concepts of human nature derived from all the relevant fields of academic inquiry and practical experience. The advantage of this approach is that it can provide an integrated ethical framework which takes into account the common good as well as the good of the individual. Human diversity is valued not only from a scientific perspective, but also as a societal good resulting in the enrichment of all.

It is sometimes argued that this integrative approach is too complex, inefficient, and slow for evaluating the potential uses of germline technology. It is much easier to contend with the concerns of only science, or religion, or economics, and not with the entire rich tapestry of the human condition. Moreover, it is argued that this more complex and complete ethical approach is unnecessary, since all the ethical approaches above might agree to applying safe and predictable germline interventions to assist individuals with lethal diseases not treatable by other means.

This argument is shortsighted. The fact that different ethical approaches reach the same conclusion at some point does not make them equally valid over time. Most predict that, once applied successfully to lethal illnesses, attempts will be made to extend the application of germline genetic interventions to other diseases or use them for enhancement purposes. At that point, the limitations of the first three ethical approaches will become all too evident. No one academic discipline or field of practical experience alone can direct us toward the best use of this powerful new technology.

I strongly argue for the development of concepts of human nature based on knowledge gathered from all the pertinent areas of human inquiry and experience. Such concepts will help us to understand more fully who we are as human beings. From this knowledge, we can conceive of who we want to become and how genetic engineering might be applied to assist us in reaching that goal.

> If you could do so safely, would you use an artificial
> chromosome to extend the lifespan of your child?

The mere addition of years is, in itself, not meaningful. Without knowing how those ten years would be lived, I would be inclined not to make such a choice. When we choose to invest our energies and resources in activities that require a great deal of effort and commitment, we do so because of the promise of long-term benefits for ourselves and others. Marriage, raising a family, and education are examples of such human activities. The addition of ten years to an eighty-year life span does not intrinsically hold the promise of such benefits; therefore I would not invest in it until the hope for a return on the investment was sound.

Ruth Hubbard:
"Germline Manipulation"

I would oppose germline interventions even if it were possible to show they are safe. The need is, at best, marginal and does not warrant the investment of time, money, or expertise necessary to perfect the technology and test it sufficiently to determine its efficacy and safety. It represents a distortion of priorities at a time when babies are sickening and dying, not because their genes are "defective," but because their families cannot muster the resources to enable them to be born, and grow up, healthy. One of the most serious problems with many of the current reproductive technologies is that they escalate the emphasis our society places on our personal "blood lines." Yet, DNA *über alles* is a most unfortunate ideology to propagate. Among other problems, it focuses our attention too exclusively on individual health, while public health is deteriorating.

The usual reasons given for trying to modify human germ cells or embryos are either specific health benefits or "enhancement." But, there is *no* way to accurately predict the effects of germline genetic engineering for a future person, much less for her or his descendants, because genes always function in concert with other factors. There is also no justification for germline engineering, because there are other ways to achieve the desired results.

With regard to health benefits, germline engineering requires in vitro fertilization (IVF), and that always produces several embryos. Each of these can be biopsied, and couples can avoid having a child with the mutation they wish to avoid by not allowing gestation of those embryos. The only situation in which this would be impossible would arise if both partners were homozygous for the identical alteration in the same gene, surely a very unusual circumstance. Such couples could use someone else's sperm, eggs, or embryos, or adopt a child. Therefore, we are not talking about condemning people to remain childless, perhaps only not to perpetuate their own DNA.

As for the notion that we need germline interventions to "enhance" the abilities we can expect to pass on to our children, I believe that people who cannot deal with the uncertainties implicit in having a child even before that child is gestated are in for trouble. Successful parenting surely requires that we be flexible enough to accept our children, whoever they are.

Germline engineering is a societal issue that involves far more than technical questions about DNA. Realistic discussions about it, therefore, need to move beyond disembodied DNA, genes, and embryos. Even just at the biological level, germline manipulations involve: hyperstimulating women's ovaries, removing their eggs, putting embryos into their womb, and conditioning that womb to accept and gestate at least one embryo and bear one baby, and often more than one baby because of the increased likelihood of a multiple pregnancy. Such risks are implicit in IVF, but it is one thing to accept them when IVF is the only way a woman can have a child that is hers biologically. It is foolhardy to accept them in the hope of germline "improvements."

Take a much simpler example. No one could have predicted that giving pregnant women diethylstilbestrol (DES) would years later produce cancers in the children they were gestating at the time. Also, it would have taken much longer to recognize this effect had the children developed more usual types of cancer.

In germline engineering, each step involves its own health and psychosocial risks, the extent and variety of which are largely unknown. A study has just been initiated in England to examine the records, collected over up to three decades, of more than 3,000 women to try to establish whether the drugs used in connection with IVF pose a cancer risk and how great the risk is likely to be. When even that is not known, surely we must face up to our ignorance about the physical, psychological, and social impacts of every step involved in germline manipulations.

Discussions about the advisability and safety of germline engineering must go beyond the technical details of how to get the right bit of DNA inserted at the right place and how to control the way it functions. To this end, they must include people familiar with the health and psychosocial aspects of ovulation, conception, gestation, birth, and raising children. Indeed, any attempts to genetically alter germ cells, embryos, or fetuses should be preceded by impact statements that consider the potential effects on health as well as the entire range of economic and psychosocial impacts on children, parents, and society.

> If you could do so safely, would you use an artificial
> chromosome to extend the lifespan of your child?

I tend to avoid all "elective" medical procedures. I would, therefore, never try to "improve" the future health or extend the life span of a "person" who hasn't even been gestated. When I think about what it takes to help a child become a responsible, contented, socially useful adult, genes are only a minor consideration. Human beings have been around for a long time. Our genes and environments have, therefore, had a chance to coadapt so that most people do just fine. A few people are born with serious disabilities, but then the job is for society to provide the support they and their families need so they can live the best and most productive lives possible. I constantly encounter people with disabilities who live good lives, and nondisabled people who don't. I would have to be mad to imagine that I am sufficiently clairvoyant to try to extend the life span of a future human being when it is just an embryo.

Gregory E. Pence:
"Maximize Parental Choice"

Almost everything that Americans believe about genetic engineering and cloning of humans is false, due to decades of titillating science fiction, sensationalistic reporting in the media, and unthinking opposition. Hence, most people's thoughts and feelings on these topics need education.

Indeed, I personally would like to ban the phrases "test tube baby," "genetic engineering," and "cloning." For the latter, I would substitute the less emotional phrase, "somatic cell genetic transfer," or SCGT.

To assume that germ cells could be modified in a human embryo and have no more risk of harm to the child than natural conception is to remove the only real, moral objection to such procedures. All the other objections to such procedures are either unjustified or surreptitiously assume the resulting child will be harmed in some way, e.g., psychologically by the prejudiced attitudes of others.

There can be no reasonable objection to parents choosing to remove a gene or cluster of genes, or to modify genes, that cause something normally regarded as bad, such as a disease or handicap. Although some disability advocates insist that there is nothing wrong with being deaf, a dwarf, or having Down's syndrome, no reasonable parent would choose to have a child with such a condition when he or she could have a normal child. Indeed, in my opinion, it might be *immoral* to choose to have such a child if one could otherwise have a normal child.

Most people object to letting parents attempt to enhance a child's genotype through germ-cell modification. Usually the hidden assumption is that it really wouldn't work—that something would go wrong—and that the child would be harmed. That takes back the assumption of this essay.

The most-repeated objection is that if society let parents make such choices, they would only want "perfect children." Such an objection assumes that ordinary people can't be trusted in creating children. It also implies that wanting the best possible genetic base for a child is a bad motive.

People have not thought this objection through. Men and women exercise choice in selecting mates and in having children. We are quite comfortable with the fact that most of the present six billion earthlings choose the mate they think is the best possible for them and their children. If exercising choice is so bad, why isn't choice about reproductive mates also a dangerous thing? (If we "allow" such a practice, will people want only "perfect" mates?)

Obviously, what you want and what you get are not the same. As for gene enhancement, it is likely that, for the next decades, we will only have the knowledge to create one trait, especially when its base requires several genes and multifactorial environmental support. As such, parents will have to choose the kind of direction they want to go and decline other directions, e.g., to their child, literary talent but not football talent.

Here is one argument for allowing children to be produced by somatic cell genetic transfer. At least here, we know the cluster of traits that the ancestor had, and many of them may have been genetically based. We may be more likely to get the desired phenotype by reproducing an existing genotype than my fiddling with germline techniques one trait at a time.

Many other objections to attempting human SCGT are based on possible psychological harm to the resulting child from prejudiced reactions of others or from misplaced expectations of parents. We should not ban a reproductive option because some people are prejudiced or misguided. Education is the correct response to prejudice or incorrect expectations, not federal bans.

I do believe that the first attempt at human SCGT should be regulated, in America by a committee such as the Recombinant Advisory Committee

(RAC) at NIH, because the first case is very important to the acceptance of a new option. Louise Brown, the first baby created by in vitro fertilization, fortunately came out healthy, but problems developed in the Baby M case where a surrogate mother was used (and hence, commercial surrogacy was criminalized in some states). So we must be as certain as possible that the first attempt to create a baby by human SCGT will come out well, both for the sake of the child and for the sake of future attempts.

All of this assumes that reproductive science could know one day that germline interventions or somatic cell genetic transfer would cause no physical harm to the resulting child. That is a big assumption. I welcome the day when it is true.

> If you could do so safely, would you use an artificial
> chromosome to extend the lifespan of your child?

Some day soon, when the opportunities arise, we will see the wisdom of allowing parents maximal choice about their future children. This is not state-controlled eugenics (which attempted to take away such choices from parents), but its opposite. If a child can be given an extra decade of life by an artificial chromosome, or 50 percent more memory through a therapy in utero, then I personally would feel *obligated* to give my future child such benefits. I believe that my child would be grateful to have been deliberately given such a benefit.

Others might disagree and choose not to do so for their children—a decision I would respect. What I fail to understand is how other people— or the federal government—could think it just to prevent me from benefiting my future children in this way, e.g., by a ban on such enhancements (perhaps from a misplaced concern for equality and social justice). I see no difference between such a ban and a similar ban on parents sending their children to computer camps in the summer: both are intended to better children, both will be done most by people with money, and both are not the business of government.

Stefan F. Winter: "Our Societal Obligation for Keeping Human Nature Untouched"

Tucholsky's words, "The essence of the sea cannot be judged upon by the nature of its drops," came to mind in 1996 as my colleagues and I at the forty-nation Council of Europe were discussing possible attempts to alter the human genome. Decades earlier, Tucholsky had reflected on the dangers of oversimplification of natural phenomena. In my view, the present global debate on germline engineering is in danger of doing just this. Europeans did, however, manage to avoid such oversimplification when, in 1997, they wrote Article 13 of the European Convention on Human Rights and Biomedicine—the first legally binding European document of its kind. It states: "An intervention seeking to modify the human genome may only be undertaken for preventive, diagnostic or therapeutic purposes and only if its aim is not to introduce any modification into the genome of any descendents."

The reason Europe created such a clear provision on this biomedical subject is that it is so much more than just a medical issue. The question posed to me for this essay implicitly considers only risks that are medical in nature, but that wrongly ignores the enormous ethical and social dimensions of this topic. And it is precisely these larger dimensions that are paramount because, with germline engineering, the scientific community would be moving away from issues of health and towards an attempt to design a "new mankind."

If germline engineering procedures were made "safe," as the question posits, more and more couples would be tempted to use them instead of natural conception. What I fear is that most such couples would be interested in *nonmedical* indications and follow a eugenic approach concerned with extending the human life span, increasing intelligence, or enhancing physical abilities.

Even ignoring that social behavior would dramatically shift from natural toward in vitro conception, a guarantee not to cross the line from medicine towards eugenics can be imagined only for preimplantation genetic diagnostic techniques (PGD) because, unlike germline interventions, they involve no alteration of the human genome, no direct intervention into human nature, and no possibility of enhancing physical or mental abilities. Moreover, even with PGD, severe ethical problems remain about the questions of what constitutes a *severe* disease and who controls the use of the technology.

Besides well-known social and ethical considerations and medical risks, the European approach to the protection of the human genome and our prohibition of germline interventions was driven by the argument that there is almost no medical need for germline gene "therapy." Admittedly, there are rare homozygous lethal conditions not amenable to PGD, and there are the arguments put forward by some authors that therapeutic enhancements such as interventions to delay the onset of age-related diseases, susceptibility to viruses such as HIV, and even cancer preventatives could be done only by germline engineering. But the question remains: do we really want artificially constructed human beings? And who is entitled to make such fundamental decisions?

Germline gene therapy requires in vitro fertilization, but IVF generally involves the fertilization of many eggs, so in most situations the likelihood of acquiring at least one healthy embryo by PGD would be high. And if there are parents opposed to PGD on ethical grounds, they remain free to use normal conception or to forego having children. From the medical point of view, despite being at high risk for bearing children with serious monogenic diseases, affected couples generally have a 50–75 percent chance of bearing healthy offspring. Only in very rare cases are they faced with a lower chance of having healthy children so, with a medical indication of a severe genetic disorder, it makes sense to focus on the reimplantation of healthy embryos instead of the insupportable risks of attempting to cure affected embryos. In those few rare cases of severe genetic disorders not amenable to PGD, for the time being medicine will be unable to provide a genetic treatment.

Other, more profound, ethical problems have been attributed to preimplantation diagnosis, however, so I believe even PGD must be judged on a case-by-case basis to insure that embryos are adequately protected and that the procedure is ethically acceptable. In each case, the appropriateness of using PGD should be judged by an ethical committee that can evaluate whether the procedure is intended for a purely medical indication.

I see no compelling arguments for the introduction of germline interventions on human beings under any circumstances. And even if the technique were "improved" so that transmission of genetic alterations to future generations could be blocked, my position on this would not soften. It is interesting that the main focus of the germline debate tends to be on the nonmedical uses, not the few rare diseases only treatable by this technique.

These general societal applications are what raise my personal fears about the future of my children. On the one hand, success in somatic gene therapy, the discovery of new genetic diseases, and the arrival of new knowledge from molecular biology will make nonmedical requests for germline interventions increasingly likely. But, on the other hand, failures in somatic gene therapy will drive researchers to think about germline intervention as an alternative. With the growing burden of increasing health care costs, it would be a dangerous temptation if germline gene interventions—although difficult and expensive at first—were some day seen as a way of controlling medical costs, because we should not forget that nonmedical possibilities are what has opened today's germline debate.

> If you could do so safely, would you use an artificial
> chromosome to extend the lifespan of your child?

My answer starts with a question: Where would we go from here? Fighting disease is one thing, playing God another. Imagine the ensuing race for immortality; imagine a world with predetermined human life spans under societal control. Such scenarios far exceed our capacity to manage the process. What if the question had been about prolonging life not for a few decades, but for one hundred or two hundred years? Is that a world in which we would want to live? I think not, so my response to the offer of germline intervention to extend the life spans of my own three children is an emphatic "No!"

I believe that my children will want to have their own children and grandchildren normally and to enjoy a natural, not an artificially determined, lifespan. But this is not an easy choice for me. As a medical doctor, I know that it seems natural to consider added longevity as a good. But notwithstanding this "dogma," I'm convinced that once germline manipulation in humans begins, there will be "no way back to paradise." I have no doubt that germline gene interventions are theoretically possible and can likely be achieved technically. But we should never apply them to human beings. The breeding of mankind would be a social nightmare in which no one could escape.

To avoid the future risks associated with the development and use of germline gene manipulations, health policy should totally ban these interventions. This has been successfully done in the Council of Europe's Convention on Human Rights and Biomedicine, and it is very encouraging that the UNESCO Declaration on the Human Genome endorsed by the United Nations in 1998 points in this same direction. But in any event, who—according to the Hippocratic Oath—could ever be certified to offer what, for the vast majority of cases, is a technique that cannot be justified medically? Do we really want a "brave new world"?

Long-Term Possibilities and Dangers

Some have asserted that altering the genetics of human germinal cells would be an assault to human dignity, others that it would lead down a slippery slope with dire consequences. What is your assessment of the eventual possibilities and dangers of human germline engineering, and what are your biggest fears about its implementation? Would humanity be better off in a distant future where no direct modification of the genetics of human germline cells were allowed, or in one where significant modification were available?

Alex Mauron:
"The Question of Purpose"

A frightening new technological gimmick has been terrorizing people for quite some time. It provides a method for manipulating individuals by actually changing the connections between their brain cells! Furthermore, people whose brain structure has been altered in this way go on to produce similar neuronal changes in other people, so that these alterations resonate through successive generations and infect ever-increasing numbers of hapless humans. People promoting this dreadful technological monstrosity claim that, in the long run, people will be "better off" with engineered brains. Now there you see the typical hubris of the scientist-technocrat. He is blind to the long-term effects of this irreversible interference with the natural order. Society is held hostage to his technological utopia. Future generations as much as present-day society are the nonconsenting victims of his supposedly benevolent intrusions. Therefore: hands off from our neurons!

This awful technology is called neuronal phenotype manipulation, a.k.a. education.

At this point, maybe you think that I am taking a cheap shot at the opponents of human germline engineering. Comparing the willful modification of genomes with the time-honored process of developing minds by teaching them may seem preposterous. And yet shouldn't we ask whether the slogan "hands off from our genome" is any different from "hands off from our brains"? Actually, I believe it is, but the difference is subtler and less obvious that many opponents of germline engineering allow.

"Playing God," eugenics, the revolutionary character of bringing human evolution under human control: Those are the core features of many arguments against germline interventions. They have in common a central assumption, namely, the special standing of the human genome. It is claimed that our genome is important in a way that everything else isn't. The genome is construed as the ontological hard core of our being, the main determinant of our individual and species characteristics, the necessary and sufficient cause that makes us us. The genome has practically become the secular equivalent of the soul.

Now that scientists and medics have replaced priests, I guess that's fair. Still, this assumption is both ironic and ill-directed. Ironic, because the same people who tirelessly warn us of the perils of genetic reductionism suddenly make the human genome the inner sanctum of humanness. Ill-directed, because it focuses attention away from what really matters, namely phenotypes. Medicine, including medical genetics, is about human illness and suffering, whose links to phenotypic characteristics are direct, while they relate to genes only in a roundabout way. This is why, in Eric Juengst's terminology,[3] phenotypic care and prevention have a moral priority over genotypic prevention. All of them are ethically legitimate if they respect patient and familial autonomy, as well as the reproductive rights of individuals and couples. However, this may be more difficult for genotypic prevention, where the rationale of a particular genetic intervention can (but need not) shift to a largely populational goal of genome cleansing. To substitute genomes for people as the legitimate receiver of medical care would go against the grain of a liberal medical ethos, because "(The) traditional emphasis on personal rather than public interests and values is central both to the intrinsic moral merit of genetic medicine and to its societal acceptance in free societies."[4] This, in effect, provides an ethical test for germline interventions: Are they primarily person centered or gene-pool centered? To the extent that germline interventions become a realistic proposition (I still need to be convinced), some will pass the test;

some, perhaps many, will not. In the end, there appears to be little basis for a wholesale rejection or acceptance of germline interventions.

This is not exactly an exciting statement. But then, to go back to neuronal phenotype manipulation, a similar conclusion would apply. This "technology" isn't exactly innocuous either. Education is fine, everybody is for it. But let us not forget that we are reaching the end of a century which, more than any other, has seen explosions of global violence in the name of nationalism, racial hatred, and ideological and religious fanaticism. In other words, propaganda, brainwashing, and groupthink are the dark doppelgängers of the very same "technology" whose bright side is called education. At the end of the day, it all depends on the purpose. If we leave aside specific techniques but consider technologies in the broadest sense, i.e., wide-ranging ensembles of theoretical knowledge, insight, practical know-how and specific tools, then the conclusion is clear. Technologies do not come with an ethical label *good* or *bad* affixed to them on a priori considerations. It all depends on the ethical evaluation of their various purposes and the ethical implications of their use. This is an extremely banal conclusion. But then, banal conclusions are sometimes true.

> If you could do so safely, would you use an artificial
> chromosome to extend the lifespan of your child?

If there were no additional risk or cost, of course I would. Can anyone seriously say No? Much of modern health care in the broadest sense has been about prolonging life, perhaps not as an explicit central goal, but certainly as a most welcome collateral benefit. I cannot see how increasing longevity could in itself be wrong. Of course, many additional questions (for instance about the quality of added life) immediately come to mind, but I presume that one talks here of prolonging life per se.

But there is a catch: "Without additional risk or cost!" Is there anything in medicine that is both risk- and cost-free? I cannot quite take the question seriously. It is like asking someone who doesn't believe in free lunches whether he is worried that a free lunch might cause him indigestion.

Rabbi Barry Freundel:
"Gene Modification Technology"

Gene modification technology is not fundamentally different from any other technology mankind has developed. It carries with it great potential for good and great potential for evil. Anything with the capacity to impact on nature will, of necessity, present both possibilities as it becomes part of human reality. As a matter of both principle and practicality, Jewish law has never sought to ban any technology. In a philosophical sense, Judaism sees the statement to Adam and Eve, "To procreate, to fill the world and to subdue it" as a positivist view of human progress. To call someone a "partner in creation with G-d" is to grant that individual one of the finest compliments Jewish thought has to offer. That which exists in this world is raw material to do G-d's work and the discovery of a new technology is simply an uncovering of another method built into creation by G-d for mankind to use in positive ways.

Further, as a matter of practicality, banning new technologies will not work. Someone, somewhere, will proceed with the technology and, precisely because he or she will be a renegade if the technology is banned, he or she is likely to use the technology in ways that are entirely unsatisfactory from a moral standpoint. Far better, then, to regulate rather than to prohibit.

There are clearly positive possibilities for genetic manipulation technology such as removal of Tay-Sachs disease or hemophilia as a threat to mankind. These uses would be seen by Judaism as fulfilling a positive meritorious imperative of Jewish law. Aesthetic considerations such as removing an inherited, disfiguring mole would also be sanctioned by Jewish law. Anything which improves the individual or the species will ultimately be viewed favorably from a Jewish law perspective.

Certainly, there are potentials for abuse in this technology. Eugenics, abusive and selfish construction of children to meet particular standards and personal fantasies, and "brave new world" scenarios are all possibilities and must be protected against. However, Judaism approaches such questions with a fundamental optimism. It believes that mankind will find ways to produce far more that is positive than is negative from its technological advances. In addition, if human beings were given free will by their Divine Creator, limiting their ability to make choices that have moral content would in itself be a denial and denigration of the special place that human beings hold in creation.

For Judaism, there is no doubt of either a practical or philosophical nature that a world that possesses this technology would be far better than a world that does not. I believe, therefore, that the traditional segments of our community would advocate for more research and more development of technological possibilities. This should be done with appropriate regulation to ensure that uses of the technology are positive and not abusive.

Even if the question is phrased to focus on human beings gaining control of their own evolution, I do not find that to be any more troubling than discussing any other human capacity to alter the natural world. I take this position as a result of Judaism's teaching that human beings are the most important part of G-d's created universe. In mystical literature, human beings come from a higher place in G-d's economy than the angels. G-d has entrusted this world to humankind's hands, and the destiny of this world has always been our responsibility and challenge. Whether or not we live up to that challenge is our calling and essential mission. If G-d has built the capacity for gene redesign into nature, then He chose for it to be available to us, and our test remains whether we will use that power wisely or poorly.

> If you could do so safely, would you use an artificial
> chromosome to extend the lifespan of your child?

I would without any doubt have the procedure done and allow the child to live for a longer period of time. In Judaism, life is a positive value. In fact, one could argue that it is an infinite value. A longer life gives a person more time to be involved in good deeds and in the tasks presented by G-d to this world as His challenge to us. Increasing life expectancy through genetic manipulation is not different than increasing life expectancy by better management of disease or by developing new surgical procedures. Any type of increase in length of life is a positive for which the provider is deemed meritorious to the highest degree. Sanctity of life for us means increasing that life to the fullest extent possible.

I am often asked to cite one Jewish teaching that impresses me above all others. In response, I point to two sentences in a work known as Ethics of the Fathers. Ethics of the Fathers is a collection of the Talmudic rabbis' favorite and most important statements about Judaism and Jewish life. In that collection there is a teaching to the effect that one hour of bliss and happiness in the World to Come is better than all of life in this world. That is a sentiment shared by many religious belief systems.

In the same context, Ethics of the Fathers states that one hour of repentance and good deeds in this world is greater than all the life in the World to Come. To my knowledge, Judaism is the only belief system that sees some type of greater value to this world than to the World to Come. For this reason the question requires little thought in order to provide an answer from a Jewish law perspective. Every hour added to someone's life comes with the possibility of doing good deeds and repentance and is, therefore, more valuable in this way than all of life in the world to come. Given that belief, one cannot answer this question except in the affirmative. I would assume that my child will share my Jewish values and would also not hesitate to affirm that this was the right decision.

Erik Parens:
"Justice and the Germline"

If we aspired to create a more just society, would germline interventions be publicly supported and esteemed?

Champions of germline interventions usually point to helping couples have healthy children. But the number of people who could not have a healthy child by some other means is minuscule. Therefore, if biotechnology companies are going to give stockholders a return on their investment, there will be pressure to sell non-health-related interventions—which, for lack of a better term, we can call "enhancements." But so what? Parents have always sought "enhancements" for their children. Why should the prospect of germline enhancements move anyone to hand wringing?

In one scenario for the future, whether one gains access to germline enhancements will be a function of one's resources. This scenario raises the question, would such limited access widen the gap between the haves and have nots? To begin thinking about that question, it is helpful to consider a crude distinction between purchasing *new tools* and purchasing *new capacities.* The privileged have always had access to new technological tools that have enabled them to increase their productivity and thus their resources. The printing press, for example, no doubt conferred a competitive advantage on those who could afford access to it. The privileged also have always had access to opportunities, such as better schools, that have enabled them to cultivate their native capacities and increase their productivity and resources. But how much one could benefit from a new tool, and how much one could benefit from the cultivation of one's capacities, was to some extent limited by one's native capacities—by one's draw in the genetic lottery.

So one of the things that might be *new* about germline enhancement would be that one's draw in the genetic lottery would not pose the same sort of limitation; to some extent, the lottery could be "rigged." The ability to buy not only tools and opportunities to cultivate one's native capacities, but also to buy new or enhanced capacities themselves, would make some individuals doubly-strong competitors for many of life's goods. Thus, there seems reason to at least think about the possibility that germline enhancements might widen the already obscene gap between those who have and those who don't.

In a different scenario for the future, everyone would have access to germline enhancements. This scenario raises the question: with respect to *which* understandings of "better" would such enhancements be undertaken? What conceptions of normality and perfection will prospective parents have in mind when they attempt to genetically "improve" their children? In a liberal society, we not only recognize but honor the right of parents to shape their children in many ways, from giving them orthodontia to giving them violin lessons. We notice, however, that giving a child straighter teeth is an intervention different in magnitude than, say, giving her lighter skin. Giving a child the opportunity to learn the violin is different in magnitude than, say, hoping to give her the capacity to be more aggressive and competitive. The magnitudes of these interventions are different enough so that it would be a mistake to rest easy in the view that there's nothing here new enough to deserve our reflection. Moreover, to the extent that such interventions will be influenced by dominant conceptions of normality, and to the extent that those conceptions are arbitrary creations of advertisers whose job is to make consumers feel that they lack something, the prospect of selling these interventions should be an occasion for reflection.

As we think about using germline interventions to shape our children, we must remember that such shaping could be used to spare some children from the suffering associated with not fitting dominant conceptions. Nobody I know thinks suffering per se is good. Children shouldn't suffer in order to be taught, or to teach anybody else, a lesson. But we should not allow our desire to ameliorate suffering in the short run to allow us to inadvertently produce more suffering in the long run.

In the short run, we might be able to reduce the suffering associated with being different by making people more the same. There is another, probably more difficult—though perhaps ultimately more humane—way of attempting to reduce such suffering. Instead of using biotechnology to change the bodies of individuals to make them better conform to dominant conceptions, we could use education to change how we think about those who are different. It would be tragic if, as we increasingly are able to change the bodies of individuals to avoid the suffering associated with being different, we are increasingly disinclined to change the complex social attitudes and conditions that produce that suffering in the first place.

I am not saying that those who aspire to create a just society should refuse to consider germline interventions. I am saying that before we embark on that project, we should try to think much harder about the long-term consequences. The question is not, do germline enhancements raise brand new ethical problems? There are no new ethical problems under the sun. The question should be, will these techniques exacerbate injustices that already plague us? Will supporting these techniques tend toward more justice or less?

> If you could do so safely, would you use an artificial
> chromosome to extend the lifespan of your child?

The prospect of life extension raises difficult questions for those concerned about justice and the germline. If my wife and I were thinking only about our child, we probably would be delighted to increase her or his life expectancy by a decade. But we are committed to thinking about not only our own children, but about their children, and about all the others with whom they will share the world.

It does not require a vivid imagination to see the probable ecological consequences of widespread extension of the human life span beyond what many biologists have discerned to be the "natural limit." If one considers galloping human population growth, dwindling forests, dying fisheries, and global warming, one sees no pressing ecological need for humans to live longer. If our moral concern extends beyond an exceedingly narrow conception of what is good for us and our children, then life extension looks like a lamentable use of extraordinary human intelligence. Many of us in the "developed" nations may be tempted to say, "Well, the *real* environmental problem is the result of those folks in the 'developing' nations having so many children. *We* only have one or two children per couple." The birth rate in the developing world is a huge problem, but equally huge is the problem that we in the developed nations are consuming limited resources at an unconscionable rate. The idea of now trying to extend our lives—and thus our opportunities to consume still more—strikes me as woefully shortsighted at best. Thus, to the kind offer of life extension for our prospective children, my wife and I would say, "Thanks, but no."

Burke K. Zimmerman:
"Human Germline Intervention:
What's the Fuss About?"

The targeted, fully controlled modification of the human genome in a fertilized embryo is technically feasible. I shall thus begin by assuming, first, that we have a detailed knowledge of the human genome, the functions encoded by each set of genes, and the variations that make us different from one another, and second, that we are able both to correct obvious genetic pathology and to select—without introducing unwanted errors or genetic artifacts—the alleles that confer a variety of known traits to our children.

Let us examine the potential uses of such methods in light of the prevailing ethical standards governing the practice of medicine, the autonomy of parents trying to provide the best possible lives for their children, and distributive justice. It is difficult to see how adding germline modification to all of the other things one now can do for one's children, and in fact that one is expected to do to bring them health, quality education, and opportunities for developing their talents, poses anything inconsistent with the ethical norms that prevail, at least in western society.

The physician has an acknowledged ethical responsibility to use whatever methods are available to treat and prevent illness or pathology in his patients. If safe and reliable germline genetic surgery on a newly fertilized embryo is available to correct a known inherited genetic pathology, then, unless other means exist to avert that pathology, the physician has a moral obligation to use this technique to try to ensure the health of the baby. Physicians have no such moral imperative, however, at least according to today's norms, to assist prospective parents in attempts to give their children added genetically determined talents or more desirable physical attributes. But neither, of course, do physicians have an ethical proscription to help people enhance themselves through cosmetic surgery, which is routinely done.

Parents are expected to give their children the best possible opportunities in life. Thus, we promote their health and education and optimize their environments to give them greater opportunities. Why, then, should this responsibility not also extend to genetic factors that may determine a child's physical and psychological attributes, including even cognitive ability? While people can slightly improve their children's odds by carefully selecting a mate, only germline intervention will permit full control of their genetic endowments. Is there some unwritten social truism that people must forever be bound to play a genetic lottery when they procreate? Would not the well-accepted principle of autonomy leave such a choice solely to the prospective parents?

Autonomy, however, is often at odds with the principle of distributive justice. Since such germline techniques are not likely to be cheap, at least in the beginning, nor to be covered by national health programs or, in the United States, by private insurance, these techniques would remain a privilege of the wealthy. It is feared that their use would only widen the gulf between existing social and economic classes. The Bell Curve, Herrnstein and Murray's widely attacked work,[5] contends that, for generations, significant selection has been skewing the gene pool between the upper and lower classes. Their arguments may be flawed, but germline methods for the privileged would guarantee such a dichotomy.

Nonetheless, to demand justice in this province when it is not applied elsewhere is inconsistent. In the United States, even minimal healthcare is not available to everyone. The distribution of wealth, privilege, and opportunity, particularly the kind that provides children with a rich environment rather than a culturally and educationally impoverished one, is grossly skewed in most of the world. In the absence of broad and serious commitments to improve distributive justice with respect to the many *existing* elements that contribute to the quality of people's lives, arguments about the inequities of germline intervention ring hollow.

Of course, the techniques of germline intervention, as with computers and other new technologies, will be steadily improved in their reliability, scope, and cost. But if this is the slippery slope, then its effect will be to make this privilege of the wealthy generally available.

I do have some worries, however. The deliberate reassortment or correction of genes that are part of us does not really enter the realm of the unknown. But, one day, someone may be tempted to try to leapfrog human evolution by attempting to design a new gene from supposed first principles. Given our dismal record in predicting the consequences of new technologies, and our perennial smugness in believing we understand far more about nature than we do, I would have grave doubts about the wisdom of such intervention, even with extensive data from animal models. While we may eventually understand how this marvelous creation, including our brain and other components, actually works, we must keep in mind that the human system is the metastable result of a long evolutionary process, and that the pieces all work together in optimized harmony. Adding new or altered components, however good our knowledge of the system, could have unpredictable consequences. This represents a risk that no one should ask an unborn child to assume.

> If you could do so safely, would you use an artificial
> chromosome to extend the lifespan of your child?

Of course I would want my child to have an additional ten years of quality life. Who wouldn't?

I am assuming that, in being offered the opportunity to extend the lifespan of my child-to-be by adding an extra chromosome pair, there were already extensive human data to show that the procedure was safe and actually slowed the aging process. Naturally, I would wish to review personally all of the data and experimental protocols used to establish both the efficacy and the outcome of the procedure. In any case, my decision would be very conservative.

But, while being convinced that the safety and reliability of the procedure would be simply a matter of stringent scientific validation, the question of how an additional chromosome would assort when it comes my offspring's turn to procreate is another matter. My decision would clearly have an important effect, not only on my son's or daughter's life but on his or her children and on all subsequent generations. Therefore, while there may not yet be human data on the next generation, I shall further assume that there are extensive animal data on the fate of such an additional chromosome throughout many generations and on its interaction with the existing set of chromosomes. If my child wishes to have children someday by someone who did not happen to get an extra chromosome, we had better be sure that a dangling unpaired chromosome is not going to cause trouble.

And if, as I was about to allow the procedure to proceed, a last-minute finding indicated a long-term downside of any sort, I would surely change my mind and, no doubt, chastise myself for not having considered such a possibiliy in the first place. But what if the news comes after his birth?

If I have acted with proper respect for the limitations of the scientific method, then my child should at least understand the basis for my decision. But if I were too conservative, and he found himself aging sooner than his contemporaries who had undergone the procedure, would he resent me one day as being an ultraconservative old fuddy-duddy unwilling to take risks? Unless of course his peers were experiencing an unexpected consequence, for example a much higher than usual cancer rate—would he then be thankful for my wisdom? On the other hand, if I chose to extend his lifespan, he would surely thank me, unless he were one of the excess cancers.

Thus, while I would use my best judgment to do right thing for my child, nothing is certain. As in all the other decisions we make in bringing up our kids, every choice is something of a crapshoot. There is, therefore, no guarantee whatsoever that the next generation would appreciate my decision, whatever it may be, as every parent of grown children knows all too well.

Paul R. Billings: "Germline Culture— The Genetics of Hubris"

One view of the twentieth century, when so many of the developments in human genetics have occurred, is that it has been humanity's most bestial—we have fought amongst ourselves more viciously and killed each other more copiously than ever before. Few wise individuals predicted that outcome, fewer still claim to understand it today; control of the forces which produced the recurrent tragedies certainly eludes us.

Another formulation of our recent past might instead emphasize changes in relationships. For instance, our relations with others have been altered by the telephone, video, E-mail, and the psychological constructs of Freud and others. Our position vis-à-vis the natural world has been reformed by travel in space, on airplanes, and in cars, by sanitation and new foods, by antibiotics, and by the investigations of science that have demonstrated human life's identity with other life forms on earth.

Some see promise in these changes, while others sense threats. Some look optimistically for new information and synergies, while others feel ever more alienated and helpless to maintain value in their lives. Change has always occurred; for some it is welcome, while for others it only bodes loss, pain, and the end of life.

When *HMS Titanic* sailed from England in 1912, the ship embodied one narrow view of humanity's relationship to the natural world. Bigger, better, more powerful than any previous boat, this vessel was unsinkable, impervious to the furies which had ravaged the lives of seafarers for all of time. *Titanic* was the quintessential product of human endeavor and the industrial revolution that had transformed many late nineteenth-century cultures. With its many decks crammed with a cross-section of the society it left landbound, *Titanic* represented the wrestling of control of ocean navigation and travel from the gods and nature, and the placing of that control firmly, safely, and forever under humans. But the intricate interaction between nature, with its complex systems, and humans, with their essential limitations, was misunderstood. The high aspirations embodied by the *Titanic* ended in still repose on the ocean floor along with the lives of over 1,500 passengers.

Though we have far more scientific information relevant to genes and genetic manipulation than ever before, our ignorance is still overwhelming. Simple concepts such as what a gene is, or how a gene's biochemical variation correlates with measurable phenotypic phenomena, turn out not to be simple. Continuing human creativity and efforts to *understand* will fill in some gaps in our knowledge, but much may remain obscure. We can hope for more useful information, for special cases that will allow our knowledge to be applied, and for serendipity that will lead to unexpected good. Moreover, by attempting to understand human genetics and gene manipulation, we may gather information useful in other pursuits or develop models that illuminate their inherent limitations.

The anthropologist Gregory Bateson once noted, "The map is not the territory." Yet a few biotechnologists armed with powerful new "weapons" against human diseases are using a new and primitive "map" to direct an assault that will affect themselves, their neighbors, and—if the germline is modified—generations to come. To suggest that even this highly-trained and specialized group can assimilate a diverse variety of inputs and viewpoints, temper their hubris to appreciate the role of fashion and biological and nonbiological complexity, appreciate the social construction of many human conditions and characteristics, and balance human needs against our wish to help and to control the unknown is more than is reasonable to expect. To implement so powerful a technology when there is no true need, so much ignorance and such diversity of opinion, and a clear forewarning that it will create more inequality and suffering for both those changed and those left out, is intervention without consent, mandate, or justification.

Are we scientists undeterred by the wisdom of the sociologist Thorstein Veblen who, when commenting on whether men and women differed in their ability to learn, suggested deferring that assessment until both had been treated equally for several generations? Will we lobby groups that can barely appreciate the implications of applying genetic "fixes" prematurely or inappropriately? Is the schism of science and other cultures, noted by C.P. Snow, about to yield a fissile energy that will humble us? What are the risks, and what are the possible gains?

I challenge myself nearly every day to know when to act despite my own failings and ignorance, and to not act as if I know things that I don't. Each day I temper myself with the Hippocratic wisdom, *primun est non nocere* (first, do no harm). I am not sure what level of assuredness would be required for the implementation of human control over the evolution and design of its DNA. Even to ask such a question, in my view, reflects both a reckless temerity and a blindness to the many ways human culture has already modified forces at work in the natural world. I do know that we are *not* at that point and that medicine's moral guide is still derived from caring for those who are sick. Genetics, like the other sciences, exists as a challenge to ignorance. Its tools are limited by rationality and generate not truth but questions, the answers to most of which are not known.

> If you could do so safely, would you use an artificial
> chromosome to extend the lifespan of your child?

The extension of life expectancy is not an unfettered "good." Otherwise, the aphorism, "Life is hell and then you die," might simply be, "The more, the merrier."

Another decade of pain, loss, frustration, poverty, torture, violence, victimization, fear, abuse, and indignation would not be relished or desired by most people. Even with today's seeming progress and relative prosperity, some choose suicide to end a life which might otherwise continue for some time. The point is that longevity is a *conditional* good, dependent on a complex array of factors. The biomedical literature on how health care consumers differentially value "life years" is one reflection of this issue's complexity.

As a physician, I have sworn to lessen individual suffering and to take measures to maintain the public's health. Even this limited responsibility is hard to satisfy, so I am grateful for its limits. As a father, I rail against the presumption that I should know best about matters pertaining to the life of my child. I would prefer not to overreach my paternal role and, instead, try simply to protect my child's life and provide what is needed for her growth.

I trust that my child would understand my wish not to presumptuously interfere with lives other than my own. Since, in the physical universe in which we shall forever live, the posed conundrum is implausible without risk or cost, it is equally unlikely that such an intervention could be reversed without impact. If a technology were actually available on such impossible terms, I might be forced to reconsider my views both on this issue and on the role of scientists as deities. But more likely, I would wonder if I next were to be sold a bridge in Brooklyn.

James Hughes: "Liberty, Equality, and Solidarity in Our Genetically Engineered Future"

If we respect people's right to bodily autonomy, we need to permit people to choose germline and enhancement genetic therapies. Most of the arguments against gene therapy are either based on uncontestable matters of faith or describe risks insufficient to justify abrogating this fundamental liberal democratic right.

Bio-Luddites reject germline therapy and insist that we preserve the genetic "patrimony" for future generations. But our grandchildren will not thank us for passing along genetic diseases for them to fix through far less effective somatic therapies. Descendants generally prefer to inherit property that has been well maintained and improved, not maintained as a historical landmark. Our grandchildren will likely appreciate being made a little smarter, stronger, and healthier before birth.

A second argument used to stall the genetic revolution is that the genome is too complex to predict the certain catastrophic consequences of our modifications. This is Luddite mysticism, a warning against hubris. The genome is undoubtedly complex, and before we allow potential parents to apply germline therapies we should understand their consequences reasonably well. But we already have certain knowledge that genetic disease and disability is a bad thing (despite the arguments of disability advocates to the contrary) and that the potential benefits of genetic enhancement are enormous. The burden of proof for the product safety of genetic therapy needs to be finite, achievable, and balanced against these known benefits. Alleged risks to descendants ten generations from now are irrelevant. Our ability to fix any mistakes will rapidly advance in every decade.

What is really at stake in this debate is whether we will find the liberal democratic road to the genetically engineered society. The late twenty-first century will be made up of humans and human-animal hybrids, augmented by genetic engineering, nanotechnology, and information technology. Some societies will delay this transition to posthuman diversity as long as possible, adhering to a rigid biofundamentalist notion of what humans and citizens are supposed to be. But the individual and collective advantages to be had from the extension of human ability will make the transition very likely. Nations that refuse to embrace genetic enhancement will find themselves at a serious disadvantage. To block this transition will require an unlikely global regime of authoritarian surveillance, since the technologies will eventually be cheap and easily hidden in small labs.

The question about genetic engineering is not whether it will occur, but whether democracies will embrace the transition and shape it with the values of liberty, equality, and solidarity. A basic principle of liberty is respect for bodily autonomy. If we allow individuals and parents to choose their own genetic course, and avoid government prohibitions of or mandates about gene therapy, the results will be diverse, dynamic, and progressive. People will choose all kinds of body types for themselves and their kids, but most will choose to be healthier, longer lived, and more able. What better guarantee and reflection of liberty than a society embracing a growing diversity of healthy, able bodies?

As to equality, a universal, publicly financed package of health services is a prerequisite for the equitable provision of genetic therapies, whether the therapies are included in the plan or purchased on the market. After we establish equitable access to basic genetic therapies, we also have a responsibility to encourage parents to provide their children all reasonable opportunities for health or abilities. Today we agonize about how strenuously to coerce parents to give their kids an education and provide them with vaccinations and necessary medicine. In the future, we will agonize about parents who deny their children routine, safe, and effective genetic enhancements for health, intelligence, and ability. Liberal democracies may avoid an absolute mandate on genetic enhancement, the way we currently permit home schooling and religious exemptions to vaccinations. But even if legal, it will still be unethical for parents to refuse to provide their child cheap, effective genetic therapy or enhancement. If the therapy involves no great cost and no risk, this act of omission will be ethically equivalent to actively robbing them of life, health, or ability.

To preserve solidarity, we need a new model of collective identity, of "transhuman" citizenship. Rights and citizenship must be redefined around the abilities to think and communicate, not around human, version 1.0, DNA. As humanity subspeciates through germline therapy, it will be best if we can remain part of the same polity, a common society of mutual obligation and tolerance, for as long as possible.

In the end, genetic therapies raise no new questions, only old political ones. Do we have a strong enough scientific and regulatory apparatus to understand the consequences of our actions? Do we have the courage to tolerate free choices and extend the boundaries of our polity? Do we have the fellow feeling to ensure the general good and secure the rights of our fellow citizens? Genetic engineering just raises the stakes on these old challenges.

> If you could do so safely, would you use an artificial
> chromosome to extend the lifespan of your child?

Yes, I would use cheap, safe, and effective therapies to enhance my children' s abilities. In fact, I believe it is a moral obligation of parents to act in their children's best interests, and by definition I think greater intelligence, health, and longevity is in their interest. We frown at the mother who drinks and smokes heavily during pregnancy, and we smile on those who take their vitamins and then work hard to stimulate their newborns physically and mentally. Why is genetic therapy morally different? This holds equally true for whether the choice is to fix a genetic disease or to enhance abilities beyond the human norm. We don't condemn parents who work to give their kids better diets or educational environments above the national average, we praise them.

I am incredulous at disability advocates who argue that correcting genetic disabilities is a form of discrimination against the disabled. Are we to deny parents the option of correct their children's retardation or infirmities? Perhaps we should then also refuse to allow parents of PKU (phenyl ketohuria) kids to put their kids on the diets that would prevent their retardation, or refuse therapy to kids with any disease since, "That's the way they were meant to be," and therapy implies we don't love them for who they are.

Many skeptics also fall back on the potential unforeseen consequences of the therapies. The standard of evidence of safety needs to be specific to the therapy, however. In fixing serious genetic disabilities in my kids, I would accept much weaker evidence of the safety and efficacy of the therapy. For cosmetic enhancements, such as for our family's obesity, I would require a much higher standard of evidence, especially if there were effective nongenetic therapies.

George Ennenga: "Would Humanity Be Better Off . . . or, What Would It Be Better For?"

We consider our historical tracts, monuments, parks, and, by extension, the global ecosystem as our common heritage. Their conservation is imperative to the common good, and their availability is held as a right. Including the human genome in this legacy and conserving it against change might seem indisputable.

However, the processes and actualities of biology are different from those of politics, society, or architecture. *Nature* and *genome* are useful as abstractions in discussion but have no biological foundation. In biology, there are only individuals that can be considered collectively as a species. The ecosystem is compounded from individuals of manifold species in complex, changing, adaptive zones. A genome is generalized from the genetic character of individuals. Changes in adaptive zones are accommodated by a concomitant response in genetic combinations of those individuals. So, while a social contract or building exists in stasis, environments and genomes evolve in dynamic mobility. The principles are change and adaptation, not conservation and stasis.

Questions of modifying our genetic character lead to considerations of our common good and our highest purpose as a species. When we appraise the common good, we must refer to John Stuart Mill. He defined the *common good* as the highest inclination for individuals in an educated society, and *right action* as that which promotes the most happiness for all. These terms differ in biology, as opposed to politics and sociology. Happiness for every species must be construed as its greatest suitability to and survivability in its adaptive zone. Insuring that suitability must be the greatest common good, for our species as well as for all others. Collectively, our suitability must be a major priority.

Yet, we live not only in a natural habitat, but mostly in our created cultural environment. Although we have evolved little genetically in the past 40,000 years, our cultural evolution has been extraordinary, indeed, earth shattering. While organic evolution changes steadily, but without clear patterns, our cultural evolution grows exponentially. The accumulated technological developments of the past 200 years only indicate how vast our cultural evolution will be in future centuries. Increasingly, we humans will slip inside our cultural environments to become their authors and their subjects. These future environments will change and, no doubt, be varied, and so we will need to be equally mobile. Assuring our suitability and harmony in these various zones must be our greatest common good, otherwise we will not be at all happy.

"Artificial Evolution" is the controlled manipulation of genetic information from one generation to the next, where the first variational step is engineered and the second selection step is insured by humankind. It is qualitatively different from natural evolution. The biotechnologies of in vitro fertilization (IVF), gene transplantation, and germline engineering are the methods of developing this loop out of evolutionary time.

Artificial Evolution will provide the way for our species to change and grow in accord with environments of the future and in accord with nature, especially including human nature. Freeman Dyson holds that, "In the next hundred years . . . we will see genetically engineered plants and animals adapted to the colonization of various asteroids and planets. . . . As humanity expands its living space away from the earth, our one species will become many, . . . some adapted to heat, others to cold, some to zero gravity, others to strong gravity, some to high pressure, others to living in the vacuum of space."

From this vantage point, it becomes critical to identify the principles of change and mobility as central to our future. If our greatest happiness and common good is to be served, our species must keep genetically apace with our cultural evolution and in harmony with future adaptive zones. Far from conserving the genome in stasis, we must activate our genetic character diligently, conscientiously, and responsibly to guarantee our suitability to expanding environments of the near and far future. Our dignity, and even our security, will be enhanced by modifying our species to fit new environments. Failing to act upon the opportunities of germline engineering would condemn our species to a static role in an otherwise dynamic universe and would greatly delimit our futures. Artificial Evolution will be our method, truly our vehicle, into those futures. It will be our way of recognizing, of honoring, and of turning to our wider universe. What higher purpose, what greater dignity for humanity might there be?

> If you could do so safely, would you use an artificial
> chromosome to extend the lifespan of your child?

It is rather like extending the party for an hour. . . . No hesitation whatsoever, given the procedural safety. My main concern would be that others, like my young daughter, did not have the same opportunity. She would no doubt feel jealousy, but hopefully appreciation and wonder as well. By extension, the ethical issues are ones of fair distribution and availability of this or any other specific procedure in our Artificial Evolution. Natural Darwinian evolution is nonprogressive, discontinuous, and without value. Our species is not part of a progressive sequence; it is no more or less important than another. But, by creating *longevity* as a human value in our offspring, or any other human value such as *useful drugs*, we are bringing value and progress to the evolutionary process. A life is more valuable to us as *longer*, but, more than that, the whole process becomes progressive and continuous to us. This added chromosome, then, would create continuity in evolutionary time and, thus, if not for extending the party for one child, but simply for itself, would be a marvel.

Jan C. Heller: "Why Human Dignity Should Not Keep Us from Genetically Engineering Our Children"

Within certain natural and cultural constraints, the ability to shape our individual and collective futures in deliberate and self-conscious ways is a distinguishing characteristic of the human species. Human germline engineering holds the potential to remove some formidable natural constraints on this ability. Would it be permissible to remove some of the cultural constraints as well?

One of these cultural constraints is the belief that there is something in the nature of being human that utterly prohibits us from engineering the human germline. That "something" is often discussed as being dignity, a quality that humans are said to enjoy because, from the Western religious view, we were created in the image of a personal deity, or, in its secular derivative, because we have the capacity to become persons. This constraint leads to a prohibition on human genetic engineering based not on the uniqueness of our genome, but on what this genome makes possible—our personhood.

Dignity, I believe, ought to be regarded as a genuine moral constraint, and thus it ought to limit what we can do in the effort to shape our futures. But it is a constraint that rationally can be applied only to certain classes of humans. It makes obvious sense to discuss the dignity of living humans. We would not think it right to kill some innocent humans so that others would enjoy a better future. It also makes sense to discuss the dignity of humans who will live in the future. We would not think it right deliberately to leave, say in a former war zone, landmines that might harm future people simply because they do not yet exist. And we even grant limited dignity to dead humans, such as when we respect their Last Wills and Testaments. However, it makes no sense to discuss the dignity of a class of humans that I call "contingent future persons." These are *people who may or may not live in the future, depending on our choices.* Future children who might have their germlines engineered are in this class of persons, assuming, of course, a sufficiently advanced technology.

The dignity of contingent future persons cannot be violated by *any* choice that brings them into existence. Indeed, they cannot be said to have dignity. This claim is based on the fact that the identity of any person is time dependent, that is, contingent on the time of its conception. Thus, if agents can control the timing of the conception of a future child, any sufficient alteration of that timing will result in a *different* child actually being born—different, that is, than the child who would have been born had the timing of conception not been altered. The same claim can be made about embryos whose genomes are altered after conception: A child with a different identity will actually be born as a result of the alteration. Could the dignity of the child who is *actually* born be violated by such technologies?

However regrettable, the answer to this question is No. Any reference to the dignity of such a child leads to an argument that becomes hopelessly circular and self-defeating. Before the child who is actually born has been conceived, it (obviously) does not yet exist as a person to whom dignity can be ascribed. All reference to its dignity must await (at least) its conception as the person it will finally be, and by that time its dignity is not in question. Said differently, because the choice we are evaluating is the very choice that will make it possible for a contingent future person to come into existence with dignity, we cannot refer to the dignity of that future person when trying to decide whether to bring it into existence.

Ethically, this means that human dignity cannot be violated by bringing a child into existence with its germline engineered. If this is true, then we can determine the permissibility of the proposed technologies only by considering their likely consequences. My hunch is that they will not be sufficiently bad to warrant a prohibition on all human germline engineering. Moreover, if there is a market for such technologies, it might be better to put incentives in place to nudge their development in certain directions and to do so in a highly-regulated environment.

> If you could do so safely, would you use an artificial
> chromosome to extend the lifespan of your child?

This question is somewhat like asking whether I would be willing, without risk or obligation, to accept, say, a large amount of money for my future child. I suspect most of us would accept this gift, just as most—assured that no additional risk or cost would be incurred—would probably agree to increase their future child's life expectancy by a decade. A more difficult question is whether I would agree to such a procedure *knowing that my spouse and I do not need the IVF (in vitro fertilization) technology to conceive a child.* That is, when such procedures become widespread, would we forego natural conception and incur the moral, emotional, and economic costs of

IVF in order to give our future child the *chance* to live an extra decade (for the artificial chromosome cannot guarantee the extra time)? Since most prospective parents will not require IVF to conceive a child, this question is the more likely one to be asked as such options become widespread.

I would first try to weigh the risk of not having *any* child using IVF against the likely statistical prospect of having a normal child conceived naturally. If I opted for IVF, I would then try to weigh the likely benefits and burdens of an extra decade. For this, I need to make a prediction about the *conditions* under which the child's extra life would be lived, say, ninety to one hundred years from its birth. Would the child be likely to enjoy good physical and mental health? If *many* people were living an extra decade of life or if the population were very large, would there be enough resources for my child? If *few* people were living an extra decade, would my child become a target of discrimination or envy? In the end, if I were using IVF in any case, I might opt to insert the artificial chromosome. However, in view of the uncertainties of IVF and of future conditions, I would not forego natural conception for a chance to give my child an extra decade of life.

Regulation and Jurisdiction

Some have advocated the development of an international policy on germline engineering and cloning. Do you think this would be preferable to a patchwork of national policies and thus worth pursuing?

Darryl Macer: "Universal Bioethics for the Human Germline"

Germline engineering and cloning technologies present a challenge to the tolerance of individual and cultural reproductive autonomy enshrined in the human right for reproductive choice. While the creation of a child by the assistance of any technology cannot be made a crime, I believe there is a need for international regulation and education to promote responsible parenting. This is based on the shared biological heritage and destiny of human beings in all "nations"; on the transitory nature of "nations" and the precedents for international law to protect humanity's common interests; and on the common perceptions and bioethical reasoning of peoples around the world—universal bioethics.

One of the arguments behind international approaches to regulate germline gene therapy is that the genome is shared by all people who have diversified from a common African ancestor over the past 100,000 years.

The germline is common property under the international conventions on human rights, and the common heritage concept is enshrined in the UNESCO Declaration on the Human Genome and Human Rights unanimously accepted by all 186 countries of UNESCO in November 1997, and by the United Nations General Assembly in 1998. Another argument based on common future interest is that because people migrate and those born as clones or with altered germlines will move across national borders, the whole world is potentially at risk.

International guidelines provide some minimum standard. Many nations will not develop their own regulations, so an international umbrella guideline is needed to protect the present and future peoples of these countries. Who has ethical interest in protecting the germline? National governments may pay health costs, but regional blocks such as the European Union may also take on this role. Human rights laws are already based in international law. All people have a common interest in the germline, so transnational guidelines are desirable, unless we want racial hygiene laws designed to protect the citizens of one country that outlaws germline therapy from the reproductive cells of people from the free-market genetic engineering state.

There are already successful transnational agreements to protect common interests and the interests of innocent parties from future technological advances. Such agreements include the law of the sea, laws against ocean dumping, conventions against biological and chemical weapons, laws against the militarization of space, declarations of human rights including those on reproductive freedom, conventions aimed at halting ozone depletion, and treaties to slow the loss of biodiversity. If we protect the commons of the sea, it is not surprising that we want to protect the commons of the human genome.

The UNESCO Declaration bans human reproductive cloning in Article 11, which generally has been supported by countries that have debated it. But this prohibition raises serious questions about reproductive autonomy by claiming that the technique is against human dignity. A similar argument also was used in the European Bioethics Convention against germline genetic engineering, but given the range of techniques that are legally supported at this time, one can certainly question whether an individual couple's reproductive choice in these matters really would be contrary to human dignity.

While it is important to adopt standards that are suitable to each society, such standards should be based on the views of the individuals in each society. At present, some countries have standards based on false assumptions of cultural uniqueness. Within even a single community, opinions differ about bioethics issues such as preimplantation diagnosis, gene therapy, and risk. But data shows that people may use the same universal principles or ideals, even if they sometimes balance them differently to arrive at different decisions. Universal bioethics does not mean identical decisions; it means that the range of decisions in any one society is similar to those found across the whole world. It is also not the same as absolute ethics, saying that there is one correct ethical decision for a given set of circumstances; rather it would say that because of our love of life and human rights, people in any society should be given some choice over decisions of their lives. If people are the same everywhere, then the same standards of bioethics may be applied everywhere, while respecting the freedom of informed choice and responsibilities to society. This is universal bioethics.

The need for discussion of the consequences of germline gene therapy and enhancement is international, but many developing countries do not possess resources to have national education programs. The success of cosmetic surgery suggests that, once it is possible, the 20–30 percent in developed countries who accept genetic engineering to improve intelligence, physique, or personality, may do so in practice, as will the majority of people in developing countries.[6]

The purpose of regulation is to avoid doing harm. At the same time, loving good also demands us to do good. To cure disease using genetic therapy is a good, and those who want to ban it should prove otherwise. Above all, we need to educate people how to exercise informed choices in medical therapy, restricting choice only if this will harm others or society in general. Regulations should postpone the general use of germline genetic therapy, reproductive cloning, or enhancement until people can make such difficult decisions more wisely, but their decisions will transcend artificial boundaries of culture or nation.

> If you could do so safely, would you use an artificial
> chromosome to extend the lifespan of your child?

No, I would not use the procedure, because I would want to see the results in reality. If the technique existed, then at least in the lifetime of the child, the technical ability would come to allow the change during his or her life time. It would be better to let children decide their own fate, because informed choice would respect their autonomy. If 99 percent of society was performing the change, however, and it was shown to be safe, then I might allow it from the beginning, in the same way I support vaccination.

Lloyd Cohen: "Multi-Jurisdiction Regulation of Germline Intervention—A Policy with Neither Virtue Nor Prospect of Success"

Leaving aside its virtues and vices for a moment, is a unified international system of regulations of germline engineering even possible? The lessons from other areas of human activity are that only some shared gains from mutual cooperation and some means of retaliation for defection permit any multinational system of regulation and restraint to succeed. The partial success stories I am aware of all involve regulation of international trade, either agreements to abstain from imposing tariffs such as the General Agreement of Tariffs and Trade and NAFTA or, alternatively, agreements to restrict sales and raise prices such as OPEC. The character of these successes is that each of the participating parties sees it as in its interest that the collective enterprise succeed, and that each is subject to sanctions from the other participants if it cheats on the agreement. Unless multinational regulation of germline engineering offers some substantial gain to the participating nations and entails some prospect of retaliation, its "success" even in the limited sense that it would result in adherence, to say nothing of whether it would serve a good end, appears highly doubtful.

The jurisdictional breadth of any regulation should correspond to the breadth of substantial interest. So, for example, Moscow, Idaho, and Moscow, Russia do not share a common set of parking regulations, because the residents of each locale are largely unaffected by the parking rules in the other. On the other hand, mercury-laced wastes from mining operations in Montana that leach into the upper reaches of the Missouri River create potential health hazards for people in Louisiana. So, as a threshold issue, we must ask what dangers are posed by germline manipulation and whether those dangers have significant cross-border manifestations.

I have heard mention of three sorts of dangers. The first is a moral objection to making decisions that affect the genetic inheritance of unknown (and unborn) others; the second is some concern with inequalities (and therefore inequities?) in access to genetic advantages; and the third is a general concern with the integrity of "the gene pool." Leaving aside, for the moment, whether there is any substance to any of these objections, there is the ancillary issue of their jurisdictional and geographical character. That is, to what extent does the weight of concern diminish with political and geographical distance?

The first two objections are of a moral/political character with which the educated layman is well familiar and have little to do with genetics per se. People in other countries may engage in practices that we find odious. Whether it be slavery, abortion, the prohibition of abortion, capitalism, or communism, our knowledge that these vile practices take place anywhere in the world distresses us, and so we seek to eliminate them. That said, offensive abortion laws in Lagos, Nigeria, distress Americans less than those in Windsor, Ontario, and both far less than those in Detroit, Michigan. So, too, with these claims of an ethical harm to others resulting from germline engineering. If Brazilians place too much emphasis on the genes that lead to success at soccer, it will trouble Americans decidedly less than if New Yorkers do so.

Beyond that, however, the presumed immorality of genetic manipulation remains largely a mystery to me. The evil done to one's issue by manipulating their genes, or alternatively the evil done to others by giving an advantage to one's own issue not available to all, seems petty indeed. As for the first, who better than the parents and grandparents to make the decision for their prospective issue? They are clearly the most reliable agents of that future person's interest. As a general matter, we trust parents to make decisions that affect the future health, character, and personality of their children. I can see nothing substantially different in the case of germline engineering that warrants a different policy.

In some sense, the opposite concern is that the parents will do too good a job, that is, that they will provide their own offspring an advantage that others with fewer financial resources will not have available. To those morbidly concerned with absolute equality of result, this may seem a substantial problem; it does not seem so to me. Far more substantial environmental and genetic advantages—through assortive mating—are already available to those with financial and other advantages. Germline manipulation would be a trivial addition to this inequality. Indeed, given the likely rapidly declining cost of genetic engineering over time, the ability to enhance the genetic virtues of one's offspring will become widely and cheaply available and thus serve to equalize the genetic endowment of human beings.

The final, and most substantial, external effect on others of genetic engineering is some transformation of the human "gene pool." Here, too, the danger seems illusory. Imagine the thoroughly implausible possibility that Brazil, for example, were to engage in germline engineering that created changes in the genotypes and phenotypes of Brazilians that the rest of us found unappealing. How different is that from what already exists? The nations of the world already differ in their gene pools to a far more substantial degree than could (in the foreseeable future) be brought about by genetic engineering. In response to this difference, in order to prevent or at least minimize the entrance of those undesirable phenotypes and genotypes into another nation's population and gene pool, the obvious policy is to restrict immigration. Why is that policy not sufficient to handle germline engineering?

But, more realistically, how likely is it that the Brazilians or anyone will transform their own gene pool in a way that we find so unattractive? Does anyone have a serious objection to eliminating Huntington's? or Tay-Sachs? or breast cancer? or to increasing intelligence?

So, in conclusion, I can see neither the prospect nor the virtue in multi-jurisdictional regulation of germline engineering. Further, while I await some more powerful argument from the other side, for the moment I see the need for precious little additional national regulation beyond that which is already applicable to medical procedures on human beings.

> If you could do so safely, would you use an artificial
> chromosome to extend the lifespan of your child?

Which part of life is being extended? If it is ten years of healthy maturity, the answer is a clear Yes. If it is ten years of senile decrepitude, the answer is a clear No. If it is ten years of childhood, the answer is less clear. If it adds to each of these periods of life proportionally, simply slowing down the growth and aging processes, the answer is a qualified Yes. I would wonder whether it slows down life in any other internal sense.

On some deeper level you are asking about preferences with respect to a *sui generis* class of genetic manipulation. All other sorts of manipulation would be directed to affect some characteristic of life, such as intelligence, health, or size. The question you pose is more fundamental dealing with life itself, not its constituent parts or character. Is life per se worth living? And, if so, is more better than less? This is a deeper question than I care to address in this forum and subject to these space limitations.

Appendix

*Select Questions from the Public to Participants
in the "Engineering the Human Germline" Symposium*

QUESTION: Am I correct, Dr. Anderson, that you're saying that the risk/reward ratio is the driving force? If so, the line you drew between enhancement and treatment is somewhat inaccurate. For instance, you might view blocking aging as an enhancement, but there's obviously considerable reward to that.

FRENCH ANDERSON: I would not consider the normal aging process a disease. The consequences of aging—namely, cancer, heart disease, stroke, and so forth—are degenerative processes that take place; those are diseases.

LEE SILVER: I think one of the ways of getting over the problem that French mentions is also a question of what you mean by *enhancement*. When parents want to give something to their children which already exists in other individuals and society, you already know how that will operate. You're talking about an alternative allele that other parents give to their children naturally, but that you can't give to your children because you don't have it. And no one wants to have an average child, of course. I don't know anybody here who would. So, is it enhancement to give your child something that other children get naturally? I would think it's very difficult to stop parents from doing that particular kind of treatment.

MICHAEL ROSE: I'd like to make a somewhat different point. I think you're tieing yourself up into all kinds of knots that arise from the medical model, which is basically inherited from Hippocrates. It's a model that's 2,500 years old. I would suggest that if you reconsider your basic biology, in terms of concepts like quantitative genetics and fitness, selection, genetic variance, and environmental variance, you would find your way out of a lot of these problems.

FRENCH ANDERSON: Is breast cancer normal?

MICHAEL ROSE: Aging is totally normal. Breast cancer is dramatically age dependent, so if you're alive over age 100 you're way overdue for mortality in terms of the normal aging pattern, to which I say: If we find something that enables us to live to be age 200, even if I'm an M.D., I'm not going to say No to it, even if it's abnormal. I mean, what can be abnormal can be fantastic.

FRENCH ANDERSON: Is breast cancer normal?

MICHAEL ROSE: In terms of the age-dependent profile, to get cancer is very normal. It's difficult to find a person over age ninety who, on autopsy, does not show some signs of cancer, some signs of tumor.

FRENCH ANDERSON: So you would say that breast cancer is normal?

MICHAEL ROSE: So are all the cancers. The older you get, the greater your chance of getting Alzheimer's; the older you get, the greater your chance of cardiovascular disease. All of these things reflect the failure of natural selection to operate at those ages. The functions we have when we are young do not betoken normality, which is a meaningless concept in biology; they instead betoken the action of natural selection to make our bodies work well.

FRENCH ANDERSON: I would say that if you think that Alzheimer's, breast cancer, and so on are normal, then you are tied up in philosophical knots that you need release from.

QUESTION: My question is about the idea of medical ethics. Informed consent is usually required for a patient. We can't even agree about whether an embryo is an individual. How in the world can we address the idea of informed consent when we make changes to the germline?

JOHN CAMPBELL: Informed consent sounds like something you could not have unless it was in advance; but I think you can.

In my examples, a change is made that is genetic but of absolutely no consequence until it is activated. The only thing that would happen would be a particular transcription factor produced in a particular cell type. The recipient has to choose whether to activate this particular gene cassette.

If people are really concerned about this issue, we could take an artificial chromosome or a segment of it and put a lock on it so that none of the genes would have any effect until a person took an artificial hormone pill to unlock the cassettes, and then the person would be able to have a new engineered phenotype. He could decide.

I don't see that there's anything that says germline engineering means that the person can't have choice. If that's important, it's a technical issue we can give to our genetic engineers and say, "That's a constraint you have to work under. A person must have a choice before he has any change made to his physical body."

LEROY HOOD: But the other point one can make is that, as Mario [Capecchi] pointed out in his talk, there has been a lot of genetic engineering practiced—therapeutic selective abortions and things like that—where there isn't any prior choice. It's something that's been done for a long time in society. So these are complicated issues, and I don't think you can categorically say we should always require informed consent. The other thing I would say is that, although you can design these reversible kinds of things, it's quite clear that if we start engineering more complicated traits, it isn't going to be possible to make all of them so easily reversible. And we are going to have to face up to this important question.

DANIEL KOSHLAND: I'm not sure informed consent is always necessary. When I was a kid I didn't have an option about whether I would go to school or not. My parents told me to go. And I told my children. My children didn't have a vote on who their mother was when I decided to have children. So I think, sometimes, to extend informed consent to the embryo is really sort of a theoretical construct.

QUESTION: We've heard a lot about safe and careful manipulation of genes and have been cautioned about the interaction of different genes. I understand that, within a given period of gene activity, certain effects could be observed and then the artificial gene might be terminated, but the interaction that took place certainly would have repercussions, and I'd like to hear more about them.

MARIO CAPECCHI: I think what you're asking is whether we will ever know what we're doing. Are the interactions so complex that we can't anticipate what's going to happen? I think we have a few of things going for us based on experience with different kinds of animal models.

That's why I promote research—you can do increasingly complex research in animals. You can start with the mouse and go to a sheep and then go to nonhuman primates and thereby test the procedures in increasingly complex animals. In terms of physiology, this is a very reasonable approach. Those kinds of measurements can be done long term, to gather the needed information.

But when we get into treatment of mental deficiencies, it may become much more difficult to predict the outcome. It's going to be a long time before we actually understand how the mind works. We have no idea. How do we get information? Where do we store it? How can we retrieve it?

All of those parameters may have to be understood before we contemplate cures for mental deficiencies. So it's a long road, and we won't have guides. We won't have animal models to rely on. Drosophila (a fruit fly) does fairly complicated manipulations, but it doesn't think. It's fairly hardwired. Mice can learn. For example, we can teach them all sorts of smells, and we can reinforce their behavior and put them through learning paradigms. But it's still a long way from cognitive recognition and identity. My guess is that we're not going to be ready for quite a while.

I want to point out one thing, however: Scientists always overestimate what they can accomplish in five years. And they always underestimate what they can do in twenty-five years, because you don't know what new developments are going to completely change the rules. Right now it may be difficult for us to think about these things. But ten years, twenty years from now, it may be a very different story.

QUESTION: My question is about somatic gene therapy. I know there are problems with diseases in the brain because you can't access the brain physically. There are blood-brain barriers. Dr. Anderson, have you found any ways of solving somatic gene therapy problems in spite of these barriers?

FRENCH ANDERSON: The question is a very astute one: How well is somatic gene therapy working? The unfortunate fact is that, with the exception of a few anecdotal cases, there is no evidence at present that there is a gene therapy protocol that helps in any disease situation.

Our bodies have spent tens of thousands of years learning how to protect themselves from having exogenous DNA get into their genomes. And so, we were all a little naive to think that if we just made a viral vector and put it into the human body, it would work. The body's done a very good job of recognizing viral sequences and, basically, inactivating them.

So the answer to your question is—not just the more obvious questions like the blood-brain barrier and so on—but the straightforward question: "Does gene therapy work?" The answer is, at this point in time, it does not work. Now, does that mean it's never going to work? Well, no. It will. And there are now some very hopeful signs in a few clinical protocols. But the fact is we have a long way to go. And to look at germline gene therapy in twenty years is probably too early. To think of artificial chromosomes being used for gene therapy in twenty years I think is definitely too early. But I agree with Mario [Capecchi], who said, "We all have a tendency to overestimate what we can do in five years and underestimate what we can do in twenty-five years." And maybe exciting things will happen fifteen, eighteen years from now, so that in twenty years these things will be possible.

Notes

Introduction

1. See U.S. Department of Health and Human Services, Centers for Disease Control and Prevention, and National Center for Chronic Disease Control and Prevention, "Assisted Reproductive Techology Success Rates," *National Summary and Fertility Clinic Reports,* vol. 3: *Western United States* (December 1997), p. 57.

2. Sammy Glick, "Splice Einstein," *New York Times Magazine,* August 23, 1998, p. 26.

Part I

1. Henry Geraedts, "SATAC Artificial Chromosomes: A 'Super Vector' for Multi-Function Genetic Engineering," paper presented at bioconference "Transgenics & Cloning: Commercial Opportunities," Washington, D.C., June 26, 1998; C.J. Farr, R.A. Bayne, D. Kipling, W. Mills, R. Critcher, and H.J. Cooke, "Generation of a Human X-derived Minichromosome Using Telomere-Associated Chromosome Fragmentation," *EMBO Journal* 14(1995):5444–54; R. Heller, K.E. Brown, C. Burgtorf, and W.R. Brown, "Mini-Chromosomes Derived from the Human Y Chromosome by Telomere Directed Chromosome Breakage," *Proceedings of the National Academy of Sciences* 93(1996):7125–30; F. Ascenzioni, P. Donini, and H.J. Lipps, "Mammalian Artificial Chromosomes— Vectors for Somatic Gene Therapy," *Cancer Letters* 118(1997):135–42.

2. L. Duan, M. Zhu, I. Ozaki, H. Zhang, D.L. Wei, and R.J. Pomerantz, "Intracellular Inhibition of HIV-1 Replication Using a Dual Protein- and RNA-Based Strategy," *Gene Therapy* 4(1997):533–43; M.A. Biasolo, A. Radaelli, L. Del Pup, E. Fanchin, C. De Giuli-Morghen, and G. Palu, "A New Antisense tRNA Construct for the Genetic Treatment of Human Immunodeficiency Virus

Type 1 Infection," *Journal of Virology* 70(1996):2154–61; M.C. Leavitt, M. Yu, O. Yamada, G. Kraus, D. Looney, E. Poeschla, and F. Wong-Staal, "Transfer of an Anti-HIV-1 Ribozyme Gene into Primary Human Lymphocytes," *Human Gene Therapy* 5(1994):1115–20; O. Yamada, M. Yu, J.K. Yee, G. Kraus, D. Looney, and F. Wong-Staal, "Intracellular Immunization of Human T Cells with a Hairpin Ribozyme Against Human Immunodeficiency Virus Type 1," *Gene Therapy* 1(1994):38–45; C. Woffendin, U. Ranga, Z. Yang, L. Xu, and G.J. Nabel, "Expression of a Protective Gene-Prolongs Survival of T cells in Human Immunodeficiency Virus-Infected Patients," *Proceedings of the National Academy of Sciences* 93(1996):2889–94; D. Bevec, B. Volc-Platzer, K. Zimmermann, M. Dobrovnik, J. Hauber, G. Veres, and E. Bohnlein, "Constitutive Expression of Chimeric Neo-Rev Response Element Transcripts Suppresses HIV-1 Replication in Human CD4+ T Lymphocytes," *Human Gene Therapy* 5(1994):193–201; J.P. Maciejewski, F.F. Weichold, N.S. Young, A. Cara, D. Zella, M.S. Reitz, Jr., and R.C. Gallo "Intracellular Expression of Antibody Fragments Directed against HIV Reverse Transcriptase Prevents HIV Infection in Vitro," *Nature Medicine* 1(1995):667–73.

3. P.J. Felsburg, R.L. Somberg, B.J. Hartnett, S.F. Suter, P.S. Henthorn, P.F. Moore, K.I. Weinberg, and H.D. Ochs, "Full Immunologic Reconstitution Following Nonconditioned Bone Marrow Transplantation for Canine X-Linked Severe Combined Immunodeficiency," *Blood* 90(1997):3214–21.

4. B. Alberts, D. Bray, J. Lewis, M. Raff, K. Roberts, and J.D. Watson, *Molecular Biology of the Cell*, 3rd ed. (New York: Garland, 1994).

5. J. Browning, J.W. Horner, M. Pettoello-Mantovani, C. Raker, S. Yurasov, R.A. DePinho, and H. Goldstein, "Mice Transgenic for Human CD4 and CCR5 Are Susceptible to HIV Infection," *Proceedings of the National Academy of Sciences* 94(1997):14637–41.

6. D.D. Duncan, A. Stupakoff, S.M. Hedrick, K.B. Marcu, and G. Siu, "A Myc-Associated Zinc Finger Protein Binding Site Is One of Four Important Functional Regions in the CD4 Promoter," *Molecular and Cellular Biology* 15(1995): 3179–86.

7. B. Alberts, D. Bray, J. Lewis, M. Raff, K. Roberts, and J.D. Watson, *Molecular Biology of the Cell*, 3rd ed. (New York: Garland, 1994).

8. K.S. Christopherson, M.R. Mark, V. Bajaj, and P.J. Godowski, "Ecdysteroid-Dependent Regulation of Genes in Mammalian Cells by a Drosophila Ecdysone Receptor and Chimeric Transactivators," *Proceedings of the National Academy of Sciences* 89(1992):6314–18.

9. G.S. Harrison, C.J. Long, T.J. Curiel, F. Maxwell, and I.H. Maxwell, "Inhibition of Human Immunodeficiency Virus-1 Production Resulting from Transduction with a Retrovirus Containing an HIV-Regulated Diphtheria Toxin A Chain Gene," *Human Gene Therapy* 3(1992):461–69.

10. M.H. Tuszynski and F.H. Gage, "Somatic Gene Therapy for Nervous System Disease," *Ciba Foundation Symposium* 196(1996):85–94, discussion 94–97; P.G. Farlie, R. Dringen, S.M. Rees, G. Kannourakis, and O. Bernard, "Bcl-2 Transgene Expression Can Protect Neurons against Developmental and

Induced Cell Death," *Proceedings of the National Academy of Sciences* 92(1995): 4397–4401; M. Cayouette and C. Gravel, "Adenovirus-Mediated Gene Transfer of Ciliary Neurotrophic Factor Can Prevent Photoreceptor Degeneration in the Retinal Degeneration (rd) Mouse," *Human Gene Therapy* 8(1997):423–30; R.M. Friedlander, V. Gagliardini, H. Hara, K.B. Fink, W. Li, G. MacDonald, M.C. Fishman, A.H. Greenberg, M.A. Moskowitz, and J. Yuan, "Expression of a Dominant Negative Mutant of Interleukin-1 Beta Converting Enzyme in Transgenic Mice Prevents Neuronal Cell Death Induced by Trophic Factor Withdrawal and Ischemic Brain Injury," *Journal of Experimental Medicine* 185 (1997):933–40.

11. W.G. Tatton, R.M. Chalmers-Redman, W.Y. Ju, J. Wadia, and N.A. Tatton, "Apoptosis in Neurodegenerative Disorders: Potential for Therapy by Modifying Gene Transcription," *Journal of Neural Transmission,* suppl. 49(1997): 245–68; M.B. Reichel, R.R. Ali, D.M. Hunt, and S.S. Bhattacharya, "Gene Therapy for Retinal Degeneration," *Ophthalmic Research* 29(1997):261–68; E. Paradis, H. Douillard, M. Koutroumanis, C. Goodyer, and A. LeBlanc, "Amyloid Beta Peptide of Alzheimer's Disease Downregulates Bcl-2 and Upregulates Bax Expression in Human Neurons," *Journal of Neuroscience* 16: 7533–39; K.A. Marshall, S.E. Daniel, N. Cairns, P. Jenner, and B. Halliwell, "Upregulation of the Anti-apoptotic Protein Bcl-2 May Be an Early Event in Neurodegeneration: Studies on Parkinson's and Incidental Lewy Body Disease," *Biochemical and Biophysical Research Communications* 240(1997):84–87; P. Jenner and C.W. Olanow, "Oxidative Stress and the Pathogenesis of Parkinson's Disease," *Neurology* 47(1996; suppl. 3):S161–70; X. Mu, J. He, D.W. Anderson, J.Q. Trojanowski, and J.E. Springer, "Altered Expression of Bcl-2 and Bax mRNA in Amyotrophic Lateral Sclerosis Spinal Cord Motor Neurons," *Annals of Neurology* 40(1996):379–86; C. Portera-Cailliau, J.C. Hedreen, D.L. Price, and V.E. Koliatsos, "Evidence for Apoptotic Cell Death in Huntington Disease and Excitotoxic Animal Models," *Journal of Neuroscience* 15(1995): 3775–87; J.Q. Huang, J.M. Trasler, S. Igdoura, J. Michaud, N. Hanal, and R.A. Gravel, ''Apoptotic Cell Death in Mouse Models of GM2 Gangliosidosis and Observations on Human Tay-Sachs and Sandhoff Diseases," *Human Molecular Genetics* 6(1997):1879–85; J. Bengzon, Z. Kokaia, E. Elmer, A. Nanobashvili, M. Kokaia, and O. Lindvall, "Apoptosis and Proliferation of Dentate Gyrus Neurons after Single and Intermittent Limbic Seizures," *Proceedings of the National Academy of Sciences* 94(1997):10432–37.

12. L. Hood and L. Rowen, "Genes, Genomes and Society," in *Genetic Secrets: Protecting Privacy and Confidentiality in the Genetic Era,* ed. Mark A. Rothstein (New Haven: Yale University Press, 1997).

13. F. Colins, "New Goals for the U.S. Human Genome Project: 1998–2003." *Science* 282(1998):682–89.

14. L.M. Smith et al., "Fluorescence Detection in Automated Sequence Analysis," *Nature* 321(1986):674–79.

15. L. Rowen et al., in *Genetics: From Genes to Genomes,* ed. Leland Hartwell and Leroy Hood (Boston: McGraw-Hill, forthcoming).

16. J.C. Venter et al., "Shotgun Sequencing of the Human Genome," *Science* 280(1998): 1540–42.

17. A.P. Blanchard and L. Hood, "Sequence to Array: Probing the Genome's Secrets," *Nature Biotechnology* 14(1996):1649.

18. S.P. Foder et al., "Multiplied Biochemical Assays with Biological Chips," *Nature* 364(1993):555–56.

19. D.G. Wang et al., "Large-Scale Identification, Mapping, and Genotyping of Single Nucleotide Polymorphisms in the Human Genome," *Science* 280(1998):1077–82.

20. F.R. Blattner et al., "The Complete Genome Sequence of *Escherichia coli* K–12," *Science* 277(1997):1453–74; R.A. Clayton et al., "The First Genome from the Third Domain of Life," *Nature* 387(1997):459–62; *C. elegans* Sequencing Consortium, "Genome Sequence of the Nematode *C. elegans*: A Platform for Investigating Biology," *Science* 282(1998):2012–17.

21. J. Gusella, personal communication, 1998.

22. I. Wilmut, A.E. Schnieke, J. McWhir, A.J. Kind, and K.H.S. Campbell, "Viable Offspring Derived from Fetal and Adult Mammalian Cells," *Nature* 385 (1997):810–13.

23. T. Wakayama, A.C.F. Perry, M. Zuccotti, K.R. Johnson, and R. Yanagimachi, "Full-Term Development of Mice from Enucleated Oocytes Injected with Cumulus Cell Nuclei," *Nature* 394(1998):369–74.

24. M.R. Capecchi, "Targeted Gene Replacement," *Scientific American* 270: 54–61.

25. M.J. Evans and M.H. Kaufman, "Establishment in Culture of Pluripotential Cells from Mouse Embryos," *Nature* 292(1981):154–56.

26. N. Sternberg and D. Hamilton, "Bacteriophage P1 Site-specific Recombination. I. Recombination between *loxP* Sites," *Journal of Molecular Biology* 150(1981):467–86.

27. M. Bunting, K.E. Bernstein, M.R. Capecchi, and K.R. Thomas, "Targeting Genes for Self-Excision in the Germline," *Genes and Development* (in press).

28. W.F. Anderson, "Human Gene Therapy: Scientific and Ethical Considerations," *Journal of Medicine and Philosophy* 10(1985):275–91.

29. W.F. Anderson, "Human Gene Therapy: Why Draw a Line?" *Journal of Medicine and Philosophy* 14(1989):681–93. W.F. Anderson, "Genetics and Human Malleability," *The Hastings Center Report* 20(1980):21–24.

30. W.F. Anderson, in *Hearings on Human Genetic Engineering before the Subcommittee on Investigations and Oversight of the Committee on Science and Technology*, 97th Congress 2nd sess., No. 170 (Washington D.C.: Government Printing Office, 1982), pp. 285–92.

31. W.F. Anderson and J.C. Fletcher, "Gene Therapy in Human Beings: When Is It Ethical to Begin?" *New England Journal of Medicine* 303(1980):1293–97.

32. Nuremburg Military Tribunal, United States versus Karl Brandt et al. ("The Medical Case"), in *Trials of War Criminals*, vol. 2. (Washington, D.C.: Government Printing Office, 1947), pp. 181–84.

33. H.K. Beecher, "Some Guiding Principles for Clinical Investigation," *Journal of the American Medical Association* 195(1966):1135–36.

34. *The Belmont Report: Ethical Principles and Guidelines for the Protection of Human Subjects in Research,* National Commission for the Protection of Human Subjects of Biomedical and Behavioral Research, DHEW publication no. [OS]78-0012 (Washington D.C.: Government Printing Office, 1978).

35. J.C. Fletcher and W.F. Anderson, "Germ-Line Gene Therapy: A New Stage of Debate," *Law, Medicine, and Health Care* 12(1992):26–39.

36. W.F. Anderson, "Human Gene Therapy," *Science* 256(1992):808–13.

37. W.F. Anderson, "Human Gene Therapy," *Nature* suppl. 392(1998): 25–30.

38. J.C. Fletcher and G. Richter, "Human Fetal Gene Therapy: Moral and Ethical Questions," *Human Gene Therapy* 7(1996):1605–14.

39. P.W. Kantoff, A.W. Flake, M.A. Eglitis, S. Scharf, S. Bond, E. Gilboa, H. Erlich, M.R. Harrison, E.D. Zanjani, and W.F. Anderson, "In utero Gene Transfer and Expression: A Sheep Transplantation Model," *Blood* 73(1989): 1066–73; D. Ekhterae, T. Crumbleholme, E. Karson, M.R. Harrison, W.F. Anderson, and E.D. Zanjani, "Retrovial Vector-Mediated Transfer of the Bacterial Neomycin Resistance Gene into Fetal and Adult Sheep and Human Hematopoietic Progenitors in vitro," *Blood* 75(1990):365–69; C.D. Porada, N. Tran, M. Eglitis, R.C. Moen, L. Troutman, A.W. Flake, Y. Zhao, W.F. Anderson, and E.D. Zanjani, "In utero Gene Therapy: Transfer and Long-Term Expression of the Bacterial *neo*ʳ Gene in Sheep after Direct Injection of Retroviral Vectors into Preimmune Fetuses," *Human Gene Therapy* 99(1998):1571–85; N. Tran, C.D. Poranda, Y. Zhao, W.F. Anderson, and E.D. Zanjani, "In utero Gene Transfer in Sheep," in preparation.

40. E.D. Zanjani and W.F. Anderson, "Prospects for in utero Human Gene Therapy," *Science* (in press).

41. C.E. Finch, *Longevity, Senescence, and the Genome* (Chicago: University of Chicago Press, 1990).

42. B. Charlesworth, *Evolution in Age-Structured Populations,* 2nd ed., (Cambridge: Cambridge University Press, 1994).

43. M.R. Rose, *Evolutionary Biology of Aging* (New York: Oxford University Press, 1991)

44. Lee M. Silver, *Remaking Eden: Cloning and Beyond in a Brave New World* (New York: Avon Books, 1997)

45. I. Wilmut, A.E. Schnieke, J. McWhir, A.J. Kind, and K.H.S. Campbell, "Viable Offspring Derived from Fetal and Adult Mammalian Cells," *Nature* 385 (1997):810–13.

46. John Maddox, "Implications of Cloning," *Nature* 380(1996):383.

47. Princeton Survey Research Associates, results of a survey conducted for *Family Circle* magazine in May 1994.

48. Sophia J. Kleegman and Sherwin A. Kaufman, *Infertility in Women* (Philadelphia: F.A. Davis, 1966).

49. Lee M. Silver, *Remaking Eden: Cloning and Beyond in a Brave New World* (New York: Avon Books, 1997)

50. I. Wilmut, A.E. Schnieke, J. McWhir, A.J. Kind, and K.H.S. Campbell, "Viable Offspring Derived from Fetal and Adult Mammalian Cells," *Nature* 385(1997):810–13.

51. J.B. Cibelli, J.B., S.L. Stice, P.J. Golueke, J.J. Kane, J. Jerry, C. Blackwell, F.A. Ponce de Leon, and J.M. Robl, "Cloned Transgenic Calves Produced from Nonquiescent Fetal Fibroblasts," *Science* 280(1998):1256–58.

52. L. Meng, J.J. Ely, R.L. Stouffer, and D.P. Wolf, "Rhesus Monkeys Produced by Nuclear Transfer," *Biology of Reproduction* 57.2(1997):454–59.

53. L. Silver, "Cloning, Ethics, and Religion," *Cambridge Quarterly Healthcare Ethics* 7(1998):168–72.

54. Ibid.

55. Although at the time of this writing, there were no publicized cases of shared genetic motherhood, there was at least one attempt at shared biological motherhood between members of a same-sex couple. On August 25, the *Mail on Sunday* (a British tabloid) reported that a lesbian couple had asked an IVF practitioner to retrieve eggs from one of them, fertilize the eggs with donor sperm, and then introduce them into the uterus of the second woman. The resulting baby would then be raised by two biological mothers—one would be her gene-mom, the other her birth-mom—who would "share in the experience of motherhood." Unfortunately for this couple, the physician took their request to his hospital's ethics review board, which ruled against it. Although this couple failed in their attempt to reach their reproductive goal, it seems likely that others have pursued the same goal with success, away from the eyes of the press and close-minded male medical personnel.

56. B. Hogan, R. Beddington, F. Costantini, and F. Lacy, *Manipulating the Mouse Embryo: A Laboratory Manual*, 2nd ed. (Cold Spring Harbor, N.Y.: Cold Spring Harbor Press, 1994).

57. M.S. Verp, H. H. Harrison, C. Ober, D. Oliveri, A.P. Amarose, V. Lindgren, and A. Talerman, "Chimerism as the Etiology of a 46,XX/46,XY Fertile True Hermaphrodite," *Fertility and Sterility* 57(1992):346–49; Veskijkul, Jinorose, and Kanchanaporn (1992).

58. W.E. Gibbons, S.A. Gitlin, S.E. Lanzendorf, R.A. Kaufmann, R.N. Slotnick, and G.D. Hodgen, "Preimplantation Genetic Diagnosis for Tay-Sachs Disease: Successful Pregnancy after Pre-embryo Biopsy and Gene Amplification by Polymerase Chain Reaction," *Fertility and Sterility* 63(1995):723–28.

59. Robert Plomin, J.C. DeFries, and G.E. McClearn, *Behavioral Genetics: A Primer*, 2nd ed. (New York: W.H. Freeman, 1990).

60. Freeman Dyson, *Imagined Worlds* (Cambridge: Harvard University Press, 1996).

61. B. Hogan, R. Beddington, F. Costantini, and F. Lacy, *Manipulating the Mouse Embryo: A Laboratory Manual*, 2nd ed. (Cold Spring Harbor, N.Y.: Cold Spring Harbor Press, 1994).

62. T. Rulicke, "Transgenic Technology: An Introduction," *International Journal of Experimental Pathology* 77(1996):243–45.

63. A.E. Schnieke, A.J. Kind, W.A. Ritchie, K. Mycock, A.R. Scott, M. Ritchie, I. Wilmut, A. Colman, and K.H. Campbell, "Human Factor IX Transgenic Sheep Produced by Transfer of Nuclei from Transfected Fetal Fibroblasts" [see comments], *Science* 278(1997):2130–33.

64. R. Liu, W.A. Paxton, S. Choe, D. Ceradini, S.R. Martin, R. Horuk, M.E. MacDonald, H. Stuhlmann, R.A. Koup, and N.R. Landau, "Homozygous Defect in HIV-1 Coreceptor Accounts for Resistance of Some Multiply-Exposed Individuals to HIV-1 Infection," *Cell* 86(1996):367–77; C. Quillent, E. Oberlin, J. Braun, D. Rousset, G. Gonzalez-Canali, P. Metais, L. Montagnier, J.L. Virelizier, F. Arenzana-Seisdedos, and A. Beretta, "HIV-1-Resistance Phenotype Conferred by Combination of Two Separate Inherited Mutations of CCR5 gene" [see comments], *Lancet* 351(1998)(9095):14–18.

65. George Turner, *Brain Child* (New York: Morrow, 1991).

66. Nancy Kress, *Beggars in Spain* (New York: Morrow, 1993).

67. Philip K. Dick, *Do Androids Dream of Electric Sheep?* (Garden City, N.Y.: Doubleday, 1968).

68. Quoted from story by David Longtin and Duane Kraemer, "Wonders of Genetics Also Carry Some Risks," *USA Today*, May 6, 1998, p. 13A.

Part II

1. This refers to experiments by Professor Kline at UCLA in 1979.

Part III

1. Glenn McGee, *The Perfect Baby* (Lanham, Md.: Rowman and Littlefield, 1997).

2. Phillip R. Sloan, ed., *Controlling Our Destinies: The Human Genome Project from Historical, Philosophical, Social, and Ethical Perspectives* (Notre Dame, Ind.: University of Notre Dame Press, 1997).

3. E.T. Juengst, "Prevention and the Goals of Genetic Medicine," *Human Gene Therapy* 16(1995):1595–1605.

4. A. Mauron, "Ethical Aspects of Germ-Line Gene Therapy," in *Proceedings of the European Network for Biomedical Ethics Symposium on "Genetics in Human Reproduction,"* Maastricht, February 1998.

5. Richard J. Herrnstein and Charles Murray, *The Bell Curve* (New York: Free Press, 1994).

6. See surveys on-line at http://www.biol.tsukuba.ac.jp/~macer/index.html.

Glossary

Allele. One of several alternative structural forms of a gene.

Chromosome. The organelle which contains the genes.

Clone. Multiple genetically identical individuals or copies of a gene; also, the act of making clones of organisms or genes.

CRE. A recombinase enzyme that causes recombination at pairs of *loxP* sites in DNA molecules. It splits the DNA molecule in the center of the *loxP* sites and rejoins the pieces. CRE can fuse two circular molecules of DNA into one or can splice out the segment of DNA between the two *loxP* sites in one DNA molecule.

DNA. Deoxyribonucleic acid. A long double-stranded polymer which is the gene molecule of all life, except for certain viruses.

Ecdysone. A steroid hormone of insects, but not of humans, that activates a certain set of insect genes by binding to and activating an ecdysone-dependent transcription factor.

E. coli. The colon bacterium *Escherichia coli* widely used in the study of microbial physiology and genetics.

Enzyme. A protein that catalyzes a specific biochemical reaction.

Exon. A coding portion of a split gene that is separated from the rest of the gene by a noncoding intron DNA sequence.

Gene. A segment of DNA coding for a single polypeptide molecule. The term is sometimes used more loosely as a particular region of the chromosome responsible for a discernible phenotypic trait.

Genetic code. The correspondence between the nucleotide sequences of gene molecules and the amino acid sequences of the protein gene product.

Genetic recombination. The exchange of segments between two chromosomes, usually a key part of the reassortment of genes during the sexual process.

Genome. The total genetic material of a cell or organism.

Genotype. The total genetic information of an organism (see Phenotype).

Heredity. Transmission of genetic traits across generations.

Heritable. A genetic trait that is passed on to descendants.

Homology. Phenotypic characters derived from a common ancestral origin.

Human Genome Project. An ongoing program to determine the nucleotide sequence of the entire human genome, expected to be completed around the year 2003.

In vitro. A biological process taking place in artificial conditions; in contrast, *in vivo* pertains to processes in a living cell or organism.

Inducible. Produced or activated in response to an external condition.

Intron. A noncoding segment of DNA located within a gene.

loxP. The DNA target site for CRE recombinase enzyme (*see* CRE).

Menopause. The cessation of ovarian and menstrual cycles at the and of a woman's fertility, usually between the ages of forty-five and fifty-five years.

Messenger RNA. An RNA molecule that is translated into a polypeptide in the process of gene expression.

Mutation. A heritable change in the structure of a gene.

Nematode. A primitive roundworm extensively studied by developmental geneticists.

Nucleic acid. A polymer of ribonucleotides (RNA) or deoxynucleotides (DNA). The sequence of its nucleotide subunits encodes genetic information.

Nucleotide. The subunits of a nucleic acid, consisting of a sugar, a phosphate, and one of four types of bases: adenine (A), guanine (G), cytosine (C), or thymine (T) (or uracil [U] in the case of RNA).

Oligonucleotide. A short DNA or RNA molecule.

Ovulation. Release of an egg from the ovary.

Phenotype. The observable biochemical, anatomical, and behavioral traits of an organism determined by its genotype in its environment.

Protein. A macromolecule comprised of one or more polymeric chains of amino acids.

Recombinant DNA. A composite molecule made by artificially joining DNA molecules from two different sources.

RNA. Ribonucleic acid. A nucleic acid with a ribose sugar backbone instead of deoxyribose as in the case of DNA and generally existing as a single chain instead of a double helix.

Superallele. An uncommon gene allele that extends a beneficial trait in a person who carries it.

Transcription. Synthesis of an RNA molecule with the corresponding base sequence of a DNA molecule, as the first step in gene expression.

Translation. Synthesis of a polypeptide with an amino acid sequence dictated by the base sequence of a messenger RNA.

Virus. Ultra-microscopic, obligatory, intracellular parasites; incapable of autonomous replication or metabolism.

Wild-type sequences. The unmutated sequence of nucleotides in a particular gene or of amino acids in a protein of a species.

X chromosome. A sex chromosome. Female mammals have two X chromosomes. Males have an X and a Y chromosome.

Index

Lou Gehrig's disease, neuronal cells
in, 14
LoxP sites, 38–41, 160
Luddites, 130

Macular degeneration, neuronal
cells in, 14
Mathematicians, recruitment of
computer scientists and applied
mathematicians into biology,
22–23
Medicine
medical genetics, 118
medical research in germline
engineering, 5
Mice
aging in, 53–54
chimeric, 65, 66
genetic engineering of, 68
mouse genomes, 23
Mill, John Stuart, 133
Model systems, human aging and, 53
Molecular biology
and biophysics, 100
and genetics, 6
Molecular genetics, 3, 58
and its application to humans, 4
Motifs, 19
Muller, Benno, 77–78
Multi-jurisdiction regulation, of
germline intervention, 142–44
Multicellular organisms, 51
Multiple Project Assurance, 91
Murderous Science (Benno), 77–78
Murray, Charles, 125
Mutant embryos and mutant genes,
32, 33

National Institutes of Health (NIH)
Human Embryo Research Panel,
91
Office of Protection from Research
Risks, 91
National Institutes of Health Recom-
binant DNA Advisory Commit-

tee (NIH–RAC), 45, 47–48, 90,
91, 112–13
Natural selection, process of, 51,
52, 54
Nature, 58
Nematodes, 23, 53, 160
Neurodegenerative diseases, 14
Neuronal phenotype manipulation,
118, 119
Nonaging human population, demo-
graphic pattern of, 49
North American Free Trade Agree-
ment (NAFTA), 142
Nuclear transfer technology
human germline gene therapy
using, 35, 36
safety and efficiency of, 68
Somatic Cell Nuclear Transfer
(SCNT), 62, 63–64
Nucleotide, 37, 160
Nuremberg Code, 44

Organization for Economic Cooperation and Development (OECD),
49, 50
Organization of Petroleum Export-
ing Countries (OPEC), 142
*Origin of the Species by Natural Selec-
tion* (Darwin), 94

Parental choices
human germline modifications
and, 99–101
maximizing, 111–13
"Parenting in an Era of Genetics"
(*Hastings Center Report*), 100
Parkinson's disease, neuronal cells
in, 14
Periodic table of chemical elements,
18–19
Periodic table of life, 19
Phenotypes, 18, 118, 143, 160
Phenyl-ketohuria (PKU), 132
Photolithography, 22
Polymorphisms, 19, 22

Henry came up behind her. "Detective?"

"Detective Sergeant Robert Martinez, sir." The detective's gaze shifted from Deirdre to Henry. His skin was dark, with the leathery texture of an aging surfer.

"Do they always send a detective out?" Henry said. "This was an accident."

"Unaccompanied death. It's not unusual. Mind if I come in the house? I have a few—"

"We'll come out," Henry said, nudging Deirdre out in front of him. He followed and slid the door firmly shut.

"Mr. Unger was a strong swimmer?" Martinez asked when they were settled at the table on the patio.

"He swam every day," Henry said. "Like clockwork. Thirty laps."

"He often swim late at night?"

"Sometimes."

Martinez shot Deirdre a questioning look.

"Sometimes," she said. "Henry would know better than me. I don't live here."

"When did you last see your father?"

"In person?" Deirdre tried to remember the last time she'd been there.

"You came up for his birthday, remember?" Henry said. "January."

"Right," Deirdre said. That had been months ago.

"And the last time you talked to him?" Detective Martinez asked.

"Last week. He asked me to come up and help him."

"Help him what?"

"Get the house ready to go on the market."

Martinez's eyebrows rose a notch. Deirdre followed his gaze up to the sagging awning over the patio, across the paving stones with their cracked cement riven with weeds, and over to the peeling paint on the frame around the sliding doors. "Was anyone with you last night?" he asked her.

"No," Deirdre said.

"Anyone see you leave your house this morning?"

"No, I don't think so. I—"

"Oh, Christ," Henry said. "You can't think—"

"What about you, sir?"

Henry's mouth hung open for a moment. "Last night? I was here. This morning? Asleep until a few hours ago. And no, no one was with me. Just my dogs."

"And when did you see your father last?"

"Last night." Henry blinked. "No. Yesterday morning. Before I left for work. I didn't get back until late. After midnight. I went straight to bed. I just assumed . . . Oh my God. You don't think he's been out there all night?"

Martinez gazed impassively back at Henry. "We'll know more when the coroner has finished examining him. Yesterday morning, when you last saw your father, how did he seem?"

"He seemed fine," Henry said. "Normal. He was griping, you know. He liked to complain. And he was hungover."

"Your father was a drinker?"

"He liked a few drinks at night. And he could get maudlin."

"Maudlin?"

"Not wallowing in self-pity or anything. Just kvetching. Short stick. Half-empty glass. But it wasn't like he was about to kill himself."

Suicide? Deirdre hadn't even considered it. After the way her father had already screwed up her life, she couldn't believe he'd arrange for her to be the one to find him. But if it wasn't suicide, and it wasn't an accident . . . "What are you suggesting?" Deirdre asked.

"What we know for sure is that your father died most likely sometime last night. It's not clear how it happened, or even where it happened. We don't know for certain that he drowned. But if he was upset—"

"I told you, he wasn't upset," Henry said.

"I'm sorry. I know this is painful."

"He was not upset," Henry said, his voice cold and emphatic.

"Was your father seeing someone?" The detective directed the question at Deirdre.

"I have no idea. Was he?" Deirdre asked Henry. Arthur rarely talked to her about his lady friends and for that she was grateful.

Henry rolled his eyes. "No. He was not seeing anyone."

"You sound sure of that."

"I live here. I knew when he was seeing someone."

"He was divorced?"

"A long time ago," Deirdre said.

"They get along?" Martinez asked.

"At a distance," Henry said.

"It couldn't have been her," Deirdre said. "She's on a retreat."

"Huh." Martinez started to get up, then paused. "Just one more thing. You say it wasn't unusual for your father to swim late at night. It seems odd that he didn't turn on the lights in the pool."

"Lights?" Henry asked.

"There are no outside lights on now," Martinez said. "Maybe you turned them off when you got here?" he asked Deirdre.

"I . . ." Had she? She'd been in such a state. Then she realized she couldn't have. "No. The light switch is inside and I couldn't get in."

"What about you?" Martinez asked Henry. "Last night when you got home? Or maybe this morning?"

"Maybe." Henry thought for a moment. "No. I'm sure I didn't."

"Hmm. Maybe the lights are on a timer and they went off automatically?"

"No," Henry said.

"And the lights are working?" When Henry shrugged, Martinez added, "Can you check?"

Henry slid open the glass doors and reached for the light switch just inside.

"Hang on." Martinez crossed the yard and stood inside the fence to the pool. "Okay, give it a try."

The lights on the patio wall above Deirdre's head came on. The light in the pool must have come on, too, because Martinez flashed a thumbs-up and called out, "Thanks."

Martinez stared out at the water, one arm across his chest, the other propping up his chin. Deirdre knew what he was mulling. Would Arthur take a nighttime swim without turning on any lights? And if he had turned them on, then who turned them off? Because by the end of his swim, he'd have been incapable of doing so.

CHAPTER 7

That's it for now," Detective Martinez said. "The investigators should be done soon. Mind if I take a quick look around inside?"

It was the second time he'd invited himself into the house. "Inside?" Deirdre said.

"Just to be thorough. Then we won't have to come back."

Henry edged Deirdre aside. "No way, José."

Deirdre cringed but Martinez barely raised an eyebrow. "Okay, then. We'll be leaving soon, but we're not done. Your father's remains should be ready to be collected tomorrow or the next day. You should line up a mortuary. They'll know how to proceed. And here." He took out a business card and gave it to Deirdre. "In case either of you needs to reach me. If you think of something." He offered a second card to Henry, who stared at it for a moment. "Or find something you think we should know about," Martinez added.

Henry took the card.

Later that night, Deirdre was curled up on the couch, Henry sprawled in Arthur's favorite chair, a leather recliner. The wind had picked up, and the occasional gust set roof tiles chattering. Deirdre put the nub of a nearly smoked-out joint between her lips, inhaled, held her breath, and handed the joint back to Henry. They'd been eating from boxes of Chinese takeout that Henry charged to Arthur's credit card.

Deirdre had called Westwood Memorial Park. Darryl Zanuck was buried there, along with Natalie Wood. The undertaker Deirdre talked to on the phone had a deep, resonant voice that reminded her of Orson Welles. Of course, he said, they'd care for Arthur's *remains*. The term seemed appropriate. What she and Henry had pulled from the pool had barely been their father. By the time the coroner and the mortuary got done with him, he'd have been examined and dissected, his fluids drained away, his hubris along with his wit and warmth. People would come to the service and say what a swell guy Arthur Unger was. As he'd once remarked of a particularly foul-tempered studio executive, *You never look as good as you do at your own funeral.*

"At least Pedro didn't say don't skip town," Henry said, taking a pull on the joint.

"The detective's name is Robert," Deirdre replied, releasing her breath. "And maybe that's just something they say in the movies." Deirdre had no intention of leaving town. She'd called Stefan and left a message saying that it might be days before she got back. He'd be on his own with the new show—hard to believe she'd installed it just twenty-four hours ago. "So I guess you didn't want him snooping around inside the house," she added.

Henry started to laugh, choking on a final drag. He sputtered as he stubbed out the butt. "No way. Not with this shit in the house. You can bet he won't find a trace of illicit substances when he comes back."

"*When* he comes back?"

"Oh, he'll be back. You bought that crap about how they send out a detective whenever there's an unaccompanied death?" Henry scowled, making a face like the petulant thirteen-year-old he'd once been.

"Poor baby. Pushed your buttons, didn't he? What's the matter, you don't like cops?"

Henry threw a pillow at her. She caught it and sank back into the couch and let her gaze wander around the room. Arthur was everywhere, from the stack of *Variety* and *Life* magazines to ashtrays that still overflowed with the remains of her father's Marlboros to a glass cart with an ice bucket and a half-empty bottle of Dewar's. She hauled herself to her feet and, unsteady without her crutch, limped over to the piano. Open on the music stand was "Rhapsody in Blue." Shelved nearby was her father's cherished collection of LPs.

She edged over to the turntable. The record on top was *Ella and Louis.* She started the machine and set the needle. Closed her eyes to listen to the piano introduction, then Armstrong's easy, bluesy voice, having *that feeling of self-pity* . . .

"We should be drinking Dad's scotch," Deirdre said, turning back to Henry.

"Help yourself."

"I didn't say I wanted any. I'm not crazy about the stuff." Besides, on top of pot, hard liquor would be a very bad idea. "But it was his drink. And this is his music."

Henry stood and offered her his hand. He lifted her off the ground, set her feet on top of his, and rocked back and forth to the music. Deirdre closed her eyes and sang along. *"A foggy day . . ."* The words were muffled in Henry's shoulder, his shirt damp with her tears. "He taught me to waltz. And the Lindy," she said.

"You were a good dancer, Deeds. All he taught me to do was smoke. And drink. And drive too fast."

"Mmm, driving too fast. I can blame him for that, too."

Henry helped Deirdre back to the couch and then sat down

again himself. He poked his chopsticks into the take-out box and took another mouthful. A Singapore noodle stuck to his chin. Deirdre imagined what he'd look like as a Chia pet with noodles instead of grass growing out of his head and started to laugh.

Henry reached across, tweezed a spear of broccoli from her take-out box, and popped it into his mouth. Brown sauce dribbled down his chin to meet the noodle.

The room started to spin. Deirdre closed her eyes, which only made her feel worse. She lurched back upright.

When the phone rang, neither Deidre nor Henry moved to answer it. The machine picked up after four rings, and their father's voice echoed into the room. "You've reached Arthur Unger . . ." Deirdre flopped over and pulled a cushion over her head. When she heard the beep, she lifted the cushion.

"Hello? Henry, Deirdre? Are you there?" *Hyello.* Deirdre recognized the slightly accented voice before he added, "It is Sy." Sy Sterling, attorney to the stars, was the closest thing Deirdre and Henry had to an uncle from the old country. "I heard the news. I cannot believe this is happening. I talked to your father just the other day. Yesterday, for Chrissake. And"—he paused; his voice turned raspy and his accent thickened—"we were saying how we had to get together. Pick up some corned beef sandwiches and go to the track."

Henry lurched from the chair, dropping the box of noodles, which exploded onto the Oriental rug. He cursed, then tripped on the rug's raveled edge halfway to the phone and cursed again. In seconds, Bear and Baby had Hoovered up the spill.

"One of you call me back as soon as you can? I am in my car right now but I will be home later. Two seven six—"

Henry finally grabbed the phone. "Sy? It's Henry." Henry sounded winded. "Thanks for calling. Yeah." He paused, nodding his head a little. "I don't know. He was in the pool when Deirdre got here this morning. The cops were here most of the day. They think he died last night." Henry listened. "Are we okay?" He looked across at Deirdre. "I guess." He listened some more. "Of course I didn't let them into the house."

Henry turned his back to Deirdre and walked toward the window. The phone cord stretched from coiled to straight until it wouldn't stretch farther. Henry stood quietly, listening, a long silence with just the occasional "Uh-huh," "Sure," "Okay."

Deirdre got up again. She limped over to the wall of bookshelves and picked up a framed photograph of all four of them, scrubbed and polished and posed against a backlit scrim of blue sky and palm trees. Ten-year-old Deirdre wore a demure black velvet dress with a white lacy collar, her hair skinned back in a ponytail. Henry, a year older, looked downright military in his little suit. What you couldn't see was that he'd been wearing flip-flops. That year he'd refused to wear real shoes.

Alongside the family portrait was a framed black-and-white photograph of eight-year-old Deirdre in a sparkly leotard and skirt of layered ruffles. Deirdre knew the ruffles were pink, and the black patent leather tap shoes had been bought a size too big for her so that she could "grow into them." More girls in similar getups stood posed behind her looking supremely bored as Deirdre danced her solo.

She turned the picture facedown on the shelf.

Behind the pictures were videocassettes, each with a handwritten label—some her mother's careful printing, others her father's scrawl. Also lined up was a row of their leather-bound movie scripts, the titles embossed in gold on the spines. Deirdre ran her hand over the leather. Gloria had let Arthur keep all their scripts when she'd walked out. She'd left behind most of her clothes and jewelry, too, along with her perfume and cosmetics. She'd probably have shed her skin and left that behind if she could have.

The shelved scripts were in chronological order. There was *Lady, Be Good*, their first movie, a remake of a 1920s silent film of the

Gershwin musical comedy that was long on jazzy score, glittery costumes, and dance numbers and short on plot. Next to it, *A Night in St. Tropez*. Deirdre opened that script and paged through hand-typed pages until she got to one of the nine-by-eleven, black-and-white glossies that were bound into the book. Carmen Miranda winked at the camera, wearing ropes of pearls and a skirt that looked like it was made of bananas.

At the end of the row were two copies of *Singing All the Way Home*, the last script her parents wrote together, and one of the last romantic musicals in an era that had been full of them.

"Really?" Henry was saying into the phone. "All right then!" Deirdre looked over at him. He was smiling. Some good news?

Deirdre pulled one of the copies of *Singing All the Way Home* off the shelf and opened it. There were no pages bound into it. Instead, tucked inside was a pocket folder that held a sheaf of papers—an unbound manuscript, carbon copies on onionskin paper. Centered on an otherwise blank first page were the words "WORKING TITLE: ONE DAMNED THING AFTER ANOTHER," and below that, "by Arthur Unger, 1985."

Deirdre turned to the next page and read.

CHAPTER 1: EXIT LAUGHING

The writing was on the wall of our office at Twentieth Century Fox when the secretary didn't show up and the phones disappeared. We were screwed. Shafted. Sucker-punched. Time to strike the set.

Deirdre smiled. She could hear her father's voice. For a moment her chest tightened and her vision blurred.

Beneath the opening paragraph, text was formatted like the slug lines and stage directions of a movie script.

INT. TWENTIETH CENTURY FOX - SCREEN-
WRITERS OFFICE - DAY (1963)

ARTHUR UNGER opens the door to his office and starts to enter. He's trim, middle-aged, wears a suit and holds his hat. Stops. He looks surprised. Dismayed.

His secretary's desk is empty. Disconnected phone wires are coiled on the floor.

ARTHUR crosses to the window, looks two stories down to a deserted studio street where a huge movie poster for Cleopatra is plastered across a wall. In front of it is an empty phone booth.

ARTHUR raises the window. Sits on the ledge.

No, I didn't jump. Two stories up? Not high enough to kill me, and damned if I was going to let the sons of bitches cripple me for life. When I went outside to use the pay phone, I swear there were vultures circling overhead. Could've been a scene out of Hitchcock, but Hitchcock worked for Universal.

Turned out hundreds of us arrived on the Fox lot that morning to find our office phone lines disconnected and our typewriters returned to Props.

It was a clever device for a screenwriter's memoir, alternating between the idiosyncratic formatting of a screenplay and straight narrative. Odd that Arthur had kept this carbon copy tucked in the cover of a movie script. Almost like he'd hidden it there.

As Deirdre flipped to the last chapter to see how far Arthur gotten, Henry's voice pulled her off the page. "All right. Uh-huh. Sure. Don't worry, I won't forget." Clearly, he was winding up the call. Deirdre put the empty script cover back on the shelf and carried the folder with the manuscript pages to her bedroom, where she slipped it into the drawer in her bedside table.

When she returned, Henry had hung up the phone. Deirdre said, "Was that Sy?"

"*Sí,*" Henry said, deadpan.

"So?" Even if it was a wildly inappropriate time to be cracking jokes, Arthur would have appreciated the old comedy routine that he'd reprise himself whenever the opportunity presented itself. It was one of the perks, he used to say, of having a friend named Sy.

"He's coming over tomorrow morning to talk about Dad's will."

"What won't you forget?"

"Huh?"

"You told him you wouldn't forget something."

"When the police come back to search the house, there shouldn't be anything here we don't want them to find." Henry went into the kitchen and came back out with a large black plastic garbage bag, into which he dumped the contents of the ashtray.

"That's a big bag for a few ashes," Deirdre said.

"There's more. Things Dad would want me to get rid of."

"What things?"

Henry's answer was cut off by the phone ringing again. Both Deirdre and Henry froze, waiting for the answering machine to kick in. After the beep, this time they heard a woman's voice: "Hey, Zelda? You there? It's Thalia."

Deirdre might not have recognized Joelen's voice, but she definitely recognized those nicknames. Zelda, the smart but painfully plain and geeky character who lusted after television's Dobie Gillis, was code for Deirdre; Thalia, the gorgeous, moneygrubbing blonde whom Dobie lusted after, was Joelen.

Deirdre reached for the phone but Henry stopped her as Joelen's voice continued. "Sy called and told us what happened. Gosh, I don't know where to begin. I just hate saying this to a machine." A pause. "I'm so sorry. I really can't believe it." There was a longer pause, then: "Listen, I don't know how long you'll be in town, and I know it's been ages since we were friends. But we were. Really good friends.

If there's anything I can do to help, all you have to do is name it. You know where I am. Same place. Call me." Joelen recited the number. Deirdre still knew it by heart. "Mom sends condolences."

Click.

"Joelen?" Henry said.

Deirdre nodded.

"Now what does she want?"

"I don't think she *wants* anything. I told you, she rang the bell this morning right before the police. She's a Realtor. She had a meeting with Dad."

"So why is she calling now?"

"She's being nice?" Deirdre yawned and stretched. The room had long ago stopped spinning and she felt drained and far too tired to try explaining to Henry the concept of *nice.* "I'm going to bed," she announced. She hoped there were clean sheets.

"I've got to take these guys out. Then I'll turn in, too." Henry pulled his leather jacket off the back of a chair. The dogs perked up and started yipping and circling him.

"And you'll take care of that?" Deirdre pointed to the deflated garbage bag that Henry had left on the floor. "And the things that Dad wanted you to throw away?"

"Oh yeah." Henry crouched and snapped a leash to each dog's collar. "Don't worry, it will all be gone by morning."

CHAPTER 8

The wind had died down and the house settled into an uneasy silence as Deirdre ferried beer bottles and leftovers to the kitchen. She carried her duffel bag into the room that was once her bedroom. The stuffy space had been taken over by Henry's bench press, weights, and an exercise bicycle. Judging from the layer of dust on them, they didn't see much use.

She opened the windows, but the air barely moved. On hot nights like this her father used to hose down the roof.

Her sliding closet door was sticky, but she managed to work it open. There, on the rack, hung some straight skirts and pleated skirts from high school, all of them much too long, with a few matching cardigan sweaters. A much shorter, swingy, navy blue tent dress that she'd worn in college hung there, too. She'd bought it because she thought it made her look like That Girl, Marlo Thomas. There was the cream-colored linen suit she'd worn to her college interviews, along with a brown trench coat that she used to wear with its broad collar turned up, its belt tied at the waist in the style of Catherine Deneuve.

Way on the end was the white two-piece dress she'd worn to her high school graduation and to the dance after. She fingered the silk brocade that had gone brittle with age. The shoes that were supposed to have been her first high heels were still in their box on the closet floor. When she'd bought them she'd been optimistic that she'd be able to take a few steps, maybe even dance. Just one more thing that was supposed to happen that never did.

Deirdre tossed her duffel bag on top of some cardboard boxes stacked in the closet. Her name was written in block letters on the sides—certainly her writing—though she had no memory of boxing anything up.

She turned. On the adjacent wall hung a large framed pencil sketch of a waif with enormous, honey-dripping eyes. The little girl held a gray kitten with its own wide teary eyes. Preadolescent Deirdre had selected this awesomely awful artist-signed (Keane) piece of '60s kitsch herself. After the accident, she'd identified with that girl and begged her parents to get her a cat. She'd made up stories, none of them with happy endings, about how the pair came to find themselves in their pitiable state. Now she limped over, took the picture down from the wall, and stuck it in the closet facing the wall.

The mattress of her trundle bed was adrift in Henry's magazines: *Rolling Stone* with U2 on the cover, something called *Spin* with a sultry Madonna, *Cycle World*. Deirdre pushed them aside, unearthing Ollie, her teddy bear. The felt that had covered his paws and nose had long ago been worn away. She pressed Ollie to her face and let his sweet, woolly smell take her back to a time well before this nightmare. Her mother would have been running her a hot bath and asking if she wanted hot cocoa to help her sleep. The bed would have been made up with freshly laundered sheets instead of two naked pillows and a stained mattress cover.

Well, there was certainly no hot cocoa now. Shrugging off her old memories, Deirdre tossed Ollie into the closet where he could have a pity party with the waif and her kitten. She took a quick shower, made the bed, and got into it. Exhausted but wired, she opened the drawer in her bedside table, pulled out Arthur's manuscript, and started to read where she'd left off.

The second chapter, titled "The Bronx Is Up," recounted his childhood. He'd grown up, the youngest son of Russian immigrants, with four brothers, none of whom Deirdre had met. She skimmed the pages, through a life story told in anecdotes, many of which she'd heard Arthur tell more than once. She paused at the sound of the front door opening and dog claws scrabbling on the floor. Henry was back.

In the next chapter, "Helluva Town," Arthur flunked out of college and landed in Manhattan, found work as an assistant stage manager and a shabby room with a shared bath in Hell's Kitchen. Late nights, he hung out in Greenwich Village. Mornings he'd get up early and write plays.

Deirdre heard the front door open and close again, then the rumble of Henry's motorcycle catching, revving, and roaring off. She wondered when he was planning to take Sy's advice and get rid of anything that they wouldn't want the police to find.

Deirdre yawned. She tried to continue reading but the words swam on the page. She slid the manuscript back in the folder and tucked it into her bedside drawer. Then she plumped up the pillows and lay back. The house was silent with the occasional comforting sounds of dogs lumbering about. She stared up at the ceiling. There was a water stain in the corner. Would she and Henry have to fix the roof and get the rooms painted? Right now she was too tired to care.

The bedside clock said it was nearly one in the morning. Deirdre turned over, bunched the pillow under her head, and closed her eyes. Maybe it had been at about this time Arthur had gone for a swim. She could see him walking to the pool, his eyes slowly adjusting to the dark. Diving in.

Was that when it had gone wrong? He'd taken a running leap from the board, hit the water, and gotten the air knocked out of him. Struggled to reach the surface, flailing in darkness, propelling himself toward what he thought was sky and smashing headlong into the cement at the bottom of the pool.

Sweat broke out across Deirdre's neck and back and she sat up, gasping for breath. She imagined Arthur hanging there, a dark shadow under the water, life seeping out of him. Her fingertips tingled and her heart beat a tattoo in her chest. She smelled chlorine and death and gagged.

Breathe, she told herself as she tried to relax, counting a slow in and out, until finally the tension eased and her lungs filled completely. Shivering, she sat there for a few moments longer before sinking back into the pillow and pulling the blanket around her. The handlebars of the exercise bike looked like shadows outlined against the window. The open closet was a dark rectangle. She started to close her eyes but that feeling, like someone was chasing her and she couldn't get away, started to take hold.

Deirdre had long known that the truly scary stuff was in her own head. Doped up on Demerol after her car accident, she'd dreamed that her limbs were scattered down a hillside and she had to convince the EMTs to collect them for her. Or that she was on the table in an operating theater, a light beating down on her from above as doctors sawed off her leg, the surrounding stadium seats filled with onlookers. Or that her father was driving her home but she had to get back to the hospital because she'd left behind her hands. Even when she knew she was dreaming, she couldn't wake herself from those dreams. The memory of that paralyzing panic was far more vivid than any memory of the accident or of anything the doctors had done to her after.

She'd learned, over time, to avoid Demerol and redirect her mind. Anchor her attention on a sensation. Like the heavy sweet smell that was in the air, maybe a gardenia or night-blooming jasmine in the yard? The scent reminded her of hairspray. Aqua Net. Connect the dots and up popped Joelen Nichol, standing in front of her bathroom mirror years ago, spraying Deirdre's hair. Deirdre remembered the feel of that cool mist drying to a tight coating like a skim of egg white on every skin surface it touched.

Joelen. Who had stood at the front door hours ago and offered Deirdre a business card before bolting out to her car. Then called to offer any help she could. So she was a Realtor, not the movie star she'd dreamed of becoming.

There was a flash. A roll of distant thunder. Then the hiss of a light rain. The rain grew steadier, and the temperature dropped a few degrees. Deirdre pulled the blanket more tightly around her and let her mind drift back to a safer place, to the morning before school in sixth grade when Joelen Nichol had walked into her life.

CHAPTER 9

The sixth-grade girls at El Rodeo set their hair in pin curls and wore blouses with Peter Pan collars and circle pins. When Joelen Nichol appeared in their midst with her reddish-brown hair poufed out around her head like spun sugar, her eyes outlined in black, and mascara clumped on her stubby eyelashes, she seemed like a seismic anomaly. Her lipstick wasn't Cherries in the Snow or Coral Bells, but instead the color of a politically incorrect "flesh tone" crayon. In a world filled with Carols and Barbaras, Pattys and Nancys, even Joelen's name was exotic.

The first day Joelen came to school, Deirdre had been waiting outside for the bell to ring, her books pressed to her chest, feeling like a tree stump growing out of the concrete. As usual, the popular girls camped out at the picnic tables, their backs to outsiders, their books on the spaces between them, sending the clear message that there was no room for anyone else to squeeze in.

Deirdre didn't see Joelen walk in from the street. What she noticed was how, one by one, like a herd of prairie dogs picking up a scent, the boys shooting hoops on the other side of the fence had paused. She noticed how oblivious Joelen seemed to the stir she was creating, leaning nonchalantly against the chain-link fence that separated the picnic tables from the playground, adjusting her cinch belt, smoothing her blouse.

Maybe because they were both outsiders, doomed to perpetual orbit around Marianne Wasserman and her circle (or coven, as Joelen liked to call them), Deirdre and Joelen became fast friends. When the bell rang and the other girls gathered up their books, Deirdre fell in beside Joelen. They walked home from school together that afternoon. From that day on, they shared their lunches and talked on the phone before bed. On weekends they had sleepovers—until the Saturday night when both their lives flew off the rails.

Deirdre turned over. It had taken her two years after the car accident before she could do that simple thing: turn over onto her injured side without aching. She'd always be uncertain on her feet without her crutch.

She closed her eyes. In her mind's eye she could walk unaided. She saw herself moving up the stairs and into the school where her friendship with Joelen had begun. She drifted through her memory of the building, down hallways and up staircases, remembering the smell of the cafeteria on fried fish day and the art room's peppermint smell of paste.

Deirdre didn't realize she'd fallen asleep until a thump yanked her awake. What time was it? Her wristwatch glowed: ten past two. She heard a shuffling sound, then a grunt. That was a person. The dogs would be growling and snarling if it were an intruder. It had to be Henry.

She tried to go back to sleep but was jarred awake by a louder thump and the sound of something being dragged. Annoyed, she grabbed her crutch and got out of bed. Paused for a moment behind the closed door and listened. She turned the knob and opened it a crack.

Henry, looking like a ninja in a black T-shirt and black pants tucked into motorcycle boots, was carrying the plastic garbage bag, which now looked to be full, from the bedroom hallway into the living room.

He disappeared into the front hall. Deirdre waited to hear the front door open and close but it didn't. Baby padded over and sniffed at Deirdre. She gave the dog a peremptory pat.

Henry reappeared. He yawned. Stretched. Turned around and scratched his head. Then he sank down on the couch and leaned back. Moments later she heard what sounded like a cow's rhythmic lowing. He was snoring.

She crept over to him. "Henry?" she said, and touched his shoulder. He collapsed a little farther onto his side, out cold.

Deirdre pulled off his boots, tilted him over onto his back, and put his feet up. Then she covered him with a plaid flannel stadium blanket that Arthur kept over the back of the couch. Warren Beatty— that was who Joelen used to say Henry resembled, and Deirdre had always been sure that Henry knew it. She'd once caught him practicing in the bathroom mirror, a Beatty-esque puckish grin morphing into a sleepy-eyed, seductive gaze. Back then he was forever pulling at his hair to get that forelock to come down over his eyes. It seemed utterly goofy and contrived to her, but girls ate it up.

These days, with his hollow cheeks and hooded eyes, his looks had sloped off into cool, sardonic Robert Mitchum territory. She pushed his dark hair off his face and brushed his forehead with a kiss.

She'd started back to bed when she noticed that Henry had left the garbage bag sitting on the floor by the front door. She went over and poked at it with her crutch. It was folded over, not tied shut. She steadied herself against the wall and leaned over to open it. Out wafted a rich, earthy smell like patchouli. Weed, packed up but not disposed of. If the police arrived early in the morning to search the house, it would be the first thing they'd trip over.

Deirdre opened the front door. The rain had stopped and the air was much cooler. Up and down the street, outside lights were on but the windows in most of the houses were dark. In the distance a siren wailed.

Get rid of it. That was easier said than done. Where? The police would easily find it if she put it out in the alley with the trash. The trunk of her car seemed the safest bet, for the moment at least.

Deirdre took her time feeling her way over the uneven paving stones, pulling the bag across the dark courtyard and out to the street. She opened her car trunk and heaved the bag inside. Then she pressed the trunk lid down until the latch clicked. At least it was out of the house. Later she'd figure out how to dispose of its contents.

She returned to the house and crawled back into bed. This time she fell asleep almost instantly.

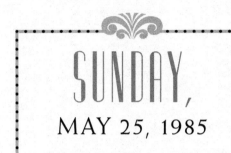

SUNDAY,

MAY 25, 1985

CHAPTER 10

The phone started ringing the next morning at eight thirty. Deirdre missed the first call and the second. The third got her out of bed. She caught the tail end of her mother leaving a message as she stumbled into the living room. ". . . I'll be there as soon as I can. By late tonight, I hope. Henry, Deirdre? I love you both."

Before Deirdre could pick up the phone, her mother hung up. Seconds later, the phone rang again. Deirdre grabbed it. "Hello?"

"Hello, Gloria?" Not her mother. A man's voice.

Deirdre took a breath. "No. This is her daughter, Deirdre."

"Ah, Deirdre. This is Lee Golden, a friend of your dad's." Deirdre knew the name. A set designer? "I just heard what happened and I wanted to reach out to you and Henry . . ." Deirdre sank into Arthur's lounge chair and held the phone away from her ear. When the phone went quiet, she thanked Lee Golden for calling and promised to let him know about funeral plans.

That was the first of a deluge of calls she took that morning.

There'd been an article about Arthur's death in the paper. Callers danced around what they really wanted to know: How on earth could Arthur have drowned during a daily regimen that he claimed kept him as fit as any thirty-year-old? Deirdre thanked each caller, took names and phone numbers, and tried to get off the phone as fast as possible. Finally she surrendered and let the answering machine pick up, half listening as message after message was recorded.

None of it woke Henry, who lay on the couch in exactly the same position Deirdre had left him the night before. Deirdre let the dogs out and filled their food and water bowls. There wasn't much in the way of people food in the house other than leftover Chinese. Desperate for coffee, Deirdre found a dust-covered percolator in one of the kitchen cabinets, along with an unopened can of Maxwell House, its sell-by date long past. Soon the pot started to rumble and pop, sending out wafts of reassuring coffee aroma.

The doorbell startled her. Her first thought: the police were back. She wasn't dressed. Hadn't even combed her hair. At least the bag with her brother's pot was no longer in the house. She waited for the doorbell to chime again but it didn't. By the time she opened the door and looked out, no one was there, but four cellophane-wrapped food baskets were lined up just outside.

One by one, Deirdre carried them into the kitchen. One was from Linney's Delicatessen. Bagels, cream cheese, lox, babka, some rugelach. The card read *Condolences from Billy and Audrey Wilder.* Arthur would have been over the moon.

She poked open the cellophane wrapping and sniffed. The smell took her back to Sunday mornings when she'd stood, holding her father's hand in front of the sloping glass deli counter at Nate'n Al's on Beverly Drive, watching the clerk hand-slice belly lox from a long filet and dollop cream cheese into a container. He'd wrap up four whole smoked, bronze-skinned butterfish, which Arthur would fry the minute he got home. She remembered the feel of warm bagels through the paper bag she carried to the car.

She hooked a bagel and took a bite. Closed her eyes. It had the perfect chewy crust, soft inside, and yeasty taste. In San Diego there was no such thing as a decent bagel, and you were lucky if you could find packaged, precut smoked salmon.

When Deirdre returned to the living room, Henry gave a phlegmy cough and turned over, his arm dropping like deadweight off the edge of the couch. He mumbled something, pushed himself up, and looked around. His expression said *Huh?*

"Morning, sunshine," Deirdre said. "Mom called."

Henry scowled. Then registered that she was eating. "What've you got there?"

"Billy Wilder's bagel." Deirdre took a bite. "Mmmmm. Delicious. Hungry?"

Henry uttered a profanity that Deirdre chose not to hear, then he rolled off the couch and stumbled toward the bathroom.

Coffee aroma reached Deirdre. She went into the kitchen for a cup and was on her way back when the phone rang again. She paused to listen to her father's greeting. *Beep.*

Another well-meaning friend of Arthur's, this time a woman, *Just calling to say how sorry I am to hear . . .*

Henry was back, standing in the doorway and scratching his crotch. "So what did Mom say?"

"She said she'll try to get here by tonight. Take a shower, then get yourself a bagel and coffee."

"Coffee? You made coffee?"

Twenty minutes later, Henry was in the kitchen pouring himself coffee and eating a bagel. The dogs started barking and swarming the front door, and seconds later the doorbell rang.

Deirdre went to answer it. Standing on the doorstep was Sy Sterling, still trim but with a toupee where for years he'd worn an elaborate comb-over. Sy dropped his briefcase and held open his arms. Deirdre choked up and let herself be folded into a soft hug, enveloped in the scents of aftershave and cigar.

When she pulled away, Sy drew a handkerchief from his trouser pocket, blew his nose, and wiped away his own tears. "Such a pair we are."

She nodded and dabbed at her eyes with a tissue. "Everyone keeps saying it, but it really doesn't seem real."

"It should not happen," Sy said, squinting at her, his eyebrows sprouting white hairs like sparklers. "Arthur swam every damned day." He shook his head and his gaze shifted over Deirdre's shoulder.

Henry had come up behind Deirdre. He held two cups of coffee. "We're still in shock," he said. He gave Sy one of the cups and took his briefcase. Deirdre closed the door behind them as Sy followed Henry inside.

"You?" Sy said, giving Deirdre a sympathetic look. "You found him."

Deirdre's throat tightened and she swallowed a hiccup.

"You should have called me right away. I could have been here for you. They took him—where?"

"To the city morgue," Henry said.

Sy shuddered. "Of course. Unattended death. There will be an autopsy. And then?"

"Westwood Memorial Park," Deirdre said.

"Good. Your father? He would want his urn next to Marilyn's. You called Gloria?"

"She's on her way," Deirdre said.

"Good, good." Sy harrumphed. "Well, of course none of this is good. But it is what it is. Come, children." He headed for the dining table. "We need to talk." He settled into the chair at the head of the table, pulled a cigar from his pocket, and chewed on it. Then he sat back, shifted the cigar to the other corner of his mouth, and chewed on it some more. In all the years Deirdre had known Sy, she'd never seen him actually light a cigar.

"I promised your father, if anything happened to him, I would be here for you. A promise I hoped I would never have to keep." He reached across the table to clasp Henry's and Deirdre's hands. The diamond in his chunky pinkie ring caught the light. "I am here for you now. You know that? Right?" He gave Deirdre's hand a squeeze and held her gaze for a few moments, then shifted his attention to Henry. For a moment his expression seemed more questioning than reassuring. Then he sat back. "So." He undid the two straps and unlatched his battered briefcase.

Sy set his cigar on the table and took out a sheaf of papers. He handed Deirdre and Henry each a packet like he was dealing cards. Deirdre looked down at hers. On the first page, it said LAST WILL AND TESTAMENT.

"Your father? He was a dreamer, but I am afraid reality had him by the short hairs," Sy said.

"Not sure I like the sound of that," Henry said. "How bad is it?"

"There is still the house. You two will own it once the will is through probate. There is a mortgage, of course, but you will be able to get quite a bit more for the house, even"—he gestured to the water-stained ceiling—"the way it is. Your father may have already lined up a broker."

"I think he did," Deirdre said.

"Did he?" Henry said, and shot Deirdre a look. She hoped he'd let Joelen sell the house for them.

"So that is good news," Sy said. "Bad news is that between Arthur's debts and his assets, there is"—he paused, searching for the word—"overlap. When the estate pays what is owed you will be left with maybe twenty-five thousand. Of course I do not charge you for my legal services, but other expenses will have to come out of that. Burial and the funeral, of course."

"But they made a fortune—" Henry said.

"Made and spent it. And I should not have to remind you that until quite recently your father had certain obligations. Financial obligations. So some of his savings?" Sy said, looking steadily at Henry, "*Pffft.*"

Henry stared back at Sy. For a moment it was a standoff.

"So," Deirdre said, "is anyone going to tell me what you're talking about?"

The dogs, who'd been lying on the rug in the living room, picked up their massive heads and started to bark, then scrambled over to the door before the bell chimed.

"Probably another fruit basket," Henry said.

The doorbell rang again, followed by a rap and a sharp voice. "Police. Please open the door. We have a warrant to search the premises."

Henry blinked. "Oh shit." He jumped to his feet, knocking over his chair, then lunged for the front hall. The dogs were in a frenzy, barking and leaping.

"Just a minute," Sy called out. "Henry, dammit, control your dogs."

Henry turned in circles, probably realizing belatedly that the garbage bag was no longer by the door where he'd left it. He shoved Baby out of the way and pulled open the door to the front closet, looking for what Deirdre knew wasn't there.

"Henry," Deirdre said sharply, gesturing her brother over. Under her breath, she said, "I got rid of it."

"Henry!" Sy said. He had one hand anchored on Bear's collar while the dog jumped up and down, oblivious. Baby was barking, standing with her paws up on the door where the finish had long ago been scratched away.

"Bear, down. Baby, down," Henry shouted. Both dogs went still. "Sit." The dogs scooted back on their haunches. Baby put her head between her paws and whined. Sy relinquished his hold on Bear and Henry grabbed the dogs' collars, one in each hand.

Multiple raps sounded on the door. Sy put a finger to his lips. He mouthed the words, *Let me do the talking*, then pulled open the door.

Four officers were on the other side. Deirdre recognized the one in the lead: Detective Sergeant Martinez.

"Officers. Can I help you?" Sy said, all traces of an accent gone.

Martinez looked past Sy to Deirdre and Henry. He glanced uneasily at the dogs. "We have a warrant to search the premises." He held up a piece of paper. "We'll need access to the garage and the cars. And, please, we'd appreciate it if you stay out of the way until we're done."

"May I see that warrant, please?" Sy asked.

"And you are?"

"Seymour Sterling." Sy took a breath and puffed out his chest, a banty prizefighter still. "I'm the family's attorney."

Henry and Deirdre nodded like a pair of bobbleheads.

Martinez handed over the paper. Sy took his time, sliding a pair of reading glasses from the inside pocket of his jacket. "Search residence," he said under his breath. "Property. Vehicles. . . ."

Deirdre's heart lurched. Would they search her car?

Sy ran his finger from line to line. "Ah, probable cause. . . ." He cleared his throat and read. "'The Beverly Hills Police Department has been conducting an investigation into the death of Arthur Unger—'" His voice dropped again and turned to a mumble. As his eyes scanned the page, the scowl on his face intensified. He stepped aside and the officers swept into the house, Martinez taking up the rear.

CHAPTER 11

Can they search my car?" Deirdre whispered to Sy once they were outside, getting settled at the patio table.

Sy gave her a narrow look. "Where is it?"

"Parked on the street."

"Then no."

At least that was a relief. But as Sy started going over the details of Arthur's will, Deirdre found herself barely able to follow. She strained to see over the bushes at the edge of the patio. The ground vibrated as the police investigators dropped item after item onto a plastic tarp spread out in the driveway. Crowbar. Tire iron. Shovel. Hedge clippers. Long-handled branch lopper. A candlestick lamp. All of them heavy blunt objects. Obviously they didn't think Arthur Unger's death had been an accident. He hadn't been taken ill. They were looking for a murder weapon.

Deirdre tried to make sense of it. Maybe Arthur had surprised an intruder. He hadn't turned on any lights, so the intruder didn't realize he was out there. Arthur could be impulsive, belligerent, especially after a few drinks. Maybe he'd confronted the person. Thrown a punch, even. The intruder would have fended him off. Picked up something readily at hand. Something heavy. Swung it at Arthur and knocked him into the pool.

"Deirdre?" Sy was saying. "Do you understand what that means?"

"I'm sorry. I zoned out."

"I said, your father named you his literary executor. You'll need to go through his personal effects. His papers, letters, memos, photographs, keepsakes. Who knows what you will find. Early drafts of movie scripts. Unpublished manuscripts. He entrusted you with deciding what to preserve."

Deirdre thought of Arthur's memoir, sitting in the drawer in her bedside table. She was having fun reading it, but did it have historical or literary merit? "I'm hardly qualified—"

"Your father thought otherwise. Just take it item by item, one step at a time. First sort and cull. Then inventory what is worthy of preserving. If you are not sure, I can help. Try to imagine someone coming along a hundred years from now, trying to understand your father's Hollywood. What you are doing: conserving his piece of it. His legacy."

"Legacy." Henry snorted a laugh.

"Okay," Sy said, "your parents were not Comden and Green. But they were not hacks, either. Their films, and even some of the projects your father worked on later alone? Among the best of a certain breed. His collected works are emblematic of an era."

"Still, Mom would make a much better judge—" Deirdre started.

"You do not get to decide. Your father selected you."

It would be no small task, going through Arthur's papers. Deirdre hadn't been in his office on the second floor of the garage in ages, but she remembered it was lined with bookshelves and file cabinets. Then there was everything in the den. More probably in his bedroom. Maybe there were storage boxes. Her mother would know where all to look. It would be a huge chore, but secretly Deirdre was pleased. Flattered that her father had entrusted her with the task. "Of course I'll want your advice—" she started.

Henry interrupted. "So there are no other assets? No life insurance?"

"No life insurance."

"What about their movies?" Henry again. "Aren't there residuals?"

"There were none back then. Who knew television would be hungry for old movies?"

Henry hunched over the table, absorbing this news.

Before the police left, a technician took Henry's and Deirdre's fingerprints. Martinez explained it was to eliminate theirs from others that they lifted. Soon after that, Deirdre and Henry walked Sy out to his car.

Henry glanced up and down the street. "So Sy, is that it? Will they be back?"

"Always, they can come back. But they will need a new warrant." Sy stopped and turned to face them. "Listen to me, both of you. If the police do come back, you call me right away." He took out a business card and wrote a phone number on the back. "In case I am not in my office or in my car, here is my home phone. Anytime."

He handed the card to Henry and winked at Deirdre. Then he got into his car and rolled down the window. "I know you, Deirdre. You are a Girl Scout. You will want to help them with their investigation. But the police are not your friends. They want to fix blame and close the case. I know you think you have nothing to hide, but believe me, we all do."

As Deirdre watched him drive off she felt a chill as a light breeze rustled the leaves overhead. "So, tyell me zis," Henry said, lowering his voice and imitating Sy's accent. He put his arm around her and squeezed harder than he needed to. "Where's that bag?"

"In my car." Deirdre crossed the street and opened the trunk.

"You might have told me you'd taken it out of the house," Henry said. "Freaked the hell out of me."

"You're welcome."

"That, too." He reached for the bag.

"Back off." Deirdre pressed down with the end of her crutch on Henry's foot. Henry yelped in pain.

Deirdre opened the bag and foraged around in it, pulling out a half-dozen twist-tied baggies of loose pills. Another contained a handful of the pot she'd already smelled, along with a packet of rolling papers. She gave all that to Henry, then rummaged some more, past papers, old clothes, and what she thought at first were telephone directories but turned out to be Motion Picture Academy Players Directories, making sure she hadn't missed anything else that was illegal.

Henry was on a slow burn. "What are you going to do with the rest of it?"

"You heard Sy. I'm Dad's literary executor. I'm going take it up to his office and start executing. Maybe I'll throw all of it away. Maybe I'll keep it all. I get to decide. You just take care of that shit"—she indicated what she'd given him—"so none of it comes back to bite us."

Henry turned and stomped back into the house.

CHAPTER 12

Deirdre lugged the bag up the driveway to the garage. The door to her father's office turned out to be unlocked, so up she went, pulling the bag step by step behind her.

As kids, she and Henry had been forbidden to so much as knock when their parents were up there working, so it felt strange to put her hand on the knob and just open the door. The little apartment exhaled stale, musty air. The walls were papered with fraying grass cloth and the ceiling was waterstained. An electric typewriter with a plastic cover sat on a metal table on one side of the room. Against a wall was a sagging pullout couch. On the table next to it Deirdre spotted a dust-free circle. That's where the candlestick lamp the police confiscated must have stood. She raised one of the bamboo shades, releasing a cloud of dust motes, then cranked open one of the louvered windows.

The floor was stacked with piles of papers and videocassettes, and below a large mirror on the opposite wall stood two-drawer metal file cabinets. Deirdre pulled open a file drawer and poked through. Contracts. Correspondence. Bills and receipts.

Sort. Cull. Inventory. As Sy had said, she'd have to take it item by item, one thing at a time. It hardly mattered where she began.

She pulled out a file at random. Telephone bills starting in 1963. That had been around the year that her parents lost their contract at Fox and started using this space as their office. *Toss.*

The unlabeled folder behind it had about a dozen black-and-white stills from a movie she didn't recognize. She set it aside. *Keep.*

Another file folder contained stock certificates. One was from the DeLorean Motor Company. Hadn't they gone bankrupt? *Ask Sy.*

On top of the file cabinet Deirdre noticed a glass ashtray from Chasen's, the celebrity hangout where her parents had dined regularly. She needed another pile for personal keepsakes. Not for any literary legacy, but because she'd always loved the restaurant with its red leather banquettes, dark corners for secret trysts, and special tables set aside for moguls and stars. Even if there'd been nothing on the menu that an eight-year-old could stomach.

Four items and already she'd started four piles. She hadn't even cracked open the closet. Make that closets—there were two of them. She'd be at this for weeks, culling the trivial from the memorable from the valuable and setting aside items that signified her father's literary life.

Deirdre went out onto the landing and retrieved the black plastic bag. She sank down on the floor beside it and started sifting through the items that Henry said their father would have wanted him to throw away. Newspaper and magazine clippings, a restaurant review for a Chinese restaurant on Beverly Drive dated 1978, empty Cuban cigar boxes. All of it: *toss.*

Next she pulled out six Motion Picture Academy Players Directories, the annual compendium that listed every Hollywood actor. She'd spent hours and hours poring over directories like these when she was stuck home recuperating after the accident. In it were pages and pages of head shots of actors, most of whom could have strolled down Rodeo Drive and not turned a single head. And yet they were all members of the Screen Actors Guild. It just brought home the formidable odds against becoming a celebrity.

These were a straight run from 1963 to 1968. Deirdre opened the 1963 directory, flipped through until she found someone she recognized—sexy, sultry Edie Adams who sang the Muriel Cigar TV commercial. That ad had ended with a sly wink and the suggestive, *Why don't you pick one up and smoke it sometime,* delivered with a sensual subtlety that Madonna never could have managed. A few pages on, there was Donna Douglas, all wide-eyed with her Elly May blond curls tamed. Annette Funicello, Deirdre's favorite Mouseketeer, looking grown-up and bland.

Tucked between two pages, Deirdre came across a snapshot. She recognized the white rippled edges as an early Polaroid. She was five years old the Christmas her father got their first instant camera. He'd snapped a picture of Deirdre with her new Tiny Tears doll, Henry, and their mother, still in their bathrobes and seated on the white "snow" carpet around their tinselly tree. Deirdre had watched breathless for what seemed like forever until the second hand on her father's watch went all the way around and he opened the camera's trapdoor. Like magic, he peeled away the film and an image bloomed.

But the person in this faded snapshot wasn't Deirdre or Henry or their mother, and there was no Christmas tree. Instead it showed an attractive young woman, her collared blouse unbuttoned halfway, kneeling on the floor beside an end table and gazing at the camera with wide, kohl-rimmed eyes worthy of Keane. A mirror in the background reflected a window with a bamboo shade, and in front of it the photographer with the camera held to his face.

Deirdre realized with a jolt that the woman was kneeling in precisely the spot where she was sitting now. She turned the picture over. On the back, in red pen, were five asterisks.

The same girl's picture, much clearer and crisper, was in the

Players Directory on the page where the snapshot had been tucked in. Second row from the top. *Melanie Hart*, the kind of white-bread, feel-good name—like Judy Garland or Hope Lange—that studios selected for young hopefuls.

Poor Melanie Hart. If she'd harbored any illusions that this photo session would lead to her big break, she'd been disappointed. Flipping the pages of the Players Directory, Deirdre found more faded Polaroid photographs, each with asterisks on the back. Her father favored buxom blondes and redheads, each of them photographed the same way, in the same spot.

Deirdre felt sick to her stomach. Her father had been taking advantage of young women who were desperate to break out in the film business. She stacked the photographs on the floor. They conjured the smell of My Sin and soiled sheets. At least her father had realized these needed to be destroyed. *Burn*. A pile she hadn't yet started.

Deirdre heard footsteps on the stairs and a moment later Henry loomed in the doorway. He had on a black leather bomber's jacket and badass cowboy boots. A motorcycle helmet—ice blue with an eagle sprouting red and yellow flames painted on it—hung from his hand. He tossed her a set of keys. "Here, so you can get in the house."

"Did you know about these?" she asked, pointing to the pile of pictures.

"Good God. I haven't been up here in ages." Henry took in the deflated garbage bag, then the Players Directories and the snapshots Deirdre had stacked on the floor. "Got to hand it to Dad. He was a pretty slick operator."

"You knew?"

Henry smirked. He picked up one of the pictures. "She doesn't look too unhappy, does she?"

"You can be such an asshole." She grabbed the picture back.

"And you can be so predictable. Dad was a jerk, but he wasn't Satan. That's how things were done in those days."

Those days. The 1960s had been a decade of upheaval in Hollywood. Her parents, along with most of Hollywood's "contract" talent, lost their jobs. From then on they worked project by project, from home, and didn't get assigned work unless some panel of studio honchos, usually decades younger than they, gave them a thumbs-up.

There had been upheaval at home, too. The car accident that crippled Deirdre had been in the fall of 1963. A year and a half later, she was finishing high school, Henry was flunking out of college, and their mother was making frequent trips to a commune in the desert.

"They knew," Henry said. "Every one of those girls knew the score."

Girls? *Women!* Deirdre wanted to shout back at him. "And I guess he was so proud of himself that he made you promise to destroy the evidence."

"You think this should be part of his legacy?" Henry poked a steel toe at the pictures. "If you'd just let me—" He leaned down and picked up one of the photographs.

"Put it down."

Henry glared at her.

"I'm telling you now, Henry, if anything disappears without my say-so, even something like that, then I'm . . . I'm . . ."

"What'll you do? Tell Mom?"

"Don't push me. Okay?"

Henry scowled and dropped the picture. "Fine. Lucky you. What on earth are you going to do with all this shit?" He didn't wait for an answer, just turned on his heel and walked out.

Good question. What *was* she going to do with all of it?

As Henry stomped down the stairs, Deirdre picked up one of the Players Directories by the spine. Shook it. More photographs rained out. The thought of what must have gone on in this room, on that couch or on the floor, made her sick to her stomach. Her father had been luring hopeful young women with promises he'd never had the clout to fulfill.

She heard the rumble of a motorcycle starting, and the floor shook as the garage door opener beneath kicked in. A minute later, the floor shuddered again as the garage door shut.

But what shook Deirdre was that one of the photographs that had dropped out wasn't another pretty stranger. It was Joelen Nichol.

Deirdre picked up the picture. Joelen had been so young. Had Deirdre been in the house while her father was out here, indulging in this sordid hobby?

Disgusted, Deirdre shoved the picture into her pocket, grabbed her crutch, and started to struggle to her feet. She was half up when the crutch tip snagged on the plastic bag, slipped, and she went down with a howl of outrage. Dammit. Damn *him*. On top of everything else, if it hadn't been for Arthur, she wouldn't have to deal with the goddamned crutch at all. In a fury she shoved away the crutch and surrendered to what she knew was a sorry bout of self-pity. The chaos, the sheer volume of it, and the sadness of the tawdry, pathetic minutiae she'd have to paw through—it was too much.

The crying jag left her with a pounding headache and an aching chest. Defeated and deflated, she dried her eyes on the hem of her T-shirt, then tried to pull herself together as she surveyed the room. The piles she'd started. The file cabinets she'd barely cracked open. None of this had to be taken care of today, or even this week.

She scooted over so she could reach her crutch and set it carefully on the carpet, realizing as she stood that the crutch had torn a hole in the plastic bag. She bent to gather up the items that threatened to spill out of it. Among them was what looked like an armful of crumpled yellow netting, brittle with age. It was wrapped around a flat wooden box. On the box's lid was a little metal shield with the word SHEFFIELD burned into it. She opened the box. Inside, set into a red flocked cardboard inset, was a knife with an old-fashioned antler grip. The blade was long and tapered. A silver cap covering the butt was engraved with the fancy initial *N*.

N for Nichol? Deirdre felt a chill creep down her back. She snapped the box shut and began to wrap it up again, her mind lurching ahead. *Toss? Keep?* That's when she realized that the decaying netting with which she was wrapping the box was the tulle skirt of a dress with a high-necked lace bodice and long sleeves. She drew back, her hand over her mouth. The yellow satin underskirt was covered with dark stains. Blood?

There should have been more blood. That was what one of the expert witnesses had testified at the inquest into Tito Acevedo's murder. On the carpet under Tito's body. On the nightgown Joelen had been wearing when she stabbed him. On the nightgown Bunny had been wearing when she said she'd cradled him as he breathed his last. Well, here was more blood: on the dress Deirdre had been convinced made her look like a movie star when she'd borrowed it from Bunny Nichol to wear it to the party the night Tito was killed.

CHAPTER 13

Deirdre dropped the dress. She'd been fast asleep, passed out in Joelen's bedroom when Bunny's final fight with Tito had turned lethal. Hadn't she?

It had been long past Deirdre's bedtime when Bunny sent her and Joelen upstairs to bed. Instead the girls had sat at the top of the stairs and watched the party wind down. Deirdre's parents had been among the first to leave, and Deirdre had run down to kiss them good night.

After the rest of the guests had gone home, after Bunny and Tito had retired, Deirdre and Joelen had padded downstairs. They smoked lipstick-stained cigarette butts left in the ashtrays and polished off the remains of pink champagne in abandoned flutes and vodka in martini glasses. They'd staggered about giggling, stuck fat black and green olives on the tips of their fingers, and gorged on leftover crab dip, pâté, and shrimp cocktail. They'd gotten slaphappy and performed a boozy duet, an a cappella "Let Me Entertain You." They twirled.

And twirled. So much that Deirdre staggered outside and puked in the bushes. After that, she lay on the grass beside Joelen and stared up at the sky. *So this is what it feels like to be drunk,* she'd thought as stars seemed to streak across the sky like meteors and the ground felt as if it were flipping her like a pancake. She rolled over and threw up again and again until there was nothing left.

She must have passed out on the lawn, because her memory of what happened after that was fragmentary at best. She did not remember going back into the house. She did not remember climbing the stairs, as she must have, to get to Joelen's bedroom. She hadn't heard Bunny and Tito fighting. She hadn't heard Joelen leave the bedroom.

All she remembered was leaving the house herself. Being guided through a dark tunnel that smelled of camphor and floor wax, down a narrow, steep staircase—not the grand staircase in the Nichols' house, which was like something you'd expect Ginger Rogers to dance down. Wondering why her father had come back to get her in the middle of the night. Shivering in her pajamas, she'd stumbled out to his car through chilly night air.

That had been the last normal walk she ever took.

She had no idea when she'd taken off the beautiful lemon-colored dress. And was this the knife that had killed Tito? How on earth had her father ended up with them both? And what was she supposed to do with them now?

Deirdre stuffed the dress and the knife back into the torn plastic bag, shoved the bag in a closet, and slammed the door shut. Then she stumped down the garage stairs and across the garden. Back in the kitchen, she washed the dust and sour smell from her hands. If only she could erase the stench that the photographs and the stained dress had left in her head. She felt like Pandora, trying to figure out what to do with what she'd found in the box.

The answering machine was flashing "Full." Deirdre half listened to the messages, intending to write down the names of people to call back when funeral plans were final. But instead she just sat there, staring at the machine and letting the voices wash over her.

Until the message that was not from a well-wisher. "This is Detective Martinez. I need to speak to Deirdre Unger." Deirdre sat forward, feeling a wave of dread. She was thoroughly rattled by what she'd found in her father's office and in no frame of mind to answer questions.

Before Deirdre could decide what to do, Detective Martinez's voice was drowned out by the dogs stampeding out of Henry's bedroom and skidding into the front hall moments before the doorbell chimed.

Detective Martinez's voice on the answering machine was giving Deirdre his telephone number as she peered out the window. A police cruiser was parked out front. She stood there, unable to answer the door, listening to her own breathing and the next message of condolence on the answering machine. Deirdre's armpits were damp, and butterflies fluttered in her stomach.

If the police do come back, you call me right away. Sy's voice came back to her. But he'd handed his card to Henry, and Henry had gone out.

At the knock at the front door, Deirdre sank down onto the floor under the window, her heart in her throat. Moments later she heard a sharp rap at the kitchen door. The dogs were going wild, racing from the front door to the kitchen. Any minute the police would come around to the back, look through the sliding glass doors, and see her cowering. Were the doors even locked? Would the police try to open them? Would they break in?

Deirdre pulled a phone book from the drawer under the phone. She found the page that began STANDISH and drew her finger down the column looking for STERLING. Was Sy even listed?

And then, just like that, the dogs stopped making their racket. The knocking stopped. Deirdre peeked out the window. Martinez and a uniformed officer were getting back into the police car. Car doors slammed.

Could it be that easy? Were they just going to give up and drive off? Deirdre drew back and waited to hear the engine start. She was still waiting minutes later when the phone rang. She didn't reach for it. It had to be Detective Martinez or the other policeman, watching the house and making the call from their car phone.

But when the answering machine picked up Deirdre heard a familiar voice after the beep. "Deirdre? Are you there? I don't know if you got my earlier message. I hope the fruit basket we sent over got there—"

Deirdre picked up the phone. "Joelen?" she whispered, even though she knew the police couldn't hear her.

"Hello?" Joelen said.

Deirdre put the receiver closer to her mouth. "Hi. I'm here. Can you hear me?"

"Yes, I . . . Is everything okay? I mean, of course it's not. But you know what I mean. Is it?"

"The police are back. They want to talk to me. I'm here all alone—"

"Do they know you're there?"

"No. Maybe. My car's parked out front."

"And they're—?"

"Sitting outside in their car. Waiting. Maybe I should just go out there and get it over with. I have nothing to hide."

Joelen laughed a not-funny laugh. "Honey, everyone has something to hide."

Deirdre thought about the yellow dress and couldn't argue the point. She heard a car pulling up in front and peered out. A bright blue van had parked behind the police cruiser. KABC-TV NEWS 7 was emblazoned on the side. A slender blonde in a dark pantsuit hopped out and went over to the window of the police car. She was chatting with Martinez's partner when a white-and-blue KNBC van pulled up and stopped across the street.

"Shit," Deirdre said. "Two news vans just pulled up."

"Okay. That's it. You need to get out of there. Now. Go out the back."

"But my car—"

"Don't take your car. I'll pick you up. Go out in the alley and start walking north. I'll be there in five."

"But what if someone—"

But Joelen had hung up. Deirdre stared at the dead handset. She remembered a moment years ago when Joelen had climbed onto the roof of her pool house and dared Deirdre to come up and join her. Henry had been there, too, and while Deirdre was screwing up her courage, Henry shoved her into the pool.

"That's what happens when you hesitate," Joelen had told her when she'd climbed out. Even now Deirdre's face grew hot, remembering how Joelen and Henry cracked up because Deirdre's white pants had turned semitransparent.

She hung up the phone, lurched to her feet, and peered outside again. A man who must have been in the first news van was filming the pantsuited woman talking into a microphone in front of the house. The passenger door of the second van opened, and a man in a suit followed by another man wearing a T-shirt and jeans and carrying a camera got out and headed up the path to the front door.

The dogs started up again. The doorbell rang. Deirdre felt as if she were under siege. Joelen was right. She had to get out of there. Now. She grabbed her jacket and messenger bag and exited through the sliding glass doors. Crossed the yard. Took a quick glance down the driveway to where the hood of the police car was just visible.

She slipped down the narrow passageway between the chain-link pool surround and the garage. Her nose tickled with a smell, ever so faint. Was something burning? It reminded her of the once pervasive metallic smoke that backyard incinerators belched decades ago before they were banned.

It wasn't until she was in the alley, enveloped in the smells of eucalyptus and garbage ripening in the metal cans lined up behind each house, that she realized she was wearing the Harley T-shirt and drawstring pants she'd slept in. She stayed close to the edge, careful that the tip of her crutch didn't skid on the layer of grit and broken glass coating the broken asphalt, checking over her shoulder to see whether the police or the TV newspeople had picked up her scent.

She was halfway up the block when a dark sedan started coming toward her, kicking up a cloud of dust. A hand waved out the window and then the car pulled up alongside Deirdre and the passenger door opened. Deirdre threw in her crutch and hopped in after it. She slammed the door and sat back, resting one hand on the dash and the other over her chest. Her heart was pounding and she was sure she was about to throw up.

"Just breathe," Joelen said, accelerating, the tires spinning on loose gravel. "Sit back and relax." The car emerged from the alley. No cruisers or media vans were there to meet them. Joelen pulled out onto the street, stopped at a corner, and turned north. "You okay?"

Deirdre took a deep breath, held it for a moment, then blew out.

"You know," Joelen went on, "you'll have to talk to them eventually. The police. They don't just give up and leave you alone. But you can do it on your own terms."

CHAPTER 14

Deirdre stared out Joelen's car window, feeling her heart slow and the sweat that coated her forehead and neck cool. Familiar and unfamiliar houses flew past. Joelen drove with her hand resting lightly on the steering wheel. She still bit her fingernails down to the quick. Though it was more than twenty years later, she didn't look all that different from the picture that her father had taken of her in his office.

"What?" Joelen asked, giving her a sideways glance. "Have I got a booger hanging out of my nose?" And, Deirdre noted, she still said exactly what she thought.

"Sorry," Deirdre said. "Didn't mean to be ogling you. It's been a crazy day. The police came this morning to search the house and the garage. Now they're back to talk to me. In the meanwhile, I found out that I'm my dad's literary executor, which means I have to deal with all of his shit. Like, one of the things he's got? Remember your mom's yellow dress?" She hadn't meant to say any of that, but there it was.

"My *mother's* yellow dress?"

"The one she let me wear to her party . . . you know, that night."

"That . . . ?" At first Joelen looked puzzled. Then, "Whoa, whoa, whoa." She pulled the car over to the curb and stopped. She turned in her seat and faced Deirdre. "What are you talking about?"

"The dress your mother let me wear to her party that night. It was in a pile of stuff that Dad wanted Henry to throw away."

"So how did your father end up with it?"

"All I know is that he did."

Joelen stared out through the windshield, her brow wrinkled, shaking her head. "I have no idea how your father got that dress," she said at last, turning back to Deirdre. "Cross my heart and hope to die."

Deirdre took a shuddering breath. "Was I there when Tito got stabbed?"

"You were in the house."

"But was I in the room?"

"Why would you think that?"

"Because the dress. It's got dark stains on it."

"And you think—?"

"I don't know what to think. I'm just asking."

Joelen held Deirdre's gaze for a long moment. "No, honey. You were not. You were fast asleep in your jammies."

"You're sure?"

"Sure as hell." Joelen looked over her shoulder and pulled away from the curb. "I was there. You were not."

Deirdre leaned back and felt the tension drain from her neck and shoulders.

After a long silence, Joelen said, "I'm sorry we didn't keep in touch."

"Me too. I tried to call. I wrote."

"I was trying to become invisible. Besides, they sent me away." Joelen stopped at Sunset, signaled right, and waited as cars streamed past.

"Where?"

"After the verdict, they sent me to juvie." She pulled into traffic. "Which wasn't really as bad as you might imagine. I met some fascinating people." She laughed. "Then the judge sent me to live with my aunt Evelyn in Des Moines, for God's sake. Not so fascinating. Fields and fields of wheat. I finished high school there. For a year I was Jennifer, so no one knew who I really was or why I was there, and I was damn well going to keep it that way. I didn't make a single friend."

"You must have gone bonkers."

"I did. A little." Joelen gave a bitter laugh. "Poor Aunt Evelyn, God bless her. She had one black-and-white television set and she had it on all the time. She was addicted to the *Price Is Right, Queen for a Day, Search for Tomorrow, Guiding Light*." Joelen rolled her eyes. "And, oh yeah, wrestling. The only books in the house were steamy romance novels. And the Bible, of course. We went to the mall every Saturday, church every Sunday." She signaled right. "Supposedly that was more therapeutic than living with my mom. I had to stay until I was eighteen."

She turned into the familiar driveway and stopped at a metal gate that hadn't been there years earlier. NO TRESPASSING and PROTECTED BY FIVE STAR SECURITY signs hung on it. Joelen rolled down the window, reached out, and pressed a button on an intercom box.

It took a while for anyone to answer. At last a man's tinny voice croaked out, "Yeah?" "Hey, it's me," Joelen said.

Slowly the gate swung open and Joelen drove through and up the winding driveway. Deirdre turned and looked over her shoulder. The gate began to swing shut.

The rest of the driveway up to the house looked familiar: a tennis court, then farther along a carport sheltered under a bank of bougainvillea. Alongside the carport a white fence surrounded a kidney-shaped pool and pool house. The driveway curved back on itself and climbed. From above Deirdre could see that the pool was half-full, and the water in it had turned a sickly green.

Joelen stopped alongside a motorcycle in a broad parking area in front of the house, just feet from the front door. Deirdre picked up her crutch and started to open the door.

"Deeds?" Joelen said. The familiar nickname that only Henry still called her brought Deirdre up short. "I heard about what happened to your leg," Joelen said, her eye on the crutch. "Tough break. I didn't find out until I got back from Iowa. I tried to call you, but you were already away at college."

Deirdre had spent the summer after she graduated from high school at UC San Diego and fallen in love with art history. She'd been desperate to get away from Beverly Hills, to meet people who didn't know her as either Joelen Nichol's onetime best friend or the crippled girl everyone pitied.

Joelen's look turned serious. "So why do the police want to talk to you?"

"All I know is Sy said if they came back, not to talk to them alone."

"Sy." Joelen blinked. "You mean, it wasn't an accident."

Deirdre looked down into her lap.

"How awful. I'm sorry," Joelen said. "But they can't think it was you."

"I don't know what they think. And I didn't want to find out when I was alone."

Joelen pushed open the car door and got out. Deirdre followed her to the columned portico. "Listen to Sy," Joelen said, "and do exactly what he tells you. I don't even want to think what might have happened to me if I hadn't."

"Is he still your mom's lawyer?"

"And friend. He's really been there for us. It's great that you've got him in your corner. And your family, too, of course. Where's your mom?"

"Living in the desert on a monastic retreat. She'll show up. Eventually."

"Here's a scary thought," Joelen said, holding the front door of the house open for Deirdre. "Marooned on a desert island with your mother and my mother. *Gilligan's Island* meets . . ."

"*Dallas,*" Deirdre said. It was a game she and Joelen used to play, and any other time Deirdre would have added on with *wearing* . . . or *eating* . . . or *singing* . . . But at that moment, Deirdre couldn't have come up with anything else clever if her life depended on it. All she wanted to do was talk to Sy.

CHAPTER 15

Deirdre stood for a moment in the massive two-story entryway. She hadn't been in this house in more than twenty years. The once uneven stucco walls of the entryway were paneled over with a light wood, like a patterned birch. The floor, once rich terra-cotta tile, was now inset with slabs of peach-colored marble. The generous staircase was carpeted in thick white pile, the wrought-iron handrail that had once wound up to the second floor replaced by opulent carved and gilded balusters. Hanging from the ceiling was a massive Lucite and crystal chandelier that would have been right at home in a Las Vegas hotel.

A young man, dark and handsome, looked down at Deirdre from the landing halfway up the stairs. Deirdre felt a jolt of recognition. Before she could process it, Joelen pulled her across the entryway and down two steps into a white-carpeted living room, its windows swathed in gauzy white. "Bunny!" Joelen called out as she headed for the door at the far end of the living room.

Deirdre remembered how weird it had seemed the first time she'd heard Joelen call her mother *Bunny* instead of *Mom*. Then it turned out to be a '60s thing. As usual, the Nichols were ahead of the curve and the Ungers were behind it.

Deirdre looked around the living room. It, too, had changed over time. Couches and ottomans that had once been covered in a floral brocade were now cream-colored linen. The white grand piano was still there, but many of the other furnishings Deirdre recalled— carved and inlaid Versailles-inspired credenzas, tables, and chairs; massive bucolic landscape paintings—were gone. She wondered if the odd combination of opulence and minimalist elegance was some interior designer's vision, or whether the furnishings had been sold off to pay bills.

One of the pieces that did remain was a towering portrait of Bunny, still hanging in an elaborate frame over the marble fireplace. She was sitting in one of the missing chairs and wearing a pale blue, diaphanous Greek goddess dress. Her black hair was brushed to the side, curls cascading over one shoulder. Standing at her knee was a very young Joelen looking like a stiff little soldier in a starched white eyelet pinafore.

Still there too, looking marooned in the half-empty room, was a white lacquered credenza that had held a stereo system. After school, Deirdre and Joelen used to hang out here and hope Tito would show up and demonstrate the fine points of tango. He'd been agile, electrically handsome, and he'd smelled of sweat and cigars and a musky cologne. Before he'd take Deirdre or Joelen in his muscular arms, he'd turn the stereo up so loud that Deirdre could literally feel the floor vibrate as the violin bow struck the strings. Then he'd stand tall, even though he wasn't all that tall, and stick his chest out, his silk shirt unbuttoned to reveal a large medal hanging from a thick gold chain against a field of dark chest hair. His stance reminded Deirdre of a toreador addressing a bull. He'd offer her his hand, and she'd let hers float down to meet it. When it did, he'd twirl her once, twice, and then whip her close in time to the musical flourish, his palm anchored firmly against her lower back and his thigh pressed hard between her legs. "Eess not about the es-teps," he'd whisper, his voice deep and intoxicatingly accented, his breath hot in her ear. "Eess about the co-NECK-shun."

Later, the memory of him pressed against her had been enough to make her go all tingly. Deirdre wondered if there were still tango records stored inside the credenza on the shelf below the sound system.

"Bunny," Joelen called out again.

The door at the far end of the living room opened, and Elenor "Bunny" Nichol entered, regal in a gold caftan, her black hair piled high on her head. At first she appeared tall, but as Deirdre got closer she seemed to shrink. Face-to-face, she was actually shorter than Deirdre.

"My dear!" Bunny held Deirdre at arm's length and took in her leg, her crutch. Like Joelen, she hadn't seen Deirdre since before she was crippled, but her gaze didn't linger. She reached for Deirdre's hand. "I heard the terrible news. I am so sorry about Arthur." Her voice was low and resonant and there was real emotion in her eyes.

"Thank you. I—" Deirdre choked and the words caught in her throat. She swallowed. "Thanks, Mrs. Nichol."

"Bunny, please. You know, your mother and I were pals. We were both chorus girls at Warner Brothers. We used to play hearts in full makeup and costume during our lunch breaks on the set." Deirdre's expression must have betrayed her because Bunny said, "Does that surprise you?"

"A little. My mother didn't have many friends." Deirdre didn't add that although her mother had once aspired to act, she had come to dismiss actresses as self-indulgent narcissists. Talking to one, she used to say, was like getting trapped in a mirror.

"Your mother was whip smart," Bunny said. In other words, never made it out of the back row whereas Bunny had quickly moved front and center. "And your father was a charmer. He made friends for both of them."

Friends? Deirdre cringed. Like the women he'd photographed up in his office? Joelen saved her from a response by saying, "Bunny, the police think someone killed Arthur and they want to question Deirdre."

The words left Deirdre momentarily stunned. It was true, of course, but she hadn't let herself think about it in such stark terms.

"Oh dear," Bunny said. "How can we—"

"She needs to call Sy Sterling," Joelen said.

"Of course," Bunny said. "Come. Use the phone in my office."

Moments later, Deirdre was sitting at the glass-topped desk in Bunny's study. Bunny knew the number and dialed for her. Joelen watched from the door.

"Attorney's office." The smoker's voice of Vera, Sy's secretary, brought back a memory of the second-floor law office in Westwood Village. Open the door with the pebble glass inset and there Vera would be at her desk, a pencil stuck in her hair and a stash of crayons and drawing paper hidden in the supply closet. The smells of Vera's cigarettes and Sy's cigars mingled in the dimly lit corridor where they used to let Deirdre ride her tricycle up and down while Sy met with Arthur in his office.

Deirdre breathed a sigh of relief when Vera put her right through. "Sy? It's Deirdre. You said to call if the police came back? Well, they did. First they called and left a message that they wanted to talk to me. Then they came to the house. When I didn't answer, they just sat out front and waited. Then TV news vans pulled up—"

"Where are you now?" Sy said, interrupting. "Are you all right?"

"I'm fine. Just rattled. My friend Joelen came and got me. I'm at her house."

"Joelen?" Sy seemed surprised. "Elenor Nichol's daughter?"

"She was my best friend in high school. Dad was supposed to meet with her to talk about selling the house." Silence on the other end of the line. "She's a Realtor now."

"I know," Sy said.

"Where should I go? I can't stay here." Deirdre swallowed, trying to tamp down the hysteria that threatened to envelop her. "What do the police want?"

"Probably just answers to routine questions. They are investigating a suspicious death. You discovered it. But I do not like them harassing you at the house. And I really do not like newspeople showing up. Schmucks, all of them." Sy's outrage was comforting. "We need to get out in front of this. Go in and talk to that detective." He must have covered the receiver because she could hear muffled voices, then, "Can you meet me in front of City Hall in about an hour? I will call you when I arrive."

Deirdre covered the receiver on her end. "Joelen, can you drive me over to City Hall? Not now. When Sy calls back in an hour."

"Of course," Joelen said.

"I'll be there," Deirdre told Sy, feeling relieved. She wasn't eager to talk to the police, but taking action, any action, felt infinitely better than waiting to be mugged.

"Can you find a scarf?" Sy asked. "Or sunglasses? Just in case reporters are hanging around. I don't want anyone to recognize you on the way in."

"Recognize me?" Deirdre asked, startled. "Why would anyone recognize me?"

"There are already news vans at your house. Who do you think they are looking for?"

"My father was just a writer, for God's sake. Why do they even care?"

"Your father drowned. And years ago he failed to save Fox Pearson from drowning."

"Who remembers him?"

"No one would except that he died with so much drama. In a swimming pool. And your father tried to save him. The press loves it when history tries to repeat itself."

CHAPTER 16

Scarf? Sunglasses? *Pffft.* Amateur hour." Bunny Nichol rubbed her hands together, wiggled her fingers, and blew on the tips. "We can do better than that." She threw open the door to her dressing room. It was half the size of the master bedroom, which itself was about the size of the entire first floor of Deirdre's house in San Diego. Out wafted the scent of orange blossoms.

Instantly Deirdre was transported back to when she and Joelen spent hours in Bunny's dressing room, sampling her skin creams and applying her lipstick—a strawberry red called Fraises des Bois—and trying on gowns and costumes. Chiffon and satin, feathers and sequins, leather and metallic lamé. Then adorning themselves with pounds of costume jewelry.

But the last thing Deirdre needed right now was a getup that drew attention to herself. "Even with a paper bag over my head I'll still be recognizable. I can't get around without this," she said, indicating her crutch.

"When I'm done with you, you'll be able to bump right into them, crutch and all, and they won't so much as blink. You'll see."

"Bunny used to be a magician's assistant," Joelen said. "She once performed with the legendary John Jasper."

"Deirdre's probably never heard of him, have you, dear?" Bunny said. "He wasn't a celebrity so much as a magician's magician. Brilliant guy. He could do anything. Make anything disappear, including the teeth right out of your mouth. He was injured doing the bullet catch onstage in Piccadilly. Died a day later. Death by misadventure. If the police had understood how the trick was done, they'd have done more investigating." She shook her head, then gave a wicked smile and a wave of her hand. "In John's early days, I was the eye candy. That's the whole point of having an assistant. To distract. Though he didn't need me. He was that damned good. But here we have the opposite problem." She pursed her lips. "We don't want you to disappear. We just want to make you appear invisible."

Invisibility. Now there was a goal worth aspiring to.

The facing walls of the dressing room were mirrored, reflecting back an infinitely repeating version of Deirdre's frazzled self. Deirdre dropped her gaze to Bunny's makeup table. It was also mirrored, and sitting on top was a gilt-framed ink-and-watercolor portrait of Bunny. She addressed the viewer with a direct gaze, a knowing gleam in her eyes, her chin resting on her curled fingers. Tendrils of silky black hair framed her face. She looked like a grown-up, worldly, and slightly naughty version of a Breck girl.

Outside the border framing Bunny's face, the illustrator had drawn a heart-shaped bottle filled with brilliant blue liquid. The word CERULEAN was lettered in gold on the bottle, and beneath it in script were the words *Fragrance for women*. The liquid in the bottle matched the brilliant blue the artist had used to color Bunny's eyes.

Bunny grabbed the framed picture and laid it facedown on the dressing table. "No one's supposed to see that," she said. "It's all very hush-hush, so you must promise me you won't tell a soul. They're not launching the product for a while yet, and I don't want to jinx it. But isn't it exciting?"

Joelen caught Deirdre's attention in the mirror and rubbed her fingers and thumb together. "Mom will be the official spokesperson."

"A little old-style Hollywood glamour," Bunny said. "Still sells. If Sophia Loren can do it, why not Elenor Nichol? I've still got it." She stood for a moment, chin up, hip cocked, admiring herself in the mirror.

"Yes, Mother dear." Joelen rolled her eyes. "Remember the last time Deirdre was here? You let her borrow that yellow dress."

"Did I?" Bunny said.

"Lace with a high neck," Deirdre said. "It was the most gorgeous dress I'd ever worn, before or since."

"Oh dear, that is a sad story." Bunny gave Deirdre a sharp, appraising look. "You could probably still get into that dress. I'm sure I could not."

Deirdre shivered at the thought of actually stepping into the torn, soiled dress. How different it would be from when she'd first put her arms through the sleeves on the night of her last sleepover.

That night, while the caterers were busy downstairs setting up for the party, Joelen and Deirdre sat and watched from the floor of this dressing room as Bunny got ready. First she "put on her face," as she called it. Foundation, then powder brushed on over it, then a darkish powder applied, she explained, to shorten her nose and accentuate cheekbones. Next Bunny did her eyes, painting a thick band of turquoise eyeliner on the lids—a trick, she said, to make her eyes look even bluer than they were. Over that, with a steady hand she painted a narrow black line that echoed Elizabeth Taylor's Cleopatra.

Joelen had stood behind her mother, brushed out her hair, and pinned it up in a silky French twist. Bunny artfully pulled out strands to frame her face. Then Joelen sprayed until the air in the dressing room was moist and heavy with scent.

One by one, Bunny had pulled cocktail dresses from the closet, holding each up to consider. Satin, lace, chiffon, some in saturated jewel tones like colors of the millefleur glass paperweight on the makeup table, others pastel, like eggs in an Easter basket.

Bunny had held up an emerald-green satin sheath. "Not my color," she said. She held the dress under Joelen's chin. Joelen looked past her mother at her own reflection in a mirror. Without a word, some agreement seemed to pass between them. Bunny unzipped the dress and held it open; Joelen took off her pants and top and stepped into it. Bunny unhooked Joelen's bra and Joelen slipped out of it and poured her breasts into the dress's boned bodice. Deirdre felt like one of the little mice who watched Cinderella's transformation as Bunny zipped Joelen into the dress, turned her to face the mirror, and pinched the fabric on either side of her narrow waist.

The overall effect was breathtaking. The intense green made Joelen's complexion glow, and the contrast set fire to the reddish streaks in her hair. Her soft, full cleavage swelled into the plunging sweetheart neckline.

Clap. Clap. Clap.

The sound had startled Deirdre. It was Tito, standing in the doorway and staring in at them. He was dressed in a formfitting black silk shirt that was open halfway down his chest.

Joelen blushed, and her hands flew up to cover her breasts. Tito strode over to her, put a finger under her chin, and waited until she raised her eyes to meet his. "Do not be ashamed. You are beautiful like your mother." He started to lean in toward her, as if he were about to give her a kiss, then turned and gave Bunny a peck on the cheek. "These young ladies," he said, winking at Deirdre, "they should come to the party." Then he strode off, leaving behind a wake of musky cologne.

"Oh, could we? Can we?" Joelen asked Bunny. "Please, please, please!"

After a few moments' hesitation, Bunny said, "Oh, all right. You girls can answer the door and take coats. Stay for a little while. But after that it's up to bed. Understood?" She set aside a few dresses for Deirdre to pick from, then left to check on the caterers.

Deirdre chose the pale yellow cocktail dress with a swishy tulle skirt and a lace bodice. With a borrowed bra of Joelen's, stuffed with Kleenex, the dress fit perfectly and made her feel like a fairy princess. By the time both girls were dressed and Joelen had finished fussing with her own and Deirdre's hair and makeup, Deirdre barely recognized the girls who looked back at them in the mirror. Joelen looked like Ann-Margret, the seductive redhead she'd seen singing "Bye, Bye, Birdie" on the *Ed Sullivan Show*. Deirdre looked like a complete stranger with dark, dramatic eyes, the lashes heavy with mascara, her lips strawberry red and glistening. Her hair was teased and lacquered, her face a smooth veneer of makeup that felt spackled on.

Deirdre and Joelen had made their way down as the first guests, including Arthur and Gloria, were arriving. Guests took turns playing the piano, and at one point Bunny urged Joelen to step up and sing "Let Me Entertain You."

"Sing out, Louise!" Bunny trilled near the end, before Joelen morphed from girlish coquette to sly seductress. When Joelen got to the part where she promised if they were *real good,* she'd make them *feel good,* not a single ice cube clinked as the room turned utterly silent. Joelen and Bunny sang the final crescendo together. Deirdre could still see the two of them standing side by side, flushed and beaming as the piano's chords reverberated. An awkward silence followed.

In the endless rehashing in the press of what happened that night, a photograph of Joelen and Bunny appeared in newspapers and magazines. It showed them standing, arm in arm in front of the white grand piano in their similarly low-cut, formfitting satin sheaths. Deirdre had been standing next to Joelen, also arm in arm, but her image had been cropped from the frame. The only evidence she'd been there was the corner of her tulle skirt and her arm, the wrist laden with borrowed rhinestone bracelets.

Joelen's question, "I wonder what happened to that dress?," brought Deirdre back to the present. Joelen raised her eyebrows at Deirdre. *Ask,* she mouthed.

But before Deirdre could form a question, Bunny swept her arms like a conductor silencing the instruments. "Magic," she said, gazing out in front of her, eyes unfocused, as if watching the word hover before her. "It's all about misdirection. Make the audience attend to what *you* want them to see. What will be compelling enough to divert their attention or, in our case, make them tune out—that is the trick."

Delicately Bunny tapped her chin with long red fingernails and stared at Deirdre in the mirror. She opened one closet door, then another, and another, finally emerging with a half-dozen garments slung over her arm. None of them were cocktail dresses. "Stand up straight. And, please, would you take off that appalling top. It's making my teeth itch."

Obediently Deirdre pulled off Henry's Harley T-shirt and stood there in her bra and drawstring pants.

"Hmmm." Bunny held up what looked like a gray cotton mechanic's jumpsuit and squinted. She pursed her lips in disapproval and dropped it on the floor. A pale purple sweatshirt minidress with a hood met the same fate. A black-and-gold floor-length African dashiki joined the pile. Next she held up what looked like a stewardess uniform—navy pencil skirt and tailored jacket. "Maybe," she said, and set it aside.

Finally Bunny considered a simple shirtwaist dress, starched and pressed gray cotton with an A-line skirt, white snaps up the front, a white collar, and short white-cuffed sleeves. She held the dress under Deirdre's chin, narrowing her eyes as she gazed into the mirror. Then she broke into a smile. "Perfect, don't you think?" She didn't wait for an answer.

Fifteen minutes later Deirdre was seated at the makeup table, wearing the dress with a pair of saggy white opaque tights and orthopedic nurse's shoes. She'd stuffed the toe of one shoe with Kleenex to keep it from falling off her smaller foot. Bunny tucked Deirdre's hair into a hairnet and secured it with a hairpin. She applied a foundation much darker than Deirdre's natural skin tone and brushed powder over it, then created hollows beneath Deirdre's eyes with dark eye shadow. Finally she gave Deirdre a pair of glasses with black plastic frames.

Deirdre put the glasses on. The lenses were clear.

"Up," Bunny commanded.

Deirdre leaned on her crutch and rose to her feet.

"Stoop," Bunny said.

Deirdre hunched over.

"Not that much. Just kind of roll your shoulders and stick your head out. Think turtle."

Deirdre adjusted her stance. The mousy woman gazing back at her from the mirror looked like a Latina version of Ruth Buzzi's bag lady from *Laugh-In*. She started to laugh. "This is ridiculous. It will never work."

"Hey, what's going on?" a man's voice called from Bunny's bedroom.

"You don't think it's going to work?" Bunny said to Deirdre. "Watch this." She handed Deirdre her crutch and led her into the bedroom, then threw open the door to the hall. Out on the landing stood the young man Deirdre had seen earlier. He was barefoot and wearing jeans and a stretched-out black T-shirt.

"What's up with you?" Joelen said.

"I . . . what? Why are you two looking at me like I did something?" he said.

"It's not what you did. It's what you're not doing," Joelen said, pushing past Deirdre.

"What are you talking about?" The man looked from Joelen to Bunny.

"See?" Bunny said, turning to Deirdre. "Not a single glance your way. It's as if you're wallpaper. I'd say the disguise is working."

"Disguise?" the man said.

Joelen took the man's hand. "Dear, meet Deirdre, my best friend all through high school. Deirdre, may I present Jackie Hutchinson. My *baby*"—her voice seemed to caress the word—"brother. Is he adorable or what?" Joelen gave him a loud wet kiss on the cheek.

"Would you cut that out?" Jackie pulled a face and made a show of wiping off the kiss. "I'm twenty-one, for God's sake."

"God help us. Just turned twenty-one," Joelen said. She chucked him under the chin and he pushed her away.

Of course Deirdre could see the resemblance. Jackie and Joelen both had Bunny's legendary electric blue eyes and heart-shaped face. But Jackie had dark curly hair, a dimpled chin, and beaky profile—not features he'd have inherited from Bunny or Bunny's late husband, Derek Hutchinson. Hutch, as he was called in the fan magazines, had a longtime starring role in a hospital-based soap opera, but he'd been much more Dr. Kildare than Ben Casey.

Recovering himself, Jackie offered Deirdre his hand. "Pleased to meet you. I'm sorry. I thought you were . . ." His voice trailed off. He seemed painfully young and he made Deirdre feel painfully old.

"Go on," Bunny said. "Say it. You thought Deirdre was the new maid."

Jackie nodded sheepishly and Joelen said, "And the prize for best disguise goes to—"

"Sorry," Jackie said.

"Don't be," Bunny said. "It's very gratifying. That's just the effect I was aiming for."

Jackie smiled a perfect toothy smile. "So my sister was your best friend?"

"From sixth grade," Deirdre said, "until . . ." Her voice trailed off.

Jackie narrowed his dark eyes at Deirdre. "Was she crazy then, too?"

"Crazy?" Joelen gave him a shove. "Look who's talking."

"Not exactly crazy," Deirdre said. "I'd say fearless. She did some pretty wild things and I followed her. So I guess I was the crazy one."

Joelen snorted a laugh. "Remember thumbing a ride home from the five-and-dime?"

"Miraculously without getting abducted." Deirdre remembered the black Cadillac that had stopped. The man had leaned across the passenger seat and opened the door and they'd hopped in. Just like that. All the way to Deirdre's house the driver lectured them about the dangers of getting into cars with strangers, explaining in graphic detail just how bad things could go. Deirdre had been relieved to get out of that car.

Joelen picked up the thread. "Hey, it was raining and we'd have been soaking wet by the time we got back. So we get a ride home and Pollyanna here insists on walking all the way back to the damned store in the downpour, so she can return the stupid lipstick she pilfered."

"*I* stole it? Ha!"

"What ha? How did it end up in your pocket?" Joelen was all wide-eyed innocence.

Passionate Pink. The tube had felt as if it were burning a hole in her pocket—once she realized it was there. "I think you know the answer to that."

"Me?" Joelen turned to Jackie. "So then she gets arrested trying to put it back!"

"I did not get arrested." Deirdre felt a flush rising from her neck to her forehead. The dweeby J.J. Newberry security guard had squeezed her arm as he dragged her to the back of the store and propelled her up a smelly staircase to an office with windows that looked down over the store's vast aisles. He'd sat her down and made her give him her name and phone number. Thankfully neither of her parents had been home to take his call. But before that asshole let Deirdre go, he made her sign a paper promising she'd never set foot in the store again. As if she would have. But the worst part was when he'd taken her picture and pinned her humiliated face to a bulletin board along with about a dozen other shoplifters.

"You must have been quite the pair," Jackie said.

"The original odd couple," Joelen said. "She was Miss Goody Two-Shoes."

"And you were"—Deirdre searched for the right comparison— "Bonnie Parker."

"Bonnie who?" Jackie said.

"He's such a child." Joelen pursed her lips. "What do you expect?"

They were quizzing Jackie on iconic rock singers, old TV shows, and more movie roles when the phone rang. For a moment, Deirdre's throat went dry. Joelen crossed the room to the bedside table and answered it.

"Sure. Okay, I'll tell her." She hung up and turned to Deirdre. "That was Sy. He's waiting for you. I'll get the car and meet you by the back door."

"Honey," said Bunny, squeezing Deirdre's hand, "it's showtime."

CHAPTER 17

Bunny packed Deirdre's jeans and T-shirt into her messenger bag and led her to the end of the hall, through a door, across a dimly lit passageway, and down a back stairway. *Mothballs. Floor wax.* Deirdre gagged on the smells as she grasped the wooden railing and slowly made her way down steeply raked steps. Her memory of her father spiriting her out of the house after Tito was killed clicked into place. Of course he hadn't led her out through a tunnel. It had been this narrow hallway.

They were halfway down the back stairs when Bunny stopped and turned to face her. "So you found the dress?"

Deirdre froze. She nodded.

In the half-light, Bunny looked tense and tired, her face showing her age. "Your father was supposed to take care of it."

"Take care—?" Deirdre didn't know what to say.

"Get rid of it."

"Because?"

"Because no one needed to know that you were there."

"I was?"

"You don't remember?" Bunny asked, and when Deirdre shook her head, she sighed. "Just as well that you don't."

"But—"

"So what are you going to do?"

"Do?"

Bunny gave an exasperated sigh. "With the dress."

From outside came the sound of a car horn tooting. Deirdre automatically looked toward the noise.

Bunny grasped Deirdre's arm, bringing her attention back. "You have no idea what you're playing with here. The last thing my daughter needs is to have things stirred up again." She squeezed Deirdre's arm so hard that it hurt. "Do you understand what I'm telling you?"

In truth, Deirdre didn't, but Bunny didn't wait for an answer. When the car horn tooted again, she released Deirdre and turned away. Deirdre followed her down the stairs. At the bottom, they emerged into a laundry room.

Joelen came in to meet them. "What's the holdup?"

"Just putting on the finishing touches," said Bunny. She opened a broom closet and pulled out a Ralph's shopping bag. Into it she stuffed Deirdre's messenger bag. She handed Deirdre the loaded shopping bag and then stood back, her brow furrowed. "Needs something more. Let me see—"

"She looks good. Just fine," Joelen said. "Let's go."

"Good isn't great and fine isn't finished," Bunny said. "Wait here. I'll be right back." She disappeared back up the stairs.

"*Good isn't great. Fine isn't finished,*" Joelen singsonged. "I stepped right into that. What can I tell you? She's a perfectionist."

Deirdre rubbed her arm where it was sore and reddened from Bunny's grip.

Moments later Bunny reappeared carrying a battered black vinyl purse. She hooked it over Deirdre's arm along with the shopping bag, smiled approval, then hustled her and Joelen out the back door to the car.

Deirdre threw the purse and shopping bag into the backseat and got in the front, her crutch across her lap. She wiped the sweat from her forehead. The too-tight underarms of her "uniform" were already damp with perspiration, and the fabric stuck to her back.

Joelen started driving down the long driveway. As she pulled the car out onto Sunset and turned south toward City Hall, Deirdre ran through the conversation she'd had in that dark stairway with Bunny.

You have no idea what you're playing with here. She'd been right about that.

"Are you okay?" Joelen asked.

"Sure," Deirdre lied. "Why?"

"I don't know. You seem . . . tense. Upset."

So you found the dress?

Your father was supposed to take care of it.

No one needed to know that you were there.

"You always were good at reading me," Deirdre said. "I guess I'm feeling anxious about talking to the police. And"—she looked down at her getup—"ridiculous. Conspicuous." She tugged at one of the sleeves. "Hot and uncomfortable."

Joelen turned the A/C up and adjusted one of the vents so the cool air blasted out at Deirdre. "Does that help?"

"Thanks. Yeah, it does."

"You're sure that's all?" Joelen gave her a concerned look.

"I guess it just seems weird."

"What?"

"You know, being back in the house with you and your mom after so many years."

"I hope not weird in a bad way."

"Your mom's the same—"

Joelen laughed. "I know. She's a tidal wave. Wouldn't want to get in her way, that's for sure. What do you think of Jackie?"

"Handsome as hell." Deirdre ran the back of her hand across her damp brow. It came away coated with dark makeup. "Sweet, actually. Is he still in school?"

"I wish." Joelen waved her hand as if she were swatting away a fly. "He barely finished high school. Not because he's not smart. He just wasn't buying what they were selling. But he's doing okay."

"Doing what?"

"Selling his favorite toys. Harleys. He's pretty good at it, too."

Deirdre remembered seeing the bike in the driveway. "Really? Where?"

"Marina del Rey. There's a dealership there that's been in business forever, and . . ."

As Joelen went on about how great the dealership was and how well Jackie was doing there, Deirdre sat in stunned silence. There was only one Harley dealership in Marina del Rey, and Henry worked there. And yet Henry claimed he hadn't heard word one about Joelen since high school?

"Sorry. I didn't mean to go on like that," Joelen said as she double-parked in front of City Hall. She put her hand on Deirdre's arm in the same spot where Bunny's squeeze had left her red. "Relax. You'll see. No one is going to bat an eyelash at you. Look, there's Sy."

Deirdre spotted him, too, sitting beyond a news team that was broadcasting from the sidewalk at the base of broad steps that led to the main entrance. The center bell tower provided the perfect back-drop for the suited man talking animatedly at the camera.

"Go on," Joelen said. "Get out. Brazen does it! Before I get a ticket for double-parking." She reached across and opened the passenger door. Hot air flooded the car. "You're in good hands. I ought to know."

A car behind them beeped. Deirdre set her crutch on the mac-adam and got out. Before she reached the sidewalk Joelen had pulled away, and for a moment Deirdre felt completely exposed. The mas-sive Spanish colonial building that housed city government as well as the police and fire departments towered before her. She adjusted her grip on her crutch and the ridiculous handbag and started past the film crew, stepping over wires that snaked back to the van. The Ralph's shopping bag banged against her side with every lurching step.

She was so close to the film crew that she could hear the young TV news commentator, his smooth mannequin face barely moving as spoke: "Scenes from this year's number-one action movie were filmed right here. But the project that started out as a vehicle for Sylvester Stallone . . ."

"Watch where you're stepping!" said a guy she assumed was a production assistant, glaring at her, his words an angry hiss.

The commentator held the mike in front of a shaggy-haired man wearing a black T-shirt tucked into belted jeans, his silver-tinted aviator glasses reflecting the sun. He chuckled, then spoke in a raspy voice: "So Sly bails. Weeks before shooting is scheduled to begin last spring, he pulls out. And we're talking about the project with Eddie. And he says, 'Enough of this. Do you guys want to make the film or just talk about it?'"

Deirdre relaxed a notch. In this celebrity-obsessed town, how hard could it be to fly under the radar? She smoothed her dress, hoisted up the sagging panty hose, affected a slightly turtle-necked slouch, and started walking toward where Sy was perched at the edge of a raised bed of pink and purple petunias, so bright that they looked artificial. People leaving the building glanced at her, but none looked twice. The hairnet made her head itchy, but she resisted the urge to scratch.

As she got closer, Sy's gaze passed over her without a flicker of recognition. It wasn't until she was three feet away that he registered her crutch, looked her full in the face, and sprang to his feet. He eyed her up and down, then looked around. "Brava," he said in a stage whisper.

"I had help."

"I imagine you did." He picked up his briefcase and cast an anxious glance in the direction of the news team. "Come on. Let's not press our luck. There is a side entrance."

Sy led Deirdre around to the side of the building where cruisers were angle parked and a sign pointing up a narrow flight of stairs said BEVERLY HILLS POLICE DEPARTMENT. He followed Deirdre up the steps and held open one of the double doors at the top.

Deirdre passed into a cool, dark interior. An outer waiting area was lined with benches—a tired-looking woman rocking a baby in a stroller sat on one of them—and smelled of burnt coffee, stale candy, and pine cleaner. Beyond another set of glass-paned double doors, uniformed police officers milled about. When an officer pushed the door open and exited, the sound of phones ringing and loud voices pulsed out.

"Does the detective know we're coming?" Deirdre asked.

"I thought we would surprise him. When you talk to him, please remember, do not offer information. Do not speculate. Just answer his questions. This is important. Do you understand me?"

"I do. Don't offer. Don't speculate. Can I change first?"

"Go."

Deirdre ducked into the ladies' room. She ripped off the hairnet and shook out her hair. Gave her scalp a good scratch. Relief! Then she changed back into her pants and T-shirt and stuffed the baggy tights and the dress and vinyl handbag into her messenger bag. She scrubbed her face using the gloppy, bubble-gum-colored soap from the dispenser. Patted her face dry with a brown paper towel that left a residue of wet cardboard smell.

When she emerged, Sy was no longer in the lobby. He was on the other side of the glass door in the midst of what looked like a heated discussion with a visibly exasperated Detective Martinez.

CHAPTER 18

Deirdre pushed through the door to the police department in time to hear Martinez reaming out Sy. "If you people are going to start playing games—"

"No one is playing games with you. She is right here," Sy said, spotting Deirdre and motioning her over. "See? Ready and willing to answer your questions."

A vein was pounding in Martinez's forehead. He gave a tense nod in Deirdre's direction and checked his watch, then turned and led her and Sy through a busy room filled with desks, down a corridor, and through a door into a small office. The interior was Spartan— just a desk, a phone, and a half-dead ficus that Deirdre found herself wanting desperately to water. A dust-coated window overlooked a eucalyptus tree behind the building.

Martinez sat at the desk and motioned for Deirdre and Sy to sit on the other side. A half-full mug of coffee sat on the desk, white ceramic with a splash of red, the motto HOMICIDE: OUR DAY BEGINS WHEN

SOMEONE ELSE'S ENDS. A second mug, filled with pens and pencils, had SUPER DADDY on it.

Martinez took out a pad and made a few initial notations. Then he leaned back in his chair and just stared at Deirdre for what seemed like forever. Taking her measure or, more likely, trying to freak her out. "You won't mind if I record this," he said, taking a cassette recorder from the desk drawer. "Then I won't have to worry about getting everything down in my notes."

"Not a problem," Sy said. "Right, Deirdre?"

Following his lead, Deirdre nodded. Martinez snapped in a fresh cassette, turned it on, and set the recorder on the desk between them. He recorded a little preamble—time, date, and who was present. Then played it and went back to recording.

"Miss Unger, thank you very much for coming in. I'll get right to the point. I need to clarify your whereabouts late Friday night and into Saturday morning."

"I've already told you, I was in the art gallery. Xeno Art. Until late. Then I went home."

"I know." Martinez gave her a tired smile. "Like I said, just to clarify and get the details correct. So you closed the gallery? When was that?"

"We're open until eight. Then I closed up. But I stayed later, prepping a new exhibit."

"Alone?"

"With the artist's assistant."

"Do you have this artist's assistant's name? Can we contact him—"

"Her. Shoshanna."

"Shoshanna . . . what?"

"I don't know her last name. But I can get her contact information for you." The assistant had been young. Brunette. With hair that hung down to her waist and a lot of makeup. *Aspiring actress* had been Deirdre's first thought. The artist had arranged for her to come help, since he was in Israel. He said she'd be at the gallery at eight but she hadn't gotten there until after ten, complaining about heavy traffic. Two hours of heavy traffic well past rush hour? It sounded lame, but Deirdre hadn't bothered to call her on it.

"Please do. And you were at the gallery with this Shoshanna until—?"

"After midnight." It was so late by the time they'd finished up that she'd been afraid her car would get ticketed for overnight parking. Too bad it hadn't.

"What about casual passersby? They'd have seen that the lights were on inside and the two of you in there hanging paintings. Maybe someone stopped in?"

"It was an installation. Not paintings." Shoes, actually. Avram Sigismund had shipped them hundreds of old shoes—looked like a Salvation Army resale store's entire stock of shoes that had been thrown in the mud and driven over a few times—along with some graffiti-covered canvas backdrops delivered to the gallery in crates. Shoshanna had a schematic that showed where the shoes, each of which was numbered, were to be placed—some on the floor, others climbing the walls, still others hanging from the ceiling. When all the shoes were in their appointed places, Deirdre hadn't been all that impressed. On top of that the gallery reeked of feet, something that the assistant called "texture" and insisted was an essential part of the concept. "And no," Deirdre added, "no one stopped in, and I doubt if anyone going past would have realized that we were there. We covered the windows."

"You covered the windows." Hearing Martinez repeat her in a deadpan, Deirdre realized how bizarre this sounded.

"The artist was quite definite." Paranoid, even. "He didn't want anyone to see his work until the show opened."

"Did that seem unusual to you?"

"I could understand it, really, especially with an installation of that nature."

"So this artist. What's his name?"

"Avram Sigismund." Deirdre spelled it for Martinez.

"He's well known?"

"He's Israeli. Up and coming." Deirdre avoided Martinez's gaze. In fact, she'd never worked with Avi (as he asked them to call him) before. Never even heard of him until just a week and a half ago when they'd agreed to clear their front gallery space and show his work. She could tell herself that it was Stefan who'd pressured her to break their long-standing policy and accept payment to mount a show, but that wouldn't have been fair. The gallery was struggling and they needed to pay their rent. It seemed like a gift when, out of the blue, Avi contacted Stefan with a proposal. He was desperate for gallery space for just two weeks to accommodate a curator from a major American museum who wanted to see his work firsthand. His work was represented by the prestigious (even she'd heard of it) Rosenfeld Gallery in Tel Aviv, but he'd never been shown in the United States. Stefan had gotten the strong sense that the museum interested in acquiring his work was the MOCA in L.A.

The whole deal had sounded slightly sketchy to Deirdre, because why couldn't he have found a gallery in the Los Angeles area to show his work? But what was there to lose when Avi was offering to pay expenses and then some, up front, in addition to a 40 percent commission when (not if) the museum purchased the work? Both she and Stefan held their noses and signed on. It was only for a few weeks, she'd told herself. Besides, they'd clear enough to bankroll shows for a half-dozen artists whose works they were eager to exhibit.

"So you were in the gallery until—"

"After midnight." How many times did he need for her to say it?

"And then?"

"I went home."

"Home?"

"To my house. I live in Imperial Beach. It's near—"

"I know where it is. Was anyone with you? Anyone drop by? Anyone who can vouch for your whereabouts?"

Vincent Price. By the time she got home, even Johnny Carson had gone to bed. The only thing on was the ending of *House of Wax.*

"No," Deirdre said, her tone sharper than she'd intended. She wasn't sure if she was annoyed because he kept asking the same thing, or because she was always alone in bed at night.

"Did you receive any telephone calls after you got home?"

"No."

"Are you sure?"

"Positive."

"What would you say if I told you that phone records show that calls were made to your home phone late that night?"

"Excuse me," Sy said. "You need a subpoena to examine my client's phone records."

"We haven't examined *her* phone records." Martinez placed a computer printout in front of her. Several lines were highlighted. "These calls were made to you from your father's phone."

Deirdre looked at the highlighted calls. She pointed to the first one, Friday at 3:12 P.M. "I was at the gallery then."

"Looks like you didn't answer this call, either," Martinez said, pointing to a call at 1:41 A.M. "You said you were home by then."

Deirdre swallowed and shifted in her seat. "I'd turned off the ringer."

"Why did you do that?"

Martinez just sat there waiting. "I was tired. It was late."

"Who would have called you so late?"

My father. Even though that was perfectly innocent, Deirdre felt beads of sweat prick from her upper lip.

"What is the relevance of this?" Sy said, saving her from having to answer. "Just because Miss Unger didn't answer her phone doesn't mean she was not at home."

Martinez leaned forward. "The coroner estimates the time of death at between midnight and three A.M. This"—he put his finger on the list—"would have been the last phone call your father made before he died. Unless"—he paused for a moment, like this thought was just now occurring to him—"unless it was someone else, calling you from your father's house."

Sy's warning came back to her. *Do not offer. Do not speculate.* Deirdre didn't say anything.

Martinez sat back. "So your story is that you left the gallery, drove home, turned off the ringer on your phone, and went to sleep?"

Close enough. Deirdre nodded.

Martinez pointed to the cassette recorder.

"That's right," Deirdre said.

"Alone?"

"Alone." She said it calmly but she wanted to scream *Yes! Alone! I live alone!*

"And you left the house again when?"

"The next morning. Saturday. Maybe at about nine."

"And you drove—"

"Straight to my father's house."

"Without stopping?"

"Without—" Then she remembered. "I stopped for gas and something to eat at a McDonald's somewhere around Mission Viejo."

"You used a credit card?"

Of course it would be nice if she had some evidence to support her claim. "Paid cash. But I think the cup and the wrapper are still in my car."

Martinez looked unimpressed.

"I probably kept the receipts," Deirdre added. She sounded confident but she wondered if she had in fact bothered to keep them. She saved every receipt, even small ones, when the expense was business related. But this trip had been personal. "I'll look."

"So you got to your father's house when?"

She'd answered that question already. Several times. "At about noon. But no one answered the door and I couldn't get in. That's why I went around to the backyard."

"Who has keys to your father's house?"

"Henry, of course. He lives there. My mom, though she'd never go there. The woman who comes in once a week and cleans for my dad." Deirdre looked over at Sy to see if he had anything to add.

"Not you?" Martinez asked.

"Not me."

"Was that a problem? Not having a set of keys."

"No. I don't visit very often."

"The last time was—?"

Was this a test? Because she'd already answered that question at the house. "January."

"Months ago. Sounds as if you and your father weren't that close."

"We got along. We just didn't spend time together."

"But you drove up to help him move."

"He asked me to. He needed help. Of course I came."

Martinez nodded and rubbed his chin. "Okay. Just a few more questions. Was your father having financial problems?"

"I don't know. He didn't talk to me about his finances and I'd never have hit him up for money."

Sy put a finger to his lips: *Just answer the question.*

"But he was putting the house up for sale."

"Right."

"Did your father have any enemies? Any ongoing disagreements with business associates or neighbors?"

"Not that I know of."

"He and your mother—?"

"Got along fine since their divorce."

He leaned forward, as if he were about to ask another question, then thought better of it. "All right. I guess that's all."

Deirdre breathed a sigh of relief. When she started to get up from her chair, the backs of her pants were stuck to her thighs.

Martinez shook Sy's hand. He offered his hand to Deirdre and held it. "Just one more thing. There was a shovel near your father's pool. Did you notice it?" He released her hand.

"A shovel?" At first Deirdre didn't remember seeing one. And then she did, lying where Henry would have backed his car right over it. "Yes. It was in the driveway. I picked it up and moved it out of the way."

"Ah. Well, that explains why we found your fingerprints on the shaft. In fact, yours are the only prints on that shovel. And there are no traces of dirt at all. Just traces of blood. Hair. Chlorine. Like it was never actually used for gardening."

Deirdre's stomach turned over and she closed her eyes.

"The blood on the blade?" Martinez continued. "It's not a particularly common blood type. AB positive. Your father is AB positive. Shall I tell you how I think the blood got there?"

She wanted to say *No, don't tell me.* But Sy's stony look kept her from saying anything.

"Sometime after midnight, your father went for a swim. His usual thirty laps. He thought he was alone, but he wasn't. Someone else was out there, and while he was swimming, that person picked up that shovel and struck him. Right here"—Martinez indicated a spot above his own right eye—"and knocked him unconscious. It would not have taken a whole lot of strength on the part of his assailant. A woman could easily have managed it." Martinez paused, then went on, "Victims of violence usually try to protect themselves. But there's no evidence that your father did that. So either he didn't see it coming, or he knew and trusted the person who attacked him."

Martinez paused for a few moments, watching Deirdre, his head tilted, like an osprey waiting for a fish to break the surface. "Which is it, do you think?"

CHAPTER 19

He thinks I killed my father," Deirdre said when she and Sy were outside in his car. She felt as if she'd been punched in the stomach.

"Not necessarily. He is considering his options." Sy put the key in the ignition and turned on the engine. The A/C started to pump cool air and the clock on the dashboard lit up. It was after four. "He is poking around to see what sparks. That is his job."

Deirdre reached out to steady herself against the dashboard. "I feel sick."

"You did fine."

"The shovel. I wasn't thinking . . . I didn't know."

"You did what anyone would have done. You picked it up and moved it. If you had killed your father, more likely you would wipe it clean, yes? What concerns me more is that no one can verify where you were when your father died. It's your word—"

"I'm sure Stefan has Shoshanna's contact information. He talked to Avi. He made the arrangements. I'll get it from him."

"Good. Do it right away. Okay?"

"As soon as I get home."

"Good. Good." Sy turned to her, a concerned expression on his face. "You did not tell me about the shovel."

"I . . ." The observation rattled her. "I barely remembered it myself, and I had no idea that it was important."

"Fair enough. But think. Is there anything else? Anything that seemed unimportant at the time? Run through the timeline of what happened that night and the next morning."

Deirdre sat back. "I worked until late. I slept at home. Alone. Yes, I turned off the phone. I wanted to get a decent night's sleep. You know how he could be."

"I do."

"I left the house around nine. Stopped to get something to eat and to pee. Found him."

"Was anyone out on the street when you arrived?"

"Not that I remember."

"Any cars that you noticed parked when you got there?"

"Just Henry's in the driveway. I moved the shovel. No one answered at the front so I went around to the back. Knocked." Deirdre closed her eyes, remembering standing on the patio as the dogs attacked the sliding glass door. "There was a glass on the table on the patio."

"One?" Sy's bushy eyebrows went up and his hairpiece shifted forward. "And then?"

"Finally Henry came to the door. Then I noticed Dad's shirt was out by the pool. That's what made me go over." She swallowed. "That's it."

Sy nodded, rubbing his chin. "You are quite sure? Deirdre, if you know anything more about your father's death, tell me." Sy returned her look with a steady gaze. "This is not the time to withhold information."

"You think I'm withholding . . . ?" Angry tears welled up. "I'm telling you everything I know. Why would I be hiding something? And you haven't asked, but no, I did not kill my father."

"Of course not." Sy put his hand on her arm. "So let me help you. I can do that."

"Like you got Joelen Nichol off?"

"Got her off?" Sy seemed taken aback for a moment. Then he gave her a wry smile. "I did not get her off. She confessed. Remember? It was the evidence supporting her confession that kept the case from going to trial, but she did not get off. She paid for what she did." Sy stared out the window for a moment, then looked back at Deirdre. "Take my advice. Focus on the present. Give the police the evidence they need to eliminate you as a suspect. Find those receipts. Get in touch with the woman who was with you in the gallery."

"Sy, even if I can't convince the police that I couldn't have been here, what motive could I have for killing my father?"

"Once the police demonstrate opportunity, motive is easy to manufacture," Sy said as he released the emergency brake, switched on the turn signal, and looked over his shoulder. "Greed. Revenge. A stupid argument gets out of hand. The police find evidence and they build a story that supports it." The turn signal ticked as Sy waited for a break in the traffic. "Your friend? Now that is a case in point."

It took a moment for her to get what he was saying. "Are you saying Joelen didn't kill Tito?"

"She was only fifteen years old. Antonio Acevedo had a history of violence. He was a bully. It was no secret that he and Bunny fought. Joelen confessed. Everyone went home happy." He backed out of the parking space and pulled into traffic. "I kept you out of trouble then. Let me keep you out of trouble now."

Sy's remark left Deirdre momentarily speechless. "Me?"

"Did the police question you? Did you have to account for your whereabouts, or give a statement about what you saw or heard?"

"I . . ."

"Well, there you go."

Deirdre was still mulling that over when Sy dropped her off in the alley behind her father's house.

"Do not forget," he said, leaning across the passenger seat to talk to her through the open car door, "find those receipts and track down Susanna."

"Shoshanna. Right away. Thanks." Deirdre closed the car door and watched Sy drive away, then pushed through the back gate. If Stefan didn't have Shoshanna's contact information, he'd certainly be able to get it from Avi. But would that be enough? Because even if she could convince the police that she'd been in the gallery when she said she was, that only accounted for her whereabouts until midnight. The drive to Los Angeles was just two and a half hours. She could have driven up, killed her father, called her own phone from her father's house, then driven back and started out again the next morning as if nothing had happened. It made no sense, but it wasn't impossible.

Deirdre was at the kitchen door, digging for her keys, when she registered an acrid smell. She looked around. Despite the deepening shadows, she could see that the door in the garage leading to her father's office was ajar. Had she left it open? Or maybe Henry had gone up after she'd left. When she started back to investigate, a flock of blackbirds perched in the upper branches of a eucalyptus tree behind the garage swooped across the yard, whistling and screeching like so many squeaky hinges. For a moment she thought she saw something move across the garage's second-floor window. She squinted up at it. Maybe Henry was up there. His car wasn't in the driveway, but it could have been parked out on the street.

That's when she noticed rivulets of smoke seeping from underneath the garage's overhead doors. She moved closer and dropped her messenger bag in the driveway. Covering her mouth and nose, she peered in through a window in the door. All she could see was a dull glow on the floor between her father's car and the bay where Henry kept his motorcycles. Something was burning.

In a panic, she reached down to throw open the garage door but stopped herself. Wouldn't that feed the fire? Maybe she could drag over the garden hose. Or was there a fire extinguisher? Her mother had bought one years ago for the kitchen.

Just as Deirdre was trying to see if a fire extinguisher was hanging on the wall inside the garage, sparks exploded like messy fireworks. She heard a *whoosh* and felt a wave of heat, and stumbled backward seconds before the window she'd been peering through splintered, pieces of glass falling and shattering on the concrete threshold. Inside, flames had sprung to life and licked up toward the ceiling.

Deirdre stood frozen for what was only a second but felt like forever. "Fire!" she screamed, as loud as she could. She banged her crutch on the door and yelled at the top of her lungs, "Fire! Fire! Fire!" Inside, the blaze had doubled. She backed away, choking on smoke. Surely if Henry was upstairs in her father's office he'd smell it now.

She had to call the fire department. She hurried as fast as she could down the driveway to the house. When she finally reached the kitchen door she realized she hadn't unlocked it and her keys were still in her bag, which was lying on the ground in front of the garage. Deirdre turned and looked back. The spot where her messenger bag lay was now completely engulfed in smoke.

Weren't there alarm boxes on the street? There'd been one a few houses down. Once upon a time, Joelen had decided it would be fun to see what happened if she pulled it.

Deirdre struggled to get out to the street, wishing a police cruiser or media van were still parked out there. She focused on the tip of her crutch, feeling the vibration up her arm each time the rubber tip connected with the sidewalk, each time she took a step, dragged her leg, and moved forward again.

The alarm box was right where she remembered, three houses down. For a second Deirdre just stood before it, panting for breath, her throat burning. Then she pulled down the handle. And waited.

Was something supposed to happen? A click? A whirr? She tried to remember, but was pretty sure that she and Joelen hadn't hung around to find out. They'd taken off running and hidden behind some bushes in a neighbor's yard.

Deirdre heard the *whump* of an explosion and turned back toward the house. Another loud pop sounded. Deirdre felt paralyzed as she watched a plume of black smoke rise, thickening and hanging over the garage like a swarm of bees. Where were the sirens? Should she rouse a neighbor? Borrow a phone? Borrow a fire extinguisher?

Finally, in the distance, she heard a siren's wail. Then another joined it. *Thank God.*

Deirdre arrived back at the house at the same time that a hook and ladder truck pulled up. "It's the garage!" she cried, pointing up the driveway, though with all the smoke *where* would have been obvious to anyone. "My brother might be up there. Please, hurry!"

Another fire truck pulled up in front of the house. Neighbors on both sides had come out of their houses and were on the sidewalks watching. A police cruiser screamed up, lights flashing, and parked sideways, closing off the end of the block.

As firefighters in dark turnout gear swarmed from the trucks, Deirdre drifted up the driveway after them. She stared up at where smoke was seeping out from between the louvers in the second-floor windows, barely able to breathe. Henry was not up there, she told herself. He couldn't be. What she'd seen had to have been the shadow of a bird. He'd told her himself he never went up to Arthur's office.

"Stay clear!" a firefighter coming up behind her barked. He was carrying a fire hose. A smaller truck and a Fire Rescue van screamed up to the house. When Deirdre looked back toward the garage, the overhead doors had been flung open and the interior was engulfed in flame. Moments later, flames shot through the roof. Heat pulsed, driving Deirdre back into the street. She was sobbing. Henry could never get out of there in one piece.

At last water gushed from the fire hoses. With the water pouring on full force, the flames were quickly tamped down. A firefighter strapped on an oxygen tank, adjusted the mask over his face, picked up an ax, and waded in through the smoke, disappearing into the shrouded stairwell. Deirdre imagined him climbing the stairs to the second floor in smoky darkness. Would he have to break down the door to her father's office, or was it unlocked as the downstairs door had been? Would he find Henry laid out on the floor? Unconscious in a closet?

She felt seconds ticking by as she waited for a yell. Or a wave from the window. A signal of some kind. Any kind.

Finally the firefighter who'd gone upstairs appeared in the doorway. He unstrapped his silver tank, shucked his coat, and wiped sweat from his face with the back of his arm. Deirdre tried to read his expression. Was he getting ready to deliver bad news?

"Deeds?" Henry's voice was loud behind her.

She whipped around. *Thank God.* "You idiot!" she screamed.

CHAPTER 20

"What happened?" Henry asked.

Deirdre gave a helpless gesture toward the garage. "It . . . I . . .
And I thought you . . ." Her voice was rising.

"What did I do now?"

It was too much. Just too much. Deirdre's world kaleidoscoped
and her legs buckled. Her crutch slipped away as she dropped to one
knee. She felt Henry lift her and put his arms around her. She buried
her face, which felt as if it were twisted into a Kabuki caricature of
anguish, against his chest.

"I'm sorry," Henry said, his warm breath on her hair. "I'm sorry."

She knew it wasn't fair. What had Henry done other than not get
himself killed? She pulled away and wiped her eyes with the back of
her hand. The hoses had cut off, and the plume of smoke rising from
the garage turned into a dark cloud that hovered overhead. Sooty
water that had been cascading past them down the driveway slowed
to a trickle.

"You scared the shit out of me. I didn't know where you were. And I thought I saw you—" She gestured toward the garage. Its siding had buckled. There was a blackened hole in the roof. A few window louvers hung from their frames like orphaned wind chimes. All it would take was a stiff breeze to send them crashing down.

"Why would I go up there?" He picked up her crutch and handed it to her. "It wasn't me. I would have gotten here sooner, but they made me park a block away."

"You scared me."

"You scared *me*. What in God's name happened?"

"I have no idea. When I got back, I smelled smoke. And then the fire exploded." Deirdre hiccuped. "I knew I couldn't get in and put it out. So I had to call. And then I couldn't get into the house." Her voice rose to a wail but she couldn't stop. "I couldn't get to a phone. I didn't know what to do. I . . ."

"It's okay." Henry put his arm around her shoulders. They watched in silence, enveloped in charred, steamy air, as firefighters brought in portable lighting and set up orange cones in front of the garage. One firefighter ventured into the garage. In his dark gear, he seemed to fade in the interior until all she could see was his flashlight beam. More firefighters followed.

Blackened cushions and the frames of yard furniture appeared as if by magic, hurled from the garage interior. One by one they landed in a welter in the driveway. A firefighter dragged out some cardboard packing boxes, one of which collapsed and disgorged what looked like sodden linens and curtains. A tire rolled out of the garage and spiraled lazily into the grass.

The sun had sunk below the horizon, and the last streaky pink clouds were cooling. Deirdre retrieved her messenger bag from the grass where firefighters had tossed it. Trampled and soaked, it seemed like the perfect metaphor for how she felt.

From the second floor, flashlight beams were visible through the openings where there had once been windows. Deirdre could only imagine how bad it was inside the office. Literary executor? Sort and cull? That was a laugh. She'd be sifting ashes. She hoped the yellow dress had been reduced to cinders, too, and she could forget about it—just like Bunny wanted her to.

A tall figure emerged from the garage, took off his heavy coat, laid it across his arm, and looked over his shoulder. Then he turned back and started walking toward Deirdre and Henry. He was flushed, and soot was streaked across his face like war paint. As he got nearer, Deirdre realized he seemed familiar. "Deirdre? Henry?" he said. "You don't remember me. Tyler Corrigan."

Tyler. Of course. He used to live across the street. A few years older than Deirdre, back then he'd reminded her of Opie with his freckles, straw-colored hair, and earnestness. She used to watch him ride his bike up and down the block, popping wheelies and spinning around. A few years after that he'd been out there doing tricks on a skateboard. His family had moved away when she was in high school.

"You're a firefighter?" Deirdre asked.

Tyler shucked a thick work glove and offered his hand. His grip was strong. "Arson investigator. But I work with the police and the fire marshal." He offered a hand to Henry.

"Hey, Tyler," Henry said, shaking his hand. "Arson?"

"It's routine for me to get involved when there's an unattended fire."

Routine. Unattended. Those were the words the police had used to explain why Deirdre's father had to be autopsied. Why a police detective had come to investigate.

"I didn't realize you guys were still living here," Tyler said.

"I still live here," Henry said.

"And my dad lives here—" Deirdre added, then caught herself. "Or at least he did. He died. Yesterday."

Tyler's look darkened. "I'm sorry. I didn't know that."

"He drowned," Deirdre said, swallowing the lump in her throat. "I drove up from San Diego to help him get ready to move and when I got here, I found him in the pool, and—" She clamped her mouth shut. She hadn't intended to say any of that, and now her eyes were stinging. Henry looked pained.

"And now this." Tyler shook his head. "I'm sorry. Your dad was a great guy."

A firefighter came up to him from behind and tapped him on the shoulder, drawing Tyler away. They exchanged a few words that Deirdre couldn't hear. When he returned, Tyler said, "They shouldn't be too much longer. Couple hours, max."

Deirdre edged closer to the open garage. Inside, a camera flash went off. Then another. Two men were crouched in the dark interior alongside the blackened hull that had been her father's car. Next to it, Henry's bikes were on their sides. "What are they doing?" she asked.

"It looks like that's where the fire started. They're documenting the point of ignition. At least no one was hurt." Tyler eyed Deirdre. "You told one of the first responders that someone was upstairs?"

Henry gave her a surprised look. "You did?"

"I told you. I thought it was you."

"Well, no one's up there now," Tyler said.

Deirdre could smell smoke, even from inside the house, long after the fire hoses had been reeled back and the hook and ladder truck had driven off. The street had been reopened, but a gray pall lingered in the air. Only Tyler was left, packing his equipment away in a fire department van parked on the street.

In the meantime, the mortuary had called. They expected the coroner to release Arthur's body the next day. What followed was a stream of questions to which Deirdre had no answers. When would they like to schedule a service? Did they want to reserve the Reposing Room? Open or closed coffin?

She promised to have answers for them in the morning, which was when she hoped her mother would be back. All she knew for sure was that her father had wanted to be cremated.

That led to more questions. Should they reserve a spot for Arthur's cremains in one of their lovely urn gardens? Or perhaps he'd prefer to reside in the columbarium?

The business of death had its own vocabulary, rife with comforting euphemisms, and every choice came with unstated price tags. Price tags came with guilt. Deirdre had no idea whether there was money in the estate for the kind of service to which Arthur would have felt entitled.

Deirdre went outside and stood alone on the lawn in front of the house, watching Tyler jot some final notes and load the van with bags of evidence—material to be analyzed, she assumed. He closed the van door, locked it, and looked over at her.

"Done," he said. His face looked grave. He opened the passenger door and threw his clipboard on the seat.

"Does it feel weird, being back here?" Deirdre asked.

"Kind of. It's a shame they did in our old house." He glanced across the street to where he'd once lived in a modest Spanish colonial with a walled garden. The property had always evoked *The Secret Garden* for Deirdre, with Tyler its Dickon, a character memorably described in the novel as looking like the god Pan with his rosy cheeks and rough curly hair, a charmer of wild animals and unhappy humans.

New owners had torn down the house Tyler had grown up in and replaced it with a house easily double its size. And in place of Dickon was this tall, gangly, competent human being who looked at her so intently that it felt as if he were x-raying her brain.

"My mom drives by and cries," Tyler said.

"Welcome to Beverly Hills," Deirdre said, "where anything that's just plain old is plain old embarrassing. Where is your family living now?"

"My parents moved to Silver Lake, but it's changing, too. And I've got an apartment in Culver City. Funky neighborhood that's staying funky for the foreseeable future."

"I'm guessing new owners will tear down our house, too. And

maybe that's not a bad thing. It's not the great house that yours was to begin with, and my dad didn't exactly improve it."

Tyler held her gaze. "I know this isn't the best time to say this, but it's good to see you again. I've thought of you often." He looked at her crutch. "I hope you don't mind my asking, but what happened?"

"Car accident."

"I didn't know. When?"

"Sixty-three. I was fifteen."

"Sixty-three." He thought for a moment. "We'd moved away the summer before. Where did it happen?"

"I don't know exactly. It was late. My father was driving me home from my friend Joelen's house. I remember rocks and thorn-bushes." Thinking about it brought back the smell of creosote and sage. The air had been thick with it as she lay on the ground and later on the stretcher. That and the pain, which everyone said you forgot but she hadn't. She folded her arms to contain the tremor in them and the tightness in her chest that the memory roused.

She went on. "For a long time I was afraid to find out. Afraid to go back. Then, when I did ask, Dad said he didn't know."

"Didn't know?"

"When I pressed, he said he forgot where it was exactly."

Tyler scrunched up his face in disbelief. "Maybe he thought he was being kind."

Maybe. But if he'd thought not knowing would make her stop thinking about it, he'd been wrong. Instead she'd become obsessed.

"Do you remember anything?" Tyler asked. "The terrain? Houses?"

"No houses. They had to carry me out of a thicket of brush and up a steep embankment. Which is weird, because Joelen lived near here on Sunset. Dad said he took a back exit"—to avoid the police—"and must have taken a wrong turn. He ended up getting so disoriented that when the car went off the road, he didn't know where he was." Back then she'd bought the story.

Tyler paused, thinking. "No houses. Thick brush. This was twenty years ago?"

"Twenty-two."

"Maybe there was some undeveloped land back then, but a slope?" He shook his head. "Farther north, maybe."

"It never made any sense to me, either. When I asked an attorney if I could find the accident report, he told me it was too late. Those records had been destroyed."

"Really? Maybe he was talking about the paper copies. In the seventies they started transferring data to fiche. But it's all still there, indexed by date. So if police responded, and you know the date of the accident, it shouldn't be hard to find."

"But Sy said—" Deirdre stopped. Of course. Sy was probably trying to protect her, too.

"You're sure you want to know? Because I can look it up for you if you want."

Could it be this easy? All she had to do was say yes? Maybe her father had been right, and as a child she'd been better off not knowing. But that was no longer the case. "Would you? I know it sounds melodramatic, but it's as if a piece of me died and I need to know where it's buried."

Tyler nodded. "Okay then. I'll see what I can find out." He took his clipboard back out of the van and handed it to her with a pen. "Here. Write down the date and time and the make of your father's car."

Her hand shook as she wrote. *10/26/63*. She stared at the numbers. For so long she'd assumed she'd never find the place that marked the line between before and after. She added *Midnight? Austin-Healey convertible.*

"Okay. I'm on it." Tyler took the clipboard back and tossed it into the car. "And if there's anything more I can do to help, all you have to do is ask."

He was being so nice. She could learn to like this man. "Seriously, thank you," she said. "Is it okay to ask what you think about this fire?"

"Unofficially?"

"Whatever you feel comfortable sharing."

"Fire in an empty structure. No one injured." He ticked the points off on his fingers. "Started in a twenty-gallon bag of potting mix."

"You're telling me the fire started in a bag of dirt?"

"What they sell as potting mix for houseplants doesn't have much ordinary dirt in it. It's shredded bark and peat moss, plus fertilizer, of course. Under the right conditions, it burns."

"My mother used to grow geraniums. She might have left behind some potting mix. But wouldn't it need a source?"

"That's exactly the question the investigators will be asking. You can't just toss a match into the bag and expect it to go up in flames. And it certainly wouldn't spontaneously combust. At the very least, it would need a sustained heat source. A hot coal. A live wire. Or a cigarette. That's what it usually turns out to be, careless disposal of smoking materials."

Deirdre groaned. How many times had she seen her father mash his cigarette in one of her mother's plant pots? It was emblematic of her parents' incompatibility that he couldn't see why his doing it bothered Gloria so much, and Gloria couldn't understand why he couldn't stop doing it just because it bothered her.

Could her father possibly have started the fire himself? "How long would it have taken to catch fire?"

"Hard to say."

"More than a day?"

Tyler frowned. "I'm not saying it's impossible, but highly unlikely. My guess? An hour; maybe as many as four. Fewer with help."

"What kind of help?"

"Accelerant. Even in charred debris, we can detect the presence of certain chemicals."

"Is there—?"

"I won't know until I've run the tests." He grinned. "It's bizarre how life turns out. I nearly flunked chemistry at Beverly and now, when I'm not in the field, they let me use an office and what's basically a chem lab in the basement of City Hall. I get paid to produce lab reports." His wry expression turned serious. "But regardless of what started the fire, once there was an open flame it could have taken only minutes for the fire to spread. Garages are typically full of flammable liquids. Gasoline, of course. Linseed oil. Turpentine."

"Could it have been an accident?"

"Most garage fires are."

"What happens if that's what it turns out to be?"

"Accidental fire? Just property damage, no one injured or killed? Usually as far as police are concerned, case closed."

But was the fire accidental? Her father's death had turned out not to be. "And what if . . . ?"

"It was deliberately set? Insurance investigators swoop in like a flock of banshees. They'll want to know whether this fire was set with an intent to defraud. They're looking for a reason not to pay out, and they're nothing if not thorough." He paused for a few seconds. "Police get involved, too. Arson is a crime."

CHAPTER 21

Later that night, long after Tyler had driven off in the fire department van, Deirdre stood with Henry outside the garage, taking in
the miserable piles of cardboard boxes and lawn furniture that had
been left heaped in the driveway. At least the crime scene tape and
orange cones were gone. The air pulsed with crickets, and a sliver
of a crescent moon hung high in a sky that shimmered in the tepid
night air.

Had the fire been deliberately set, and if so, was it a firebug who
liked to watch things burn, or someone whose aim was to destroy her
father's garage and office and its contents? And if so, how could it *not*
be connected to her father's death?

"Promise you won't bite my head off if I ask you something,"
Deirdre said to Henry.

"What?"

She turned to face him. "First, promise."

"How can I promise if I don't know what you're going to ask?"

"Did you set this fire?"

"Did I . . ." Henry's mouth fell open. "Deirdre, how could—"

"Just answer the question. Did you?"

He glared at her. "Idiot."

"That's not an answer."

Henry paused. Then said emphatically, "No."

She stared hard at him. Used to be she could tell when he was lying. Now he seemed completely opaque. "Do you know anything about how it started?" she asked.

"No. I do not. Do you?"

She entered the garage and shined a flashlight beam across the floor. Prints from the patterned soles of rubber boots tracked through the soot, and water still dripped overhead. "Here's where it started." She shined the beam on a spot on the floor.

Henry crouched over the lighted area. He ran his finger through ashes, sniffed at them, and pulled a face.

"Tyler told me that was why they were taking so many pictures right there," Deirdre said. "He said it could have been started by accident, something like careless disposal of smoking materials. Or it could have been set."

"Why would anyone set fire to Dad's garage?" Henry said, taking the flashlight from Deirdre. "Your friend Tyler have any theories about that?"

"Why would anyone kill Dad?" she said. Henry glanced up at her, then back at the floor. "What do you have against Tyler, anyway?"

"Wasn't he the one in high school who made a big deal about there being no ROTC? He was always Mr. Straight Arrow."

"That's it? That was twenty years ago." It amazed her, the old tapes that were still running in his head. Did any of them ever outrun who they'd been in high school?

Henry walked over to where one of his motorcycles was tipped over on its side. He ran the flashlight beam across the skim of ash that now coated its twisted flank. The leather seat had been burned away, revealing bits of charred yellow foam. He shook his head. "Shit."

"That's it? Just 'shit'?"

"Hey, it's just a bike." He shrugged. "And it's insured. So's Dad's car. And the garage, too, for that matter. They're just things. Not like it got one of us or the dogs."

Someone would have to call the insurance company—and as usual that someone would end up being her. Deirdre stared up at the ceiling where the fire had burned through. A huge cleanup lay ahead of them. Any records that her father had kept up there, like their homeowner's insurance policy, had probably gone up in flames along with financial records and whatever "literary estate" he'd left for her to execute. *Execute* seemed the apt term, since that was pretty much what the fire had already done to it.

"Don't even think about going up there now," Henry said.

"I want to know how bad it is." What she really wanted to know was whether anyone had been messing around with her father's papers after she'd left and before the fire started.

"It's late," Henry went on, "and besides, there's no electricity. You don't know if it's even safe to walk around. The insurance adjuster is coming over first thing in the morning. At least wait until after the inspection—"

"You actually called the insurance company?" Deirdre said, astonished.

"You know, you're completely batshit," Henry said. "Believe it or not, I do plenty of things without you or Mom telling me I'm supposed to and then pecking me to death until they're done."

Deirdre yawned. She could feel the adrenaline that had been fueling her drain away. "I think you enjoy being pecked at. I just never thought you'd figure out where to call. Especially when most of Dad's records are probably up there." She kissed Henry lightly on the cheek. He reeked of smoke. She realized she did, too. Her clothing.

Her hair. Even her skin smelled charred. "Seriously, thank you," she said. "The truth is, I'm exhausted. What I need more than anything right now is a hot shower and my pillow. Maybe a drink to help me pass out."

"Take your shower. I'll uncork some wine," Henry said.

Ten minutes later Deirdre was in her bathroom. When the water was hot enough, she peeled off her shirt and pants and underwear and stepped into the shower, holding on to the grab bar that her parents had had installed after her accident. Smoke-scented steam filled the air as she shampooed her hair and soaped her body, then closed her eyes, letting the water pulse against her back. She couldn't help thinking about what she'd find when she went up to her father's office in the light of day and took in the destruction.

She stepped out of the shower, dried off, and put on clean underpants—her last pair—and one of her father's soft chambray shirts, the tail of which grazed the backs of her knees. Then she scooped her clothing from the floor and carried it out to the little back room off the kitchen. She was about to stuff her pants into the washing machine when she noticed a piece of paper sticking out of the pocket. She eased it out. Staring back at her from the faded snapshot was the ghost image of Joelen Nichol, on her knees in front of the window in Deirdre's father's office. The other Polaroid snapshots of young aspiring actresses had probably gone up in smoke.

Henry was right. Joelen did not look unhappy. Far from it. The corners of her mouth were curled in a bemused Mona Lisa smile, as if she were taking the photographer's measure every bit as much as he was taking hers.

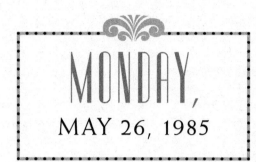

MONDAY,
MAY 26, 1985

CHAPTER 22

Before dawn, the heat broke with a crash of thunder. Deirdre had fallen asleep nearly the instant her head hit the pillow, leaving the glass of wine Henry poured for her untouched on the bedside table.

She lay awake, the quilt pulled up to her chin, listening to the steady thrum of rain. Her stomach turned queasy as she imagined water pouring into her father's office through the damaged roof and windows. Hope grew fainter by the minute that any of her father's papers could be salvaged.

When the rain let up and the sky lightened to gunmetal gray, she got out of bed. It was barely six. She pulled on her extra pair of dark leggings. In the closet she found a pair of once soft, now stiff fringed suede boots that she'd worn in college. She put them on and looked in the mirror. With her father's long work shirt, now wrinkled; her wild hair; and those boots, all she needed was a flower painted on her cheek and love beads.

In the living room, she found the flashlight that she'd used the night before and let herself out through the sliding glass door. The tip of her crutch left the lawn punctuated with a trail of tiny puddles of standing water.

The door to the garage was open, and the base of the staircase up to her father's office was dark. Even though Deirdre knew the electricity wasn't working, she tried the switch. When nothing happened, she turned on the flashlight and climbed the steps, pushing off with her crutch from each riser and taking shallow breaths of rank, smoky air.

She couldn't remember whether she'd locked the door to her father's office when she'd stormed off yesterday, her anger boiling over at the pictures her father had taken. It was ajar when she reached the top of the stairs. Swelled with moisture, the door creaked when she pushed it open. At least the firefighters hadn't had to break it down.

Her father's office was a monochromatic, ash-coated gray as daylight seeped in through empty window frames that would soon have to be boarded over. A section of ceiling had collapsed, and the floor was blackened where the fire had burned through from beneath. Several file cabinet drawers hung open, their contents strewn across the floor in a sodden mess.

But not everything had been damaged. The cover on the electric typewriter was barely singed, and the pullout couch was soaked but not burned at all. For the next hour, Deirdre worked her way around the room, sticking to the edges for safety's sake, taking a mental inventory of what had survived and what had not, prioritizing what she'd deal with after the insurance adjuster had assessed the damage. Everything on the bookshelves on one wall had been burned, and the shelves themselves had come down. But the shelves on the opposite wall were still in place. The first book she pulled down from one of those shelves was wet but probably salvageable.

Anything left in the middle of the floor had been reduced to cinders. Deirdre poked her crutch into the floorboards, carefully testing, before she shifted her weight and moved closer. The spines of the Players Directories had survived, but the pages were curled into ashes, oddly beautiful, like petals of a fragile, slate gray rose. One of the cigar boxes had survived, as had Arthur's Chasen's ashtray.

Deirdre crouched and reached across with her crutch to nudge the ashtray closer. Several marbles, disturbed by the crutch, rolled over as well. She examined them closely: they weren't marbles at all, but equal-sized turquoise beads, all of them blackened on one side. Poking around, she found more. Eight in all. She dropped them into her pocket.

Finally, Deirdre circled around to the closet door. It hung open a few inches, and Deirdre suspected that the firefighters had looked in the closet for a victim. The wood had swelled so much that she could barely wrench it the rest of the way open. Moisture and smoky stink seemed to have settled in the interior. There was the plastic bag, sitting where she'd left it.

She took out the bag, shaking off the moisture that had pooled on top. Opening it, she shined the light inside. The dress that was bundled around the knife was unscathed.

It was only later, when she'd left her father's office and was feeling her way down the dark stairway, carrying away with her the plastic bag, that she started to wonder: Why would firefighters have taken it upon themselves to open and empty out file drawers? Because, as far as she knew, she'd been the last person to set foot in her father's office before the fire, and she was certain that she'd left every one of the file drawers closed with its files intact.

CHAPTER 23

Baby and Bear greeted Deirdre as she crossed the yard. Henry opened the sliding glass door for her. It was just eight o'clock.

"What are you doing up?" Deirdre asked. She smelled coffee.

Henry held his finger to his lips and whispered, "What were you doing up in Dad's office?"

"Why are we whispering?" she whispered back.

"Mom's here."

"Mom?" Deirdre followed his gaze toward the kitchen. So she'd finally shown up.

"What were you doing up there?" Henry grabbed her arm. "You couldn't wait until after the insurance adjuster—"

She wrenched free. "Henry, I needed to see. Turns out Dad's file cabinets are open and papers are all over the floor. Someone's been up there."

"The firefighters were up there."

"Throwing around his files? How likely is that?"

"And what's that?" He was looking at the plastic bag that held the yellow dress and the knife.

Deirdre ignored the question and headed for her bedroom. She dumped the bag in the back of her closet, then closed herself in the bathroom and washed her hands and face, trying to erase the smell of smoke that clung to her like a second skin.

When she emerged, she recognized a new smell. Bacon? That seemed impossible; her mother had long ago given up eating meat. Deirdre's stomach rumbled anyway. She was starving. She headed for the kitchen.

From the back Deirdre recognized the slender figure standing at the stove, wearing a saffron-colored turban, loose-fitting cotton pants, and a linen top. "Hi, Mom."

Her mother turned around, fork in her hand. The turban framed her pale, shiny face, the skin stretched taut. She tilted her head and gave a sympathetic smile. "Hello, darling." Crow's-feet fanned at the corners of her eyes.

Deirdre said, "I'm glad you came."

"Of course I came. I'm sorry it took so long. I had car trouble. And then . . ." Her mother put down the fork and turned off the burner. She approached Deirdre and placed a warm hand on the side of her face. "Well, never mind my woes. It's nothing compared to what's been going on around here." She fingered the collar of the chambray shirt that had been Arthur's and her eyes filled with tears. "I'm so sorry about Daddy. I know you must be very sad, too."

Sadness was just one of the emotions in the mix, Deirdre thought, blinking back her own tears. She'd barely begun to sort out the other feelings.

Her mother kissed her on the forehead. "Isn't it just like him? Couldn't die like a normal person. Had to make a production out of it." She wrapped her arms around Deirdre and rocked her, not something Deirdre could remember her mother ever having done. She'd never been one for kissing boo-boos. Instead she'd clap her hands and assure Deirdre she was fine, even when it was obvious that she was not.

Gloria held her at arm's length and gently tucked a lock of hair behind Deirdre's ear. "And yet life goes on, doesn't it?" There. That was more like it. "Act four. Act five. Your father always insisted that a really good story makes you care about what's going to happen to the characters after the movie ends."

"He was full of good advice," Deirdre said.

"For everyone but himself."

The doorbell rang. Henry went to answer it.

"I hope that's not another reporter," Deirdre said. "They were camped outside yesterday, and the police have been—"

She was interrupted by Henry's return. Following him was a woman about Deirdre's age with a mane of shoulder-length, lion-colored, perfectly layered hair. She had on brown work boots and a raincoat and carried a hard hat and a clipboard, a sturdy canvas bag, and a walking stick.

"Mom? Deirdre?" Henry said. "This is the insurance adjuster."

"Sondra Dray," the woman said. Her canvas satchel thunked on the floor when she set it down to shake hands with Gloria and then Deirdre. The thick belt on her coat was hung with tools—a heavy-duty flashlight, a tape measure, a pry bar. "I was just telling Mr. Unger"—*Mr. Unger?* Deirdre's stomach turned over, and it was a moment before she realized Sondra meant Henry, not Arthur—"that I'll need at least a few hours to complete my inventory. The sooner I get started, the sooner I'll be done."

"Here, I'll take that." Henry picked up the satchel and led her out through the kitchen door.

"Your brother can be a gentleman when he feels like it," Gloria said.

"He can also be a jerk."

"That," her mother said, "is not news." She returned to the stove and turned the burner back on.

"You're cooking?"

"Now don't you start with me," Gloria said, shaking a fork at Deirdre. "Your brother's already been there. I may not be a gourmet chef, but I've always been able to put together a perfectly serviceable breakfast. I could have been a short-order cook."

Deirdre snorted a laugh. "I'm not questioning your competence. But bacon? You once told me it has more carcinogens, ounce for ounce, than tobacco."

"Not this bacon. This"—Gloria lifted a strip of what looked like pink-and-white rubber—"is soy based. Nothing toxic in it. And it doesn't taste bad as long as you forget that it's supposed to be bacon." She glanced sideways at Deirdre. "Don't look at me like that. I do remember what bacon tastes like. And yes, I do miss it."

The truth was, whatever it was that her mother was cooking, it smelled yummy. Deirdre's mouth watered.

Gloria went on, "I also brought organic eggs and whole-grain bread. Or I have granola, too. Would you rather have that?"

"Just bread." Her mother's granola was so healthy it tasted like wood chips. Deirdre opened the bag of bread and put two slices in the toaster.

"Your brother told me what happened. About your finding him." Gloria shuddered. "About the police."

"Someone killed him. And the police actually think it could have been me."

"That's ridiculous." Gloria looked out toward the pool. "Whatever else you can say about the police, they are not complete fools. Why would they think you killed him? It's absurd. You got along. Unlike plenty of other folks who might have wanted to kill your father at one time or another. Myself included."

Her mother was always so definite, regardless of whether her opinion was informed or not. For once Deirdre found that reassuring. "You weren't here," Deirdre said. "You have an alibi."

Her mother lifted a strip and checked the underside. Then she removed strip after strip of soy bacon from the pan and laid them on a paper towel. "I'm glad you called Sy."

"He talked to you?" Deirdre asked.

"Henry told me."

"Sy went with me to talk to the police."

"He's the real deal. Defended Timothy Leary. Emily Harris. Patty Hearst."

"Joelen Nichol."

"Joelen Nichol." Her mother broke an egg into the pan. It sizzled and spat. She lowered the heat. "I hear she's turned up again."

"Mom, Sy said something to me that I didn't understand. He said he helped me stay out of trouble then. And I got the impression he was talking about the night Joelen's mother's boyfriend was killed."

Her mother's hand froze in midair above the egg carton. "One egg or two?"

"Two."

"So what is she doing?"

"Joelen? She's living with Bunny—again or still, I don't know which. Selling real estate. Dad had an appointment to talk to her about putting the house on the market."

"He did, did he?" Gloria broke the second egg into the pan.

"Sounds like you're surprised that he'd hire her."

"With all the Realtors to choose from? Yes."

"I thought you were friends with her mother."

Gloria tucked a wisp of hair into her turban. "Friends? Me and Elenor Nichol? Whatever gave you that idea?"

Deirdre took in her mother's makeup-free face, baggy clothing, and battered leather sandals with rubber-tire soles. The only hint of vanity was the turban hiding her shorn hair. The idea that her mother and Elenor Nichol had been bosom buddies was preposterous.

"Something she said. When reporters and police showed up here, Joelen drove me over there and Bunny helped me dress up so I wouldn't be recognized. She said you were chorus girls together at Warner Brothers."

Gloria gave a shrug, allowing that it was true. "We worked at the same studio, along with a lot of other people."

"You and Daddy went to her parties."

"Us and half of Hollywood." Gloria bit her lip and poked at the eggs, breaking one of the yolks. "Poor thing. After the scandal, she had quite a lot to deal with. I think your father helped her out where he could. Got her a cameo in *Towering Inferno*. He was one of her many admirers." She stated that last part as if it were just a fact. "It was a mistake, letting you stay over there whenever you wanted to. I was . . . distracted."

It struck Deirdre, not for the first time, that her mother's transformation—from wisecracking broad who took her scotch straight on the rocks and bought tailored suits from the same exclusive designer as Pat Nixon, to New Age acolyte in sackcloth—had always felt like some kind of penance. But neither the old chic-but-prickly Gloria Unger nor this new dowdy-but-outwardly-serene version had even the slightest bit in common with Bunny Nichol. And Bunny was shrewd enough to know that. So why pretend otherwise?

Gloria shook the pan, loosening the eggs, and with a practiced gesture flipped them. Smiled. She reached into the overhead cupboard and pulled down a plate. Deirdre got out some silverware and a napkin and sat at the kitchen table while her mother slid the eggs onto the plate along with strips of soy bacon and the toast, which had popped. "Bon appétit!"

Deirdre picked up a piece of the soy bacon and nibbled on it. Salty. Sweet. Crisp, not greasy. Not awful at all, just odd. She stuffed the entire piece into her mouth and chased it with a bite of egg. "Did you know that Dad named me his literary executor?"

"I did." Her mother went to the sink and ran the water. "He asked if I thought it was a good idea." She shot Deirdre a quick glance as she scrubbed the pan. "I know. Not something you'd have volunteered for. Don't panic. I'm here to help. We can take a quick first pass through his papers—shouldn't take more than a day or two if we put our minds to it. With the fire, there's less to deal with."

That was an understatement. Deirdre dragged a piece of wheat toast through the yolk and put it in her mouth.

Gloria picked up a dish towel. Leaning with her back against the sink, she started drying the pan. "Have you and Henry made plans for the funeral?"

"I talked to the mortuary, but I didn't know what to say about a service. The coroner is supposed to release Dad's body today."

"Right," her mother said, drying her hands, snapping the dish towel and folding it smartly. "Finish your breakfast. Then get me the phone number of the funeral home and find me your father's Rolodex. We'll schedule a service for day after tomorrow. Keep it simple. Tasteful. I'll get some of his friends to say a few words. I'll have food delivered to the house for after. And after it's all over, how about the three of us drive out to Paradise Cove? Scatter your father's ashes in the sea. He always said he was part fish. Then I'll take you and Henry to Holiday House. I haven't been back there in ages. We can order cracked crab and champagne and sit out on the patio and toast your father's memory."

Gratitude pulsed through Deirdre. Henry had called the insurance company. Her mother was offering to organize the funeral and help sort through Arthur's papers. At least she wasn't going to be on her own acting out the role of the dutiful daughter, something she'd never been very good at anyway.

"Holiday House. That sounds perfect," she said. And it did. Her father would have loved to see them toasting him, the consummate celebrity wannabe, at the storied celebrity hangout. It was where JFK and Marilyn, Liz and Eddie, Frankie and Ava had supposedly shared intimate tête-à-têtes and then slipped off to the attached no-tell motel. Its ultramodern design of glass and steel and stone and spectacular view would have made it a tourist attraction if the maître d' hadn't courteously but firmly barred anyone who smacked of tourist or, even worse, paparazzi. Deirdre had a soft spot for it as well. She'd once handled the sale of a photograph by Man Ray of a weather-beaten shipwreck washed up on a stretch of beach that could only be viewed from the Holiday House patio.

"That's it then. Decided," Gloria said with a wry smile. She sat at the kitchen table opposite Deirdre, took a deep breath, and bowed her head. Her lips moved in a whisper as she rubbed together the thumb and fingers of her left hand. This was Gloria's way of maintaining her cherished tranquility, reciting a mantra and fingering the string of prayer beads that for years she'd worn wrapped around her wrist. Portable valium, Arthur used to call them. One hundred and eight beads, four lapis lazuli and the rest turquoise.

Only now there was no string of beads wrapped around Gloria's wrist.

CHAPTER 24

Missing something?" Deirdre reached across the kitchen table for her mother's hand and dropped two of the beads she'd found among the ashes on the floor of her father's garage office into Gloria's up-turned palm. "Three guesses where I found them."

Her mother's eyes snapped open, but she didn't say anything.

"You weren't late because you had car trouble. You were here yesterday. It was you I saw up there in the window before the fire, wasn't it?"

Gloria pursed her lips and rubbed her fingers together. "Along the road to truth, there are only two mistakes you can make. Not starting. And not going all the way."

Serenity could be so irritating. "Did you set the fire?"

Gloria reared back as if she'd been slapped. "Of course I did not set the goddamn fire. Do you think I'd have been up in your father's office if I had?"

That, at least, made some sense. "Then what were you doing up there? And why didn't you come in? You could have at least—" What? Shown up? Said hello? Been there for Deirdre and Henry?

"I'm sorry. I'm so sorry. I—" Gloria moved to embrace her.

"Sorry?" Deirdre sobbed and pushed her away. "You never think of anyone but yourself."

Her mother held up her hands and backed off. "Okay. Fair enough. You have every right to be angry. Let me try to explain. I got back yesterday." She swallowed. "And actually I did call. I called because I wanted to be sure you and Henry weren't going to be here when I arrived."

Deirdre felt her jaw drop. "Because?"

"Because . . ." Tension drained from her mother's face. "Deirdre, I knew you'd be going through your father's papers. I was trying to protect you and your brother from what you might find."

"I don't need protecting. And Henry certainly doesn't. And why now? How long's it been since I've seen you? Months? And then only because I drove to Twentynine Palms." Her mother flinched, but Deirdre kept going. "Besides, if you were trying to protect us, that train left the station a good long time ago."

"Deirdre, Deirdre. Don't." Her mother gave her a long, mournful look. "Holding on to anger is like holding on to a hot coal."

"Spare me the bumper stickers. Why were you up in his office?"

"Deirdre, your father never meant to hurt you."

"What were you looking for? His creepy snapshots?"

Gloria blinked. "Snapshots?"

"You didn't know? He was bringing young women, some of them just teenagers, up to his office and taking their pictures. And I can only imagine what else."

"Teenagers?" Creases deepened between her mother's eyes. "I don't believe it."

"The photographs got destroyed in the fire, but I saved one of them." Deirdre went into the laundry room and got the Polaroid she'd left on the shelf. She slammed it down on the kitchen table.

Her mother recoiled. "Oh my." She stared at the photograph for a moment, then across at Deirdre. "Joelen Nichol."

"She's the only one I recognized." Deirdre turned the picture over to show her the asterisks written on the back. "He even rated them. See?"

"And you think your father would . . . with your best friend? You can't seriously believe that." Gloria took the picture from Deirdre and held Joelen's face under the light. "She was a beautiful girl, wasn't she? And I don't doubt that she was"—she paused for a moment—"precocious, in some respects. Frankly, I wasn't thrilled that you and she were such close friends. But I had no idea that anything like this was going on." She put the picture down on the table and looked hard at Deirdre. "I don't know everything that your father was getting up to. I didn't want to know because I was leaving him, and it would have been just one more thing to be furious about, and I knew enough already. It would have been like drinking poison and wanting *him* to die." Realizing what she'd said, Gloria shook her head. "I don't mean that literally, of course. I'd never have wanted him to . . . I mean . . . I just meant that metaphorically. But here's the thing. Joelen was still a teenager when this picture was taken. And whatever else Arthur may have been, he was not a pedophile."

CHAPTER 25

I'm back." At the sound of Henry's voice, Gloria shot up from the kitchen table. The dogs tumbled into the room and swarmed at her feet. She reached over to the counter for two pieces of raw soy bacon. They'd barely hit the floor before the dogs had scarfed them up.

"Is the insurance adjuster done out there?" Gloria asked Henry.

"She's done with the garage downstairs. Other than the bikes and the car, there wasn't a whole lot more to claim. Now she's upstairs, working on the office." Henry helped himself to a piece of fake bacon. Sniffed. Took a bite. Chewed. Pulled a face. "What *is* this?"

"It's healthy," Deirdre said. "Mom brought it."

"It's weird," he said, snagging a second piece.

"When your brother was a toddler, he ate carpet backing," Gloria said. "A real connoisseur of kapok."

"Ah! So *that's* what this tastes like," Henry said, popping the last piece into his mouth. "Sondra says they won't be able to begin processing the claim without a copy of the official incident report. One of us has to go to City Hall and request it. Even with that, the bureaucracy can take weeks to spit out the report . . . *unless* it's goosed along by someone on the inside." Henry eyed Deirdre. "Know anyone who might be able to help?"

"I do not *know*"—Deirdre drew quote marks in the air—"Tyler Corrigan."

"Tyler?" Gloria said. "The boy who lived across the street?"

"Used to show off for Deirdre," Henry said. "He was kind of a prick."

"He was a nice boy," her mother said. "Delivered our newspaper for a while."

"He's the city's lead arson investigator," Henry said, "and Sondra says he's the one who signs off on cases."

"So now we're a case?" Deirdre said. Henry's fixation on Tyler was starting to annoy her. "How is *Sondra* doing?"

"She's up there," Henry said, "literally picking the place apart. Talking into a cassette recorder and making an inventory of everything that got damaged, from the carpet to the toilet paper dispenser. It's like watching an autopsy. Slow. Painstaking. Messy."

"I'll bet," Deirdre said, sniffing at her own fingers. She didn't know if that was the soy bacon or barbecued prayer beads that she smelled.

"She's got rubber gloves and baggies that go over her boots. The smell and the heat got to me right away, but she's oblivious. Girl knows how to travel—she's got water in her backpack and a very long straw." Henry poured himself a cup of coffee and sat at the table. "So what were you two talking about?"

"Those photographs that were stuck in the Players Directories that Dad wanted you to throw away? There's only one that didn't get incinerated." Deirdre turned it over so he could see Joelen's face.

For a few moments, the only sounds in the room were Baby's claws clicking across the floor and a chuffing as she sniffed, ever hopeful, at the floor where bacon had landed. Deirdre waited until she couldn't any longer. "Recognize her?"

Henry raised his eyebrows and smirked, allowing that he did.

Deirdre turned the picture over to show him the asterisks. "Mom says Dad didn't write those."

Henry picked up the snapshot. "Really?" He and Gloria exchanged a look.

"What?" Deirdre said.

"*What* what?" Henry said.

"Don't give me that. I'm not blind. What's up with you two?"

Gloria said, "Henry, your sister thinks your father was responsible for that." She pointed to the photograph.

"And the others like it," Deirdre said.

"He was responsible." Henry stared impassively at Gloria. "A regular trailblazer."

"Henry—" Gloria started.

"And what do you know about it?" Henry said, cutting her off. "You were on *the path*." *The path* was the term that their mother used for her cleansing journey to what she called self-awakening. It had started long before she left Arthur, and even though Deirdre knew Gloria had needed to do something to preserve her own sanity, like Henry she resented the way Gloria had spun herself a protective cocoon.

Gloria reared back. "And look what you were on your way to, Henry." She spread her arms and looked around. "Still living with your father in a house that's literally falling down around you."

"It wasn't my fault that I got thrown out of school. My roommate—"

"Right. He's the one who made you stop going to classes. Did he make you give up music and wreck your car, too?"

"Oh, remind me again, how much did you pay for that car?"

Deirdre knew from experience that they were just getting warmed up. "Stop it!" she said, standing so fast that her chair tipped over backward. She snatched the photograph from Henry, nabbed her crutch, walked her plate to the sink, and dropped it in with a clatter. Across the room, her messenger bag hung from a hook by the back door. She grabbed it. It was still damp and weighed almost nothing. All that was in it was her keys and wallet. She slipped the photograph in, too, and headed for the door.

"Where are you going?" Gloria asked.

"Out."

"Go to City Hall, why don't you," Henry said, "and file the request for the form we need."

The last thing Deirdre felt like doing at that moment was agreeing with Henry, but it was actually a good suggestion. She paused, the door open. "What's it called?"

"An incident report," Henry said. "And remember to charm Tyler, won't you?"

Deirdre stepped outside and slammed the door behind her. She clumped down the back steps, out the driveway, and into the street to her car. She'd started the engine when she realized a ticket was stuck to her windshield. She got out and snagged it. *Overnight parking* was checked. There was an envelope for remitting her twenty-five-dollar fine. *Damn.* She got back into the car, jammed the ticket in her glove compartment, and took off.

Charm Tyler. She glanced at her reflection in her rearview mirror. Eyes wild. Skin blotchy. Hair a rat's nest. On top of that, her outfit—those ridiculous boots and her father's shirt—made her look as if she were on her way to a Halloween party. She needed to pull herself together if she was going to get anywhere in the charm department.

It had been many years since Deirdre had shopped for clothes or gotten her hair cut in Beverly Hills. She parked in the lot behind the stores on Little Santa Monica near Beverly Drive and fed some coins into the meter. Across the street was the park where she used to stand and wave at trains that rode through. If she was lucky, someone hanging out of the last car, a real red caboose, would wave back at her. That was even better than getting a semi on the freeway to toot its air horn at you.

Walking along Little Santa Monica, feeling as if she were throwing a dart at a map, she stopped in front of Latour's Hair Salon. A small WALK-INS WELCOME sign was in the window. She pushed open the heavy wood door and stepped inside.

A spectrally thin young woman in a black turtleneck and fringed leather vest stood at the front desk, talking on the phone. Her gaze flickered over Deirdre and then away. It was the same dismissive look the clerk at Jax had given her when she was in high school and ventured into the elegant store where the popular girls at school bought their straight skirts and shells and matching Geistex sweaters. Back then, Deirdre had turned tail and fled. Didn't matter that she had saved up enough from babysitting to pay for any of their outfits.

Now she held her ground. Behind the counter, stations on facing walls were half-full of customers and the air was laden with the sewer-gas smell of perms.

Finally the receptionist got off the phone. She gave Deirdre a brittle smile. "Do you have an appointment?"

"Do I need one? I'd like to get my hair cut." Quite deliberately Deirdre laid her crutch on the desk.

The woman looked startled for a moment, then turned and buried her nose in an appointment ledger. "Cut? Blow-dry?"

"Please."

An hour later, Deirdre emerged from the salon, her hair cut short and layered, just framing her face, the bangs poufy and saucily blown to the side. She caught glimpses of her new self reflected in store windows as she continued to Rodeo Drive. For so many years she'd cursed her curls and now they were in style. The chambray shirt and boots, on the other hand, had to go.

She entered a new shopping complex with a glass atrium. She couldn't remember what had been at that address when she was growing up—maybe Uncle Bernie's, the toy store with a lemonade tree in the back. Now it was home to Gucci, Giorgio, and Chanel. They made Jax look like J.J. Newberry.

Farther down the street Deirdre passed boutique after boutique. Finally she entered a dancewear store and bought a dark purple scoop-necked leotard, black leggings, and a flowy white silk shirt that grazed her knees. She passed on the slouchy pink leg warmers the Jennifer Beals–look-alike salesgirl tried to foist on her.

Next door, among Indian bedspreads, Moroccan leather hand-bags, and feathered earrings, she found a suede belt with a brightly enameled buckle and a long Indian scarf in reds and pinks. A few doors down was a consignment shop with a GOING OUT OF BUSINESS, LOST OUR LEASE sign. There Deirdre found a whole row of what looked like brand-new Keds. She bought two pairs in white—she always had to buy two pairs of shoes because one foot was now two sizes smaller than the other.

She ducked into the consignment shop's makeshift dress-ing room—sheets hung from a clothesline in a back corner of the store—and stripped off her clothes, then assembled her new outfit. She fluffed her newly shorn hair with her fingers, cocked her hip, and examined her reflection in the mirror. *Locked and loaded.*

She was ready to find Tyler Corrigan.

CHAPTER 26

City Hall was nearby, but just a little too far for Deirdre to walk there and back with her bad leg. So she drove the few blocks over and parked in a handicapped spot in front. This time no news crews were there filming.

She climbed the long, broad front staircase, though there was probably a handicapped entrance at ground level. She caught her reflection in the glass of the door just before she pushed it open. The hair was cute and bouncy, the shirt elegant and casual, the sneakers a hint that she wasn't taking herself too seriously.

Cool air oozed out as she stepped into the lobby, a magnificent Spanish Renaissance two-story entryway with terrazzo floors, white marble walls, and a coffered ceiling. The vast space hummed with a steady flow of uniformed officers, men and the occasional woman in business suits carrying thick briefcases, and lost-looking citizens who were probably there to file for tax abatements, report for jury duty, or, like her, request a copy of an official document.

It was past noon, and the soy bacon and eggs seemed a long time ago. Deirdre bought a granola bar from a newsstand tucked incongruously in the corner under a massive California state flag and wolfed it down. She chased it with a stick of Dentyne, hoping to dispel the miasma of perfumed conditioner and hair gel that felt as if it were floating in a thick cloud around her head.

She had no desire to run into Detective Martinez, so she made her way quickly down the hall, following the signs to Public Records. The room had linoleum, not terrazzo, on the floor, and its walls were painted mustard yellow. Six rows of folding chairs took up half the space, most of the seats taken. A man wearing a bright green golf shirt and sunglasses on top of his bald head brushed past her on his way to the door. "Good luck," he said. "Effing incompetence. An hour and a half wasted."

The number 110 flashed over a counter with a bank of clerk's stations. Deirdre took a number from the feeder—*142*. She found the Request for Records form on one of the shelves, stood in the back, and started to fill it out. Her name. Address. She checked the box beside "Incident Report," then wrote in the date and time of the fire, the address, and a description. When she finished, the number counter had crept up to 112. Two harried clerks seemed to be actually serving customers. Several others were on phones, another hunched over his desk, all of them studiously avoiding eye contact with the thirty-plus impatient citizens sitting and standing beyond the safe barrier of the counter.

Clearly, she had plenty of time to kill. Tyler had said his office was next to some kind of lab in the basement. Deirdre left the waiting area and wandered back through the hall to the atrium lobby. There she found the elevators, their outer sliding doors elaborate wrought-iron grillwork. She stepped inside one and pressed B. The elevator descended two floors and slid open to reveal a basement hallway.

Paint the color of wet sand peeled on the walls. Two rows of Wanted posters—all men—hung on the bulletin board across the hall. The air was cooler and clammier than on the main floor, and Deirdre wondered if that was a whiff of formaldehyde under a layer of Pine-Sol. Signs pointed one way to Maintenance and the elevator, the other way to the restrooms, Arson Investigation, Crime Lab, and Records Storage.

Deirdre followed the sign pointing toward Arson Investigation, continuing to a door with a pebbled glass inset stenciled with the words ARSON UNIT. She was about to reach for the knob when the door opened. A man she didn't recognize came out. He held the door for her.

The Arson Unit was a single room, mostly bare with a half-dozen desks crowded in, surrounded by shelves and file cabinets. A folding table against a wall was loaded with pamphlets. On the side wall was pinned a massive gray-and-green topographic map with colored pushpins stuck in it.

Tyler was sitting at a desk under a high window by the back wall. He was engrossed in some typewritten pages, switching between writing in pen and highlighting with a yellow marker. Deirdre headed his way. When she was within reaching distance, she said, "Tyler?"

He looked up. "Deirdre!" He shoved the papers he'd been working on into a file folder and stood, grazing his head on one of the pipes that ran overhead. "Hey. I was just thinking about you." His eyes widened. "You look . . . different."

Deirdre felt a flush creep up her neck. "I hope it's an okay different."

"Very okay. I was"—he shot a guilty look at the closed file folder—"just working on your case. Report's almost finished."

"I thought it takes weeks."

"Who told you that?"

"Our claims adjuster."

"I guess it can take that long to get processed once I file it. But the analysis—well, we know pretty much what we're dealing with. Most of the time, anyway."

"As in now?"

He nodded.

"So? Tell me. You can tell me, can't you? What started the fire?"

Tyler sat. Deirdre could feel herself trembling as she waited for his answer.

"I can tell you what we know," he said. "The fire started right where we originally thought it did. In a bag of potting mix."

"Right. Probably left over from years ago when Mom was still living there."

Tyler gave her an uneasy look. "You said your mother grew geraniums?"

"Scented geraniums," Deirdre said, wondering where this was going.

"The thing is, the concentration of ammonium nitrate in that potting mix is much too high. It would have burned the roots of her plants. Even amateur horticulturists know that. Maybe your father bought it?"

"Not likely," Deirdre said. There was only one way her father messed around with potting mix. "Were there any cigarette butts in it?"

"There were. But they're not what started the fire."

Deirdre took a deep breath. "So what are you saying?"

"It looks like someone tried to make it appear as if the fire was caused by careless disposal of smoking materials. So we'd find the cigarette butts and stop looking for what really fueled the fire."

"Which was?"

"Good old-fashioned kerosene." Tyler gave her a long, somber look.

Arson. Deirdre dropped into the chair opposite his desk. It wasn't unexpected, but still the certainty of the verdict knocked the air out of her. Someone had set fire to her father's garage. Someone had killed her father. "Who? Why?"

"Those are questions for the police."

Deirdre tried to put it together. Cigarette butts stuck into kerosene-laced potting mix that her mother never would have purchased. Whoever did that knew her father was a smoker who stubbed out his cigarettes wherever happened to be convenient. "Could it have been set up in advance?" she asked.

"Probably was. It would be simple. Lace the mix with kerosene. Wait till there's no one around, sneak in, and put the bag in the garage. Poke a few burning cigarettes into it and let nature take its course. Might have taken a few minutes or a few hours to really get going, but it was a pretty sure bet that eventually it would."

Only whoever it was had miscalculated. The house might have been empty, but their mother was in the garage's second-floor office. While Deirdre was pulling the alarm, Gloria must have bolted and then tried to hide the fact that she'd been there. Deirdre never would have known if she hadn't found the prayer beads.

"So there's no way it could have been an accident?" Deirdre said. She knew she was grasping at straws.

"An accidental kerosene spill at just the right moment? How likely is that?" Tyler paused. "You can be sure that the insurance company will bring in a professional investigator to see if the fire was set for financial gain."

Deirdre groaned. "Here we go. They'll think one of us did it."

"Maybe. But fire damage doesn't add value to a property you're about to sell. So what would you have stood to gain?"

Deirdre thought about it. If the fire wasn't set for financial gain, then why? Pure malice? Why target just the garage? Unless that was the point, maybe to destroy what was in the garage, including whatever her mother was up there trying to keep Deirdre and Henry from finding.

"Well, thank you for telling me," Deirdre said. She started to get up.

"Deirdre, there's more. I found your accident report." Tyler's solemn tone and grave expression dropped her back into the chair. She swallowed hard and waited for him to go on.

"The records from 1963 are all on microfiche, so it should have been easy to find. And it would have been . . . if the accident had been in Beverly Hills. But it wasn't."

Not in Beverly Hills. That meant that her father hadn't been driving her home from Joelen's house. He'd been driving . . . where? Deirdre sat back and took a deep, shuddering breath.

"Once I was sure the report wasn't in our records, I called a buddy over at the LAPD. They've got a huge repository. Good thing there's not many Austin-Healey convertibles out there to get into traffic accidents. He found it and sent me a copy." He opened his desk drawer, drew out two grainy faxes, and laid them on the desk in front of Deirdre.

She leaned forward. Across the top in capital letters were the words *POLICE INCIDENT REPORT*. Below that:

```
Crash investigator: TROOPER MITCHELL


Vehicle # [1] Year [1957] Make [AUHE]
Model [CV]
```

Deirdre ran her fingers across the letters. This was the footprint she'd been sure she'd never find.

Then she read the next line.

```
Driver [DEIRDRE UNGER] [F] [15] of [BEVERLY
HILLS, CA]
```

It felt as if the floor had opened up under her and she was in free fall. There had to be some mistake. "This has my name as the driver." When Tyler just nodded, she said, "But how could that be? I remember riding in the *passenger* seat. The top was down. I was thrown from the car. It was cold. I . . . . I can remember all kinds of details."

"You thought you were in Beverly Hills."

"I did . . . and I didn't. I wanted to believe that, but it never made any sense. Even with a detour in the wrong direction, it just wasn't right. But this? This is completely insane."

"I'm sorry. I know it's not what you expected."

Deirdre gripped the arm of the chair. *She'd driven the car off the road. Not her father.* "I'm just trying to understand."

For a minute, Tyler didn't say anything, giving her time to absorb the shock. Then he said, "You wanted to know where it happened." He turned to the second stapled sheet and pointed to a paragraph in the middle of the page.

Deirdre pulled the faxed sheets closer and read.

Narrative: V1 DRIVER WAS DRIVING EAST ON MULHOLLAND. V1 CRASHED INTO A GUARDRAIL LOCATED AT APPROXIMATELY 10536 MULHOL-LAND DRIVE. DRIVER EJECTED FROM THE CAR. DRIVER TRANSPORTED TO NORTHRIDGE HOSPITAL. THE CRASH REMAINS UNDER INVESTIGATION AND CHARGES ARE PENDING.

Deirdre shook her head, and then shook it again. *Mulholland Drive?* It was at least five miles from the Nichols' house, and in the opposite direction from home.

Tyler went over to the map on the wall. He stuck a white pushpin at a curve on a road highlighted in yellow, a road that snaked along the crest of the finely drawn, crenellated landscape that was the Santa Monica Mountains. "You're not the only one who's wiped out there. There's a reason they call that spot Suicide Bend."

Deirdre read aloud the final line of the report. "'The crash remains under investigation and charges are pending.' What does that mean?"

"You were never charged?"

"I don't remembering being charged. But I don't remember driv-ing, either." Maybe this was what Sy had meant when he said he'd kept her out of trouble *then*. No charges.

She walked up to the map and stared at the white pushpin. She hadn't driven that stretch in many years, but she knew it well. After she'd mastered driving in the flats between Santa Monica and Sunset, her father had taken her into the canyons for serious driving lessons. There, she'd learned to start from a dead stop on a steep incline without rolling backward. To take curves, downshifting first, judging how well the road was banked to determine how much to decelerate going in and how fast she could accelerate coming out. Always, always, her father reminded her, *stay in control and stay in your goddamned lane.*

Driving Mulholland was the ultimate test. In her mind's eye Deirdre could run the curves and straightaways of the infamous road that was known as "the snake," catching glimpses of the vast and usually smog-skimmed San Fernando Valley unfurling to the northwest.

With her finger she traced the yellow-highlighted road. She tried to envision the spot, right at a sharp elbow. Was this where her father had always cautioned her to respect the signage and slow the hell down? Where he'd once made her pull over and hike twenty minutes down a steep embankment until they reached a Dodge Dart lying in the scrub, its blue paint nearly rusted away? Nearby, in a dry streambed, a red Porsche had lain on its back, looking like the empty carapace of a stranded beetle. Deirdre had peered into the car through the broken windshield, fully expecting to find a skeleton sitting at the wheel. But the car's interior had been stripped, filled only with a tangle of vines and what she later realized was poison oak. Surely her father had been trying to convey a lesson about the dire consequences of reckless driving, but what stayed with Deirdre, even now, was the brutal beauty of the landscape and the power of time.

Maybe she'd been going too fast that night. Maybe she'd been blinded by oncoming headlights. Swerved to avoid another driver? Skidded on a gravel spill?

But why had she been there at all, and where on earth had she thought she was going?

CHAPTER 27

Deirdre left Tyler's office feeling numb. She barely registered his parting words: "Call me if there's anything more I can do." He added, "Anytime." *Really?* And then, as if he'd read her mind, he'd written his home and office phone numbers on the accident report and repeated, "Anytime."

She sleepwalked from City Hall out to her car, nearly missing a step off the curb. When she settled into her car, she gripped the steering wheel tightly, holding on to the present as if it were a life preserver as piece by piece her memories bumped up, at last, against facts. She'd gone for so many years assuming she'd never know exactly where the car had crashed, and now, just like that, she had the answer.

So much for the fantasy that her father had taken a wrong turn leaving the Nichols' estate. One thing was clear. She hadn't been taken to Northridge Hospital because of their trauma unit. She'd been taken there because it was the closest hospital.

So where had it come from, her vivid memory of her father helping her down the Nichols' dark back stairs and out to the car? Of curling up on the passenger seat, shivering with cold because the top was down and she was wearing only her pajamas? Of her father's voice telling her to "sleep tight," followed by a kiss on her forehead? Of feeling so sick and dizzy when the car started to move that she'd had to close her eyes? Had she simply imagined her father's silhouette at the wheel?

She closed her eyes now. Were her memories of what came next as tainted? The sound of metal on metal at the moment of collision. She didn't remember being airborne, only the bone-jarring impact as she landed. The horrifying sound of her femur cracking. And then pain. Pain so intense she was afraid to move. Afraid to look.

She'd heard a groan in the dark, and her name: "Deirdre?" If it hadn't been her father's voice, then whose was it?

She must have passed out because the next thing she remembered was pebbles and grit hitting her face. Footsteps scrabbling. Hands reaching for her. She'd tried to reach back.

"It's a girl," a man's voice had called out. "She's hurt bad. Better call an ambulance, quick. I'm afraid to move her."

A motorcycle revved in the distance, somewhere above her, and roared off. Then quiet enveloped her. Crickets. The rustling of a breeze through tree branches. And pain, still so much pain.

The voice that called to her from somewhere in the dark as she lay on the embankment, trying not to lose consciousness as she waited for help, could not have been her father's. The labored breathing must have been her own.

She'd heard the first siren, a cry, deep in the night. She imagined pulling it toward her, reeling it in like a hawk caught on a fishing line. Finally, bright lights. Voices. The crunch of feet on unstable hillside. A reassuring hand on her shoulder. Gentle pressure. Antiseptic smell. Then pain like lightning seared through her as she was jostled and lifted, brush pulling at her clothing and snagging in her hair. That was her own voice that she heard, screaming into the night.

"It's going to be all right." A woman's voice. "We have to get you out of here. I know you're hurt. This should help. Hold still. Just a pinch." She'd felt a prick on her arm and slowly, gradually, she disconnected. The pain took shape and pulsed in front of her as the stretcher was lifted, more like heat lightning than jagged spikes, a phantom that grew ever more transparent with each step closer to the light. To the street.

"Deirdre . . ." A man's voice. She'd strained to see behind her, but her head was too heavy and it hurt too much to move. Finally she floated into the ambulance, from noise to stillness, from shadow to bright. The slam of the doors was muffled, and she was in another world of whiteness and stainless steel and blood.

The next morning Deirdre had woken up heavily sedated and still in pain. Her head ached and dark circles under her bloodshot eyes made it look as if she'd been punched in the face. Her father sat grim-faced by her bed. He'd emerged from the accident unscathed. He'd been belted in—that's what he told her. She hadn't.

At the knock on the window, Deirdre jolted out of the past. A woman in a dark uniform was peering in at her through the windshield. A meter maid.

The last thing she needed was another parking ticket. Deirdre rolled down the window and called out, "Thank you! I was just leaving." As she backed out, she realized she still had the accident report clutched in her hand, along with her number 142 from the Records Office.

The night Tito was killed she might have gotten into her father's car and, upset and disoriented, ended up on Mulholland. Now she drove there deliberately. It was all she could do to keep from blowing through stop sign after stop sign as she crossed the empty intersections between residential blocks, driving north on Beverly.

Could her fifteen-year-old self have driven off in her father's car? Her gut said *no way.* Drive without a driver's license? Not the good girl who'd detour a half block to avoid jaywalking. Who'd never been tardy to school, never ventured into the school hallway without a pass, never borrowed a library book she hadn't returned. Not the girl who'd walked all the way back to J.J. Newberry in the rain to return a tube of Passionate Pink lipstick that her best friend had slipped into her pocket.

No. She'd never have taken off in her father's car, not unless she'd been running from the devil himself. And no matter how drunk she'd been, she'd have remembered that.

By the time Deirdre was above Sunset her grip on the wheel had loosened. The mystique of Mulholland Drive had spawned urban legends: tales of a headless hitchhiker, of a depraved sex maniac with a hook for an arm who stalked couples necking in their cars at the overlooks, of a phantom Ferrari that led motorists off cliffs. As if the road's twists and turns weren't hairy enough, many a driver saw bodies hanging among the dangling boughs of willow trees that lined Mulholland's edges. It didn't help that the Mafia really had used the road's steep banks to dispose of corpses.

It would take some of the fun out of it, driving an automatic. But with only one good leg, operating a stick shift was impossible. It was like trying to hitchhike without a thumb. She passed a grassy park and kept on going. There was the gate that her father told her led to what had once been Jimmy Cagney's estate. A driveway that disappeared into the bushes led to the home of Mel Torme. Arborvitae lined the driveway to Charlton Heston's estate.

By the time Deirdre reached the turn onto Mulholland she was calm. In the zone. She waited at the stop sign as a motorcycle flew past. Then another. Mulholland was dangerous for motorcycles, and yet this was where they all came to be challenged.

She flipped on the radio. As if summoned from the underworld, there was Mötley Crüe. *Shout! Shout! Shout!* The pounding beat filled the car. Deirdre's heart kicked into gear as she turned and accelerated, her tires spitting gravel. She pictured the overlook where she was headed. Grasping the wheel with two hands, she eased into the first curve, the Valley rising before her. She accelerated past the entrance to Coldwater Canyon Park, then took the next curve a bit too fast and felt the rear wheels start to slide toward a rock face.

Adrenaline pulsed in her ears along with the Crüe's sinister chant. She amped the volume until she could feel the bass drums and snares vibrating through the steering column. Under her, the road undulated and straightened, tilting and righting itself. Mentally she tracked her path as she beat the steering wheel with the heel of her hand. She sped past one overlook, then another. She knew she was getting near where Tyler had stuck the white pushpin in the map.

Belatedly, she registered the 10 mph hard right arrow and skid marks all over the road. She was already into the turn before she realized what was happening. The car slew sideways. *Turn into it, turn into it!* Her father's voice rang in her head. *Steer in the direction of the skid!*

It was too late for a tidy recovery. The car slid backward, toward a cluster of motorcycles parked at the overlook. Deirdre pumped the brakes, praying that the tires would gain traction. In her rearview mirror, she watched the bikers leap out of the way, like fleas off a dog's back, as the car fishtailed to a halt, a cloud of dust blooming around her.

CHAPTER 28

Thank God Deirdre had missed the bikers. Missed the bikes. Not to mention missed smashing into the guardrail and going over the edge. Heart hammering, she peeled her fingers off the steering wheel for the second time that day, bashed the radio into silence, and killed the engine. A green-and-white sign at the edge of the parking area read SUICIDE BEND OVERLOOK.

This was the spot where she'd crashed twenty-two years ago.

Emerging from the dust in front of her was a guy with a blue bandanna tied Indian style over his forehead. He had on a black leather jacket that might, in another lifetime, possibly have zipped over his paunch. He stomped over to her car until his presence filled the windshield, flicked a cigarette on the ground, and crushed it with the sole of a tooled black cowboy boot, then folded his arms across his chest and glared at her.

Deirdre reached for her crutch, opened the door, and got out. "Sorry, sorry!" She held up a hand in surrender. "Is everyone okay?"

The big biker took off his mirrored aviator glasses. His hair was nearly all gray and pulled back into a long, thin ponytail. "You act as if you want to get killed," he said, his voice a gravelly John Wayne imitation.

Deirdre relaxed a notch. It was a line from *Gunfight at the O.K. Corral*, a movie John Wayne wasn't in. She even knew Doc Holliday's deadpan response: *Maybe I do.* But now was not the time to show off.

"Nice wheels," the big biker went on, stepping over to her Mercedes and stroking its fender. "Can it do any other tricks?"

The other dudes who'd gathered around cracked up. Deirdre's face burned.

"Hey, you okay?" one of them asked. "Maybe you'd better sit a spell."

"Thanks," she said. "I'm fine. Just stupid."

That earned nods all around. Then, one by one, they got on their bikes and took off. Last to leave was the guy who'd greeted her, revving a whole lot louder than he needed to and shooting a cloud of soot out the tailpipe. "Let's be careful out there," he shouted to her over the din. *Hill Street Blues.* "I wouldn't want to find your pretty little bumper hanging from one of these trees." Sounded like that line he'd written all by himself. He put his glasses back on and roared off. *Into the sunset*, only it was well past high noon.

A skim of fine dust had settled over Deirdre's car. With her finger, she wrote on the front fender: JERK. What she should have scrawled there was DAMNED LUCKY THIS TIME. Her rear wheels were just a few feet from a forty-five-degree drop. She leaned against the guardrail, waiting for her heart to stop pounding. Her mother's string of prayer beads would have come in handy. Her white sneakers were streaked with dust and she felt ridiculous in her new outfit with her perfect hair.

Two cars sped past. Then a bike. The sweat coating Deirdre's face cooled as she turned and gazed out past trees and scrub and into the omnipresent haze that settled over Sherman Oaks, turning landmarks, if there'd been any, into smudges.

A sharp smell wafted from the surrounding chaparral. For a moment it took her back to when she'd been carried from the underbrush. She remembered staring up at a moon that seemed to be caught in tree branches.

But she didn't remember hearing the sounds that she heard now, thunks and clangs like dull wind chimes, from beyond the edge of the overlook. She stood and turned to get a better look. There really was a car bumper hanging from a branch of one of the trees growing on the embankment. Sunlight reflected off its dull chrome. The remnants of a bumper sticker, REAGAN in blue block letters under a wave of stars and stripes, came in and out of view as the bumper twisted in the breeze. Other branches were hung with hubcaps and license plates. One sagged under the weight of a car's dented front grille with a Volkswagen W in the middle.

At the tree's base, maybe fifteen feet down a scrubby incline, lay bouquets of flowers, one merely wilted, the rest virtually mummified, along with framed photographs and stuffed toys, including a teddy bear that looked like her Ollie. But not Ollie, of course.

As Tyler had said, there was a reason this spot was called Suicide Bend. Nailed to the tree's thick trunk was a plank of wood hand-lettered in red paint: SLOW DOWN OR REST IN PEACE.

All the way back to the house, Deirdre seethed. She scolded herself for driving so stupidly and putting her own and others' lives at risk. She was no longer fifteen years old. She was also furious that all these years she'd allowed herself to be convinced that there was no way to find out where she'd crashed. That she'd been blind to the fact that she'd been driving. What else didn't she know?

She parked the car in front of the house and went inside, slamming the door behind her. "Mom? Henry?" she called out.

"Hello, dear! In here." Her mother's reedy voice came from the den.

Deirdre stomped in. "Did you know?" she said.

"Oh good. You're back." Gloria looked up from the legal pad on which she'd been writing. Scattered about at her feet were video-cassettes of the movies she and Arthur had written. The VCR was going—Fred Astaire in top hat and tails danced his way across the tabletops of a French sidewalk café.

Gloria paused the video and put the pad on the desk. "Just in time to help us put together a list of clips for a montage to show at the memorial service."

Deirdre put her hands on her hips. "Did you know?"

Her mother blinked. Then frowned. "Goodness. What did you do to your hair?"

Immediately Deirdre felt twelve years old. She could just barely stop herself from shooting back, *And what did you do to your hair? Since when is shaving your head a fashion statement?* It was so aggravating that her mother still had the power to push her buttons.

Deirdre leaned forward on her crutch. "I just found out that every-thing I thought I knew about what happened to me the night of the car accident that did this to me"—she lifted the crutch—"is a lie."

Her mother's jaw dropped but she didn't say anything.

"Deirdre? What is this all about?" Deirdre jerked around, recog-nizing the deep, gravelly voice with just a hint of an Eastern Euro-pean accent. Sy Sterling rose from the wing chair.

"What about you? Did you know, too?" Deirdre threw the words at him. "Because you're the one who kept telling me there was no way to find out where the accident happened. Turns out it's ridiculously easy."

"I did try to find out for you," Sy said. "The record wasn't there."

"It was there. In the Los Angeles Police Department records."

Gloria turned to Sy. "What on earth is she talking about?"

"See for yourself." Deirdre tossed the report on the desk. "Since when is Mulholland Drive on the way from the Nichols' house to ours? And who made up the fiction that it was Daddy driving—"

"Whoa, whoa, whoa." Sy held up his hands. "Slow down. Sit."

Deirdre didn't want to sit but she did, perched on the edge of the chair opposite her father's desk. Sy came around behind the desk and put his hand on her mother's shoulder. "Okay, then. Let me see what you have here." He slipped on reading glasses and picked up the report. As he read, his scowl darkened. At last he handed it to Gloria.

"See," Deirdre said. "That's the official report of my accident. One person in the car. Not two. I was driving, on Mulholland Drive. And all this time—"

"You were not driving that car." Her mother's hand trembled as she stared at the report. "I don't care what this says." She tossed the paper back on the desk.

"Then what happened? Dad drove up to Mulholland for a joy-ride? Crashed the car and then abandoned me?"

Gloria and Sy looked at each other, but neither of them spoke.

"The police thought I was driving. I didn't have a driver's license, I got into an accident, but charges against me were never filed. Was that your magic?" Deirdre stared at Sy. "Was that the trouble you said you kept me out of?"

Sy didn't answer, just raised his eyebrows, allowing that there might be some truth to that.

"And there's more," Deirdre went on. "Yesterday, very early in the morning, around two A.M. or so, before you came over to read us the will, I woke up and found Henry dragging a bag out of my father's bedroom. A bag of things that he said Dad would have wanted him to get rid of. There were snapshots of young women in there. Lots of them. One of the girls"—she stared hard at Sy—"and she *was* just a girl, was Joelen Nichol."

"Christ," Sy said. He seemed dismayed but not particularly sur-prised.

"Know what else I found in that bag?" The words came tumbling out. Now that she'd started, she couldn't stop herself. "A dress. The dress I was wearing at the party earlier that night. The night Tito was killed. So here's what I want to know: How did the dress get covered in blood? And how did my father end up with it?"

Sy hesitated, gazing out into space, his face blank. "This is news to me." Deirdre remembered that her father always said Sy was a brilliant poker player, but a moment's hesitation was his tell.

Well, if Sy wasn't going to spill, Deirdre would. "I also found a knife." Sy's eyes widened. "A carving knife with a bone handle. Something else that Henry said Dad wanted him to get rid of."

"And you think—" Sy started. Now he looked genuinely bewildered.

"I don't know what to think." Tears welled up behind Deirdre's eyes. She clenched her jaw to keep them from spilling over. "But I'm starting to wonder. What if the police don't have the real knife that killed Tito, and what if my father did? And what if I wasn't asleep when it happened?" She looked from her mother to Sy and back again. "Why won't anyone tell me the truth?"

"No one is trying to torture you," Sy said. "We would all like to know exactly what happened. Maybe if your father had written about it, we would know." He paused for a moment, looking directly at Deirdre, so intently that she wondered if he knew about her father's memoir.

Gloria got up from the desk and came around to Deirdre. She took her hand and held it between hers. "I'm so sorry that you've had to go through so much pain and confusion. And it's so unfair that it's all getting dredged up again."

"I didn't kill Tito," Deirdre said in a small voice.

Her mother stood back. "Of course you didn't."

"Did I?" Deirdre asked Sy.

This time there was no hesitation. "You did not. Of that you can be absolutely certain."

"How do you know?" Deirdre said.

"Because I was there," Sy said.

CHAPTER 29

Sy returned to the wing chair and sank into it, his face receding into shadows. He closed his eyes for a moment and tented his fingers over his belt buckle. Then his eyes opened and he glanced across at Gloria, who was still standing behind Deirdre with her arms around her. Some kind of message seemed to pass between them.

"All right," Sy said. "Well then. I was hoping it would never come to this, but here we are and so it is. As you know, I have for a very long time been Elenor Nichol's personal attorney. I am also her friend. She called me that night. Very late. She called and asked me"—he gave a tired smile and shook his head—"make that *commanded* me to come over right away. She said something terrible had happened to Tito.

"I told her to call an ambulance. She said it was too late for that. She needed me to be there when she called the police. So of course I dressed and went right over. As I was driving up the driveway to the house, I passed a car pulling out. It was dark, and I could not see who was driving. But it was a sports car with the top down. Naturally I assumed it was your father. And when I learned what had happened, and that you had been in the house, I further assumed that he had come to get you out of there before all hell broke loose. That is what I thought until just now when you showed me the accident report. I still find it difficult to believe that you were driving that car."

"The dress? The knife? Why did my father have them?"

"I'm afraid that is something I do not know. This is what I do know. When I got there, Bunny took me up to her bedroom. Tito was on the floor. Dead, of course. Bunny said they had had a terrible fight. Worse than usual. Trying to placate him, she had told him that she was pregnant. She thought that would make him happy. Instead, he exploded. Punched her in the stomach. Tried to choke her. Tito knew it could not be his child. He was sterile."

"Elenor Nichol killed Tito?" Deirdre asked.

"That is what she told me. And right away I thought, 'self-defense.' I did not doubt it for a moment, and I am sure I could have persuaded a jury. Police had been called to the house before. Newspapers had printed photographs of them fighting in a nightclub. On top of that, Antonio Acevedo had a long, well-documented history of violence. If Bunny had been charged, I would have tried to make the jury aware of the rumors that he had his last girlfriend disposed of. Elenor Nichol would have come across as a sympathetic victim. Desperate. And—"

Gloria said, "And an accomplished actress." The bitterness in her tone took Deirdre aback.

"Of course she is," Sy said. "But this did not seem like an act. She was agitated. In acute distress, emotionally and physically. Her neck was red and her vocal cords were so badly bruised that she could barely speak."

A chill ran down Deirdre's back. Why on earth had she and Joelen been allowed to hang out all those long afternoons with just Tito in the house?

"I placed the call to the police," Sy went on. "While we waited for them to get there, I prepared Bunny for the questions they would ask.

I told her that I had seen your father's car pulling out when I arrived. She said she had called Arthur to come get you. That you had been sound asleep and knew nothing about what happened. We agreed, the police didn't need to know that you'd been there.

"The police came. Examined the body. They were about to start questioning Bunny when Joelen made a rather dramatic appearance. She staggered into the room, unsteady on her feet, slurring her words. Bunny told me later that she had given Joelen a sedative, but apparently it had not knocked her out. Slurred speech or not, there was no question about what she said. 'I did not mean to kill him.' The police took it as a confession."

"Bunny didn't contradict her?" Deirdre said.

Sy shook his head and pressed his lips together. "After that, things moved quickly. One of the officers read Joelen her rights. They tried to cuff her but Bunny broke down, sobbing and screaming at them to stop. After all, Joelen was just a child.

"Finally Bunny calmed down and the police let her find a coat for Joelen to put on. And that was classic Bunny—always thinking about how things would look, and she was absolutely right. Photographers were already assembled outside the house, of course, just waiting for her to come out. God knows how they knew." Sy stood, stepped to the window, and looked out. He pulled a handkerchief from his pocket and blew his nose. "Very next day, first thing Bunny did was get a security gate. Too bad she had not installed it earlier."

"What did you think?" Gloria asked. "They can't both have killed him."

"What I thought? *Pffft.* What difference did it make? The police heard Joelen's confession. I did my job. I told them both to stop talking." He gave a world-weary grimace. "That is about the best an attorney can do in a situation like that."

"Why would Arthur have ended up with the knife that killed Tito?" Gloria asked.

Sy pondered for a moment, working his lips in and out. "We don't know that it's the same knife." He turned to Deirdre. "Where is it now?"

"I threw it away." The lie popped out without a moment's hesitation.

"You did, did you?" Sy said. Deirdre could see the skepticism in his eyes.

"Day before yesterday. I tossed it into a neighbor's garbage can."

"Hmm. And what about the dress?"

"Destroyed in the fire."

"And—" The sound of the front door opening stopped him.

"Henry?" her mother called out. To Deirdre, she said in a quiet voice, "Let's discuss this some other time. All right?"

A moment later Henry walked into the den, his motorcycle helmet hanging from his hand. He looked from Gloria to Sy to Deirdre. "Who died now?"

"Just your father," Gloria said. She and Sy exchanged a look, and they both eyed Deirdre. *Later.* She'd already gotten the message. "Henry, you're back in time to help us call around and let people know about the memorial service."

Henry looked Deirdre up and down. "Wow. So you pulled out all the stops. How'd it go at City Hall? Did you get Tyler to spill?"

Deirdre felt exhausted and drained. She took a breath. They were all watching her. "He says it was arson."

"Arson? But that's absurd," Gloria said.

"The fire started in a big bag of potting mix, but it was the wrong kind. Too much nitrate, or something like that. He said you'd never have used it for growing geraniums. There were cigarette butts in it. And kerosene."

Henry's gaze shifted toward the garage. "So does this mean the insurance claim gets tied up?"

"It means somebody deliberately set fire to the garage," Deirdre said.

"Henry's right," Sy said. "This will surely tie up any kind of settlement. The insurance company will send in an investigator, and the police will be back, too, asking the obvious question: Was the fire connected to your father's death?"

The logic was inescapable. A death that turned out to be murder. Two days later, a fire that turned out to be arson. How could they not think there was a connection?

"What should we do?" Gloria asked.

"There's nothing to do," Sy said. He crossed to the television and unpaused the VCR. A jazz trumpet blared and on the screen, Fred Astaire twirled, scooped up a silver tray with demitasse cups on it, and gracefully leaped off the table without losing a cup. "Just sit tight and try to give Arthur a proper send-off."

CHAPTER 30

It's only a movie. It's only a movie. That was what Deirdre used to whisper to herself as she tried to drown out the sound of her parents arguing. She'd repeated those same words to get her through round after round of torturous physical therapy.

It's only a movie, she told herself now, as she made phone call after phone call, working her way through a list of Arthur's friends and associates, telling everyone that Arthur's memorial service had been scheduled for Wednesday, day after tomorrow. *I hope you'll be able to make it. We'll have sandwiches at the house after if you can drop by.* She tried not to think about when the police and insurance investigators would descend next.

Henry worked the other phone line while Gloria cleaned the house. After about an hour, Gloria put out a platter of tuna fish sandwiches and the three of them took a break to eat. Deirdre tossed her leftover crusts to the dogs and then went back to making calls.

Meanwhile, Sy went out for a case of Arthur's favorite scotch and bags of ice. When he came back, he stood beside Deirdre and leaned close. "I noticed," he said under his breath. "You did not seem worried about what the police might find out in the alley when they come back." It smelled as if he'd helped himself to a nip of the liquor he'd purchased.

Deirdre had forgotten her lie, so it took her a moment to realize that he was talking about the knife. Flustered, she started to dig herself in deeper. "I took it up the alley and buried it in a bag of grass clippings."

"Grass clippings? You're sure about that?" When she mustered a weak response, he held up his hands. "No. It's better that I am ignorant. But try not to forget, I am much better at sussing out lies than you are at telling them."

Deirdre's face grew hot. Henry, who was standing in the doorway, must have overheard that because he guffawed.

"Henry," Sy said, "that goes for you, too."

The smirk wiped itself off Henry's face. Abruptly, he turned and walked away.

Sy turned back to Deirdre. "And you really do need to find that person who helped you with the exhibit Friday night in the gallery. If she verifies your account, the police will back off. If you do not . . ."

Sy's tone shook Deirdre into action. She called Stefan at the gallery. "Did you talk to Avram?"

"I've tried, believe me. But . . ."

"But?"

"When I call the number he gave us, I get a recorded message that isn't in English. At first I thought it was just a problem with international connections, but—"

"There has to be a way to reach him. Stefan, this is serious. His assistant is the only person who can vouch for where I was that night."

"I get that. But listen, I think we have a problem. I tried calling some other galleries, thinking maybe one of the other dealers might know how to reach him. Not one of them has ever heard of Avram Sigismund."

Deirdre felt like a stone sank in the pit of her stomach. "I thought you checked him out."

"I did. His portfolio seemed solid. His sales records in Europe looked good. But it was all a sham. On top of everything else, the last check he wrote us bounced."

"I don't understand. Why—?"

"And you know what else? Turns out I could have stayed at the gallery that night and worked on the exhibit with you after all. That journalist I was supposed to meet? She stood me up."

"Stood you up?" Deirdre felt numb.

"Didn't even call to apologize. Can you believe it? I drove all the way down to Coronado, waited at the bar at the golf course for over an hour."

It didn't require much paranoia to wonder if someone had gone to a lot of trouble to ensure that no one could vouch for Deirdre's whereabouts that night. Then she herself had sealed the deal by picking up that shovel from the driveway and leaving her fingerprints on the shaft.

By the time Deirdre hung up the phone, her hands were sweaty. When Detective Martinez returned, she'd have to explain to him that she had no idea how to reach the person who was in the gallery with her until late Friday night. That the artist whose show Deirdre had been preparing to open could not be reached and might not, in fact, exist. That she and Stefan had been conned by cartons of smelly old shoes and the promise of payment up front.

CHAPTER 31

That night, Deirdre had dinner with her mother and Henry at Hamburger Hamlet. Then they drove to Hollywood Boulevard for sundaes at C.C. Brown's, where the booths were like church pews and they served mammoth scoops of ice cream in chilled tin cups with thick hot fudge and crispy whole almonds, a pitcher of extra fudge sauce on the side. Deirdre would have preferred the small, elegant sundaes served with a single amaretto cookie at Wil Wright's, but Brown's had been her father's favorite and Wil Wright's had closed.

Later, when Deirdre got in bed, she thought about how readily Sy had seen through her lies. Knew full well that she hadn't gotten rid of the knife. She wondered if he knew that Arthur had been working on a memoir. It seemed so unlikely that Arthur would have kept that from his oldest friend and closest confidant.

Deirdre pulled the manuscript out of the drawer in her bedside table. *One Damned Thing After Another*—not only was it the perfect title for Arthur's memoir, but it also described precisely what her life had turned into since the moment she'd agreed to help him get his house ready to go on the market. She paged through the beginning, skimming past what she'd already read. In the next section, Arthur wrote about arriving in Hollywood and rapidly blowing through his savings. Broke, he'd holed up on a friend's couch. Crashed some cocktail parties. Made connections and bullshitted his way into some low-level jobs, working with other talented newcomers. Met and fallen in love with a chorus girl. Born Gertrude Wolkind, she'd changed her name to Gloria Walker. The truth was, she was a whole lot smarter than she was sprightly, and soon she'd quit dancing and started to work with Arthur. *Helping him write* was how Arthur saw it.

From the moment Arthur started collaborating with Gloria, his luck changed. Deirdre had intended to skim the pages—after all, she'd heard most of the stories many times over. But she found herself caught up in her father's storytelling.

In one chapter he told how he and Gloria talked their way into getting assigned their first movie script. Gloria stole a copy of the Academy Award–winning screenplay for *Casablanca* from the studio library and they cribbed shamelessly from it for story structure and formatting. When their script passed muster, they had their first movie credit and their career took off.

From there on, Arthur's memoir read like a movie with Hollywood's greats in supporting roles and a bit player holding the camera. In one scene Spyros Skouras, the head of Fox, rose from his breakfast in a rage, jowls quivering, spewing incomprehensible English and crumbs of half-chewed toast at Arthur. A few chapters later, Arthur was in the dressing room with a half-dressed Marilyn Monroe, resisting her advances while coaxing her into costume and out onto the soundstage to deliver a knockout performance of "Heatwave." He claimed to have held Marilyn's hand and offered this advice:

Keep trying. Hold on, baby. And always, always, always believe in yourself, because if you don't, who will? Head up, chin high. Most of all keep smiling, because life's a beautiful thing and there's so much to smile about.

Could that have been Arthur? Sensitive, supportive? It sounded more like lines he'd written. Or was Deirdre's view of her father tainted, warped by the angry adolescent girl she still had snarking away inside her?

As she read on, what came across was how much her father adored everything about the movie business. And despite the prism through which Arthur saw the past—selective memory colored by an over-sized ego—it was clear that he and Gloria were much in demand in those heady early years when they churned out hit after hit.

Every so often, Arthur would mention Deirdre or Henry, and when he did it was with blind affection and pure delight. In the bitterness that had built up over the last twenty-plus years, Deirdre had forgotten how unabashedly gaga he'd been about his kids. Forgotten the many times he'd taken her to the studio to show her around but also to show her off. First they'd have lunch, sitting at a corner table in the cavernous studio commissary, surrounded by actors and actresses in full makeup and extraordinary getups. Then they'd walk over to one of the vast soundstages where invariably a movie was being shot. Deirdre had to be careful not to trip on the cables that crisscrossed the floor, and she got goose bumps remembering how absolutely still and silent she had to be the moment a voice boomed, "Quiet on set!" The painted backdrops that looked so phony in person were somehow rendered utterly believable through the magic of filming.

She was near the end of the manuscript, tired and ready to turn out the light when she read these words: *There are parties and there are parties, but the shindigs at Elenor Nichol's house were legendary. Why did it have to be that night of all nights that our attorney finagled an invite there for us to mingle with the crème de la crème of Hollywood's most glamorous?*

A chill passed through Deirdre as she read on.

The setting was out of a movie script. Liveried attendants valet-parked the Jaguars and Mercedes that pulled up at the end of the driveway. Gloria and I got out of my six-year-old Austin-Healey feeling like pikers. We waited for a golf cart to ferry us up to the house.

Tuxedoed waiters, most of them out-of-work actors, glided about with silver trays bearing champagne flutes of Dom Pérignon and shots of Chivas and Glenlivet. The crowd included stars and studio executives, a heady mix of staggering beauty—men and women both—and arrogant power. The men swaggered about, bravado masquerading as brains. Oscar Levant seemed permanently ensconced at the piano, completely brilliant and completely soused, per usual. Needless to say, writers like Gloria and me, a dime a dozen in Hollywood, were in short supply. Most of the folks there were under the illusion that actors and directors made up lines as they went along, so who needed writers, anyway?

Bunny, as Elenor Nichol was known, though there was nothing remotely soft or cuddly about her, reigned over all. Queen of wanton amorous fire, that night she wore a crimson dress with a plunging neckline and ropes of pearls that couldn't hold a candle to the luminescence of her skin. With her swelling bosom and round bottom, her sultry voice somewhere between a purr and a snarl, she had every man in that house salivating, including yours truly. But no one dared to make a pass at her—not with Tito Acevedo watching her every move like a dyspeptic guard dog.

Thug. Bully. Gigolo. Goon. Those were just a few of the labels hung on Tito—never to his face, of course. Supposedly he used to be errand boy for Mafia boss "Sam the Cigar" Giancana in Vegas before shifting his base of operations to Hollywood. Here, rumor had it, he threatened to castrate the director of Bunny's last film when he got what Tito deemed a bit too chummy. On top of that, he fancied himself a player and took meetings, reading scripts and throwing around wads of cash. A crass charmer, he'd have made a great character in a B-movie. In real life, he was a black hole of pure nastiness. Everyone gave him a wide berth.

That night, Tito glowered silently from the shadows beside a mas-

sive potted palm in the corner of Bunny's palatial living room. He was doing a second-rate Humphrey Bogart imitation, his eyes half-closed, pinching the end of his cigarette between his thumb and forefinger behind a cupped hand.

Like the cigarette he was smoking, it turned out Tito Acevedo was on a slow burn.

Deirdre paged ahead, looking for but failing to find any mention of her or Joelen at the party. Like Oscar Levant, Arthur would have been plenty "soused" himself with all that high-class booze floating around, more than a few rungs up from his usual Dewar's. Finally she found her own name.

Gloria and I had long ago bailed and were home sleeping it off when the phone rang. I was thinking, Christ almighty, who calls at two in the morning? I almost didn't pick up. But then I did.

"Arthur? It's Bunny." Her voice didn't sound soft or sultry—more midway between outraged and petrified. "Get Deirdre."

Get Deirdre? For a crazy moment I was thinking: great title. Then I realized my daughter was sleeping over at Bunny's house. I'd seen her at the party, she and Bunny's daughter all dressed up and parading around like grown-ups.

I sat bolt upright, wide awake. "What's wrong?"

"Something's happened," she said.

"To Deirdre? Is she all right?"

"She's fine. But you've got to get her away from here before they come." Before I could ask who "they" were, she hung up. Talk about your cliffhanger ending.

I slapped some water on my face, threw on some clothes, and drove over there as fast as I could. Up Bunny's long driveway to the big white house that had been lit up like a stage set hours earlier but now had just a single light on in an upstairs window.

Before I could knock, Bunny pulled open the front door. It was

dark, but I could see she looked pale, her face puffy and teary-eyed.
She had a nasty bruise under one eye and her lip was split. She wore a
flowing peignoir that, it only occurred to me later, looked like a leftover
costume from her movie Black Lace.

I followed her up the stairs into what I realized right away was
her daughter's bedroom. Pink walls. Twin beds. One of the beds was
empty. Lying facedown on the other was Tito Acevedo.

I could smell the blood that had soaked into the quilt under Tito.
The soundtrack, high-pitched squeals, turned out to be a pair of thor-
oughly spooked guinea pigs. Bunny's daughter, Joelen, was huddled in
a corner by their cage. She was hugging a pillow and leaning against
the wall. Her eyes were shut tight. At first I thought she was asleep.

I looked around for Deirdre. Thank God she wasn't there.

When I reached for Tito's wrist to feel for a pulse, Bunny stopped
me. "He's dead, for Chrissake. Can't you see that? Help me move him."
Imperious as ever.

Deirdre read on. Her father had helped Bunny wrap Tito in the
quilt. They'd pulled him off the bed and dragged him down the hall
to the master bedroom, where they'd rolled him over onto the floor.
That must have been where the news photographers later snapped
pictures of what was supposedly the crime scene. Deirdre clearly remembered a shot of a cop sitting at the edge of Bunny's satin-covered
bed, staring down at the dead man.

What happened? Who killed him? When I asked Bunny Nichol, she
showed me a knife. "Recognize this?" she wanted to know.

Of course I recognized it. The last time I'd seen it was in a drawer
in the buffet in my own dining room. It had been a wedding present. So
what was it doing here?

I was desperate to take the knife from her. At the same time, I was afraid
to touch it. The thought of how it had been used made me sick to my stom-
ach. I know I've seen too many cop shows, but I was worried about leaving

my fingerprints on top of those of the killer. At the same time, I realized it was too late to worry about fine points like that. The arms of my jacket and my trousers were already stained with Tito's blood.

Bunny said not to worry. She'd get rid of the quilt from her daughter's bedroom that we'd just dragged Tito in on. And she'd "take care" of the knife. Then she showed me a dress she said my daughter had worn to the party earlier that night. It was covered in blood too. I stared at it, too stunned and frankly afraid to ask the obvious question. Bunny promised me she'd take care of the dress, too. That the police would never know.

Know what? I wanted to ask.

If I didn't tell, she said, she wouldn't tell, and she'd keep these items somewhere safe. She called them her "little insurance policy."

I asked her what in God's name she meant by that. She blew up. What happened was my fault as much as it was hers. If I'd been a better father, and so on and so on. I had no idea what she was going on about.

Finally she calmed down and said, "If you know what's good for you, you'll forget we had this little talk."

Even at the time it sounded like a line of dialogue from one of her movies. But then, the whole situation felt like it was out of a movie. Everything except for Tito Acevedo, who was not pretending to be dead. And my daughter, who was somewhere in the house, needing me to get her out of there.

I asked Bunny where Deirdre was. Her answer stunned me to my core: "Shouldn't you be asking, where's Henry?"

Deirdre felt her jaw drop. What on earth had Henry had to do with what happened that night?

Apparently Arthur had had the same reaction.

I was about to ask what my son had to do with any of this when I heard a car outside on the gravel. I looked out the window. Headlights. Taillights. Then I realized I was looking at my own car driving away.

Bunny was beside me, looking out, too. "If you want to protect our children," she said, coming down hard on our, *"you'll go home and never breathe a word of this to anyone."*

I thought about that as I walked home, hoping the police wouldn't stop me for loitering even though I was moving as fast as I could. I was praying that when I got back to the house I'd find Deirdre safe and sound, asleep in bed.

Fortunately, it was not very far. Unfortunately, my daughter was not there. Neither was Henry.

That was the end, the very last typed line. Below it were hand-written notes, scrawled at the bottom of the manuscript's final text and on the back of the page.

Gloria New Age. Deirdre knew what that would be about.

Talk That Talk. Deirdre recognized the title of the movie that had been her father's one and only attempt at directing.

Baby boy. She had no idea what that referred to.

Sy trust. That was underlined twice.

Jack Nicholson, Robert De Niro, Harrison Ford, Maximilian Schell.

The list made Deirdre smile. Arthur was considering A-list actors to play himself.

Deirdre gathered up the manuscript pages and was about to slide them back into the folder when she realized something was stuck in one of its pockets. A small envelope. She slipped from it a greeting card. The front was printed with a ring of flowers circling a baby-carrying stork. Inside was a handwritten message:

Congratulations! It's a baby.

That's all. No name. No date. No six pounds eleven ounces. No return address on the envelope. Just a postmark: Beverly Hills, May 11, 1964. Six months after Deirdre's accident. Six months after Antonio Acevedo was killed.

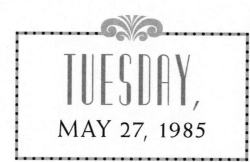

TUESDAY,
MAY 27, 1985

CHAPTER 32

At four thirty in the morning, Deirdre lay awake in the dark, mulling over what her father had written. There was some comfort in knowing that she had not, after all, been at the wheel of her father's car when it crashed. But her father hadn't been driving either. It was Henry who'd led her from the house. Henry who'd driven her up to Mulholland and crashed the car into the guardrail. For some reason he'd been at the Nichols' house, too, the night Tito was killed.

And what about the dress and the knife? What kind of "insurance" was Bunny buying for herself by holding on to them, and how did her father end up getting them back?

Deirdre got out of bed, pulled out the torn plastic bag she'd stashed in the closet, and took out the dress. Unwrapped the knife. Examined the flourishy initial engraved in the silver cap at the end of the bone handle. Was it *N* for *Nichol?* Or—she rotated the knife 180 degrees—*U* for *Unger?*

And what about the dress? As she smoothed it out on the floor, brittle bits of netting broke away. Were the brownish stains on it blood? They could as easily be cocktail sauce or red wine. She and Joelen had gorged on both after the party, then thrown up.

Deirdre sniffed at the stains, but after all these years the only smell was of dust and decay. There was no telling what had made them. Or was there? Would Tyler, with his chemistry lab, be able to identify the stains? He'd offered to help. Urged her to call on him "anytime." Did that mean it was okay to call at five in the morning? Would he write her off as a crazy nut job? She hoped not.

She crept into the kitchen, where she'd left her bag by the back door. In it was the report of her accident on which Tyler had written his phone numbers. She dialed the one marked "Home" and held her breath.

"Corrigan," Tyler said, picking up on the third ring. His voice was thick.

"Tyler? I'm sorry, it's—"

Before she could give her name, he said, "Deirdre! Hang on." She heard muffled sounds on the other end, then he came back on the line. "Are you okay? Is everything all right?"

It didn't sound as if he was writing her off. "I'm sorry to call at this ridiculous time, but you did say that if I needed anything it was okay to call anytime."

He yawned. "Said it and meant it."

"The thing is, I'm not sure this is something you're allowed to do. I found a very old dress and was hoping that you might examine it and tell me whether the stains on it are blood. Off the record, of course. Just as a favor."

"So you think the stains could be blood?" He said it in what sounded like a cop voice: *Just the facts, ma'am.*

Had she been right to trust him? After all, she hadn't seen him in more than twenty years and they'd hardly had what you'd call a relationship. Why *was* he so eager to help her, anyway? And why was she so ready to trust a virtual stranger when she couldn't trust her own mother, whose prayer beads she'd found in her father's office? Or her brother, who'd never admitted that he was responsible for the accident that crippled her and who seemed to have a vested interest in burying her father's secrets? Even Sy made her feel apprehensive, though she couldn't put her finger on why.

Any of them could have purchased a shovel and used it to bash her father in the head during his midnight swim. Even if Arthur had seen one of them in the yard, he'd never have expected to be attacked. Any of them could have arranged for a mythical Israeli artist and a no-show news reporter to ensure that Deirdre didn't have an alibi.

"Sorry, Deirdre," Tyler said, "but I have to ask. Does this have anything to do with the fire?" It was a fair question, and he sounded like a real person asking it. She relaxed a notch.

"The stain is old. Really old. From twenty years ago. So I can't imagine how it could be connected to the fire," she said with a twinge of guilt. Because it was just possible that the fire had been set in order to destroy items in Arthur's office, that dress among them.

"Okay then. Sure. It's not complicated. I'll bring over my own test kit and you can do the test yourself."

"That would be great," Deirdre said, feeling as if a heavy weight had lifted.

"How about later this morning? I could come to your house—"

"No," Deirdre said, louder than she'd intended. She heard the dogs stirring in Henry's bedroom. "Sorry. My family is already stressed out, and I'd rather they not know about this."

"Then how about I meet you somewhere and we can do it right now?"

"Now? Really?"

"Sure. I'm awake." He yawned again.

"Sorry."

"No need to apologize. I'm glad you called. Where do you want to meet?"

Where? She hadn't gotten that far. Somewhere nearby. "You know the fountain on the corner of Santa Monica and Wilshire, across from Trader Vic's? Will that work?"

"We should be able to find a spot there that's dark enough to see the reaction. Assuming you don't mind crawling around a bit under some bushes."

It wouldn't be the first time she'd crawled around under those bushes. She and Henry used to play hide-and-seek in that park, but never at five in the morning.

"Meet you there in thirty minutes," Tyler said.

"Thirty minutes." Deirdre couldn't believe how easy this was turning out to be. "Thank you so much."

"If you want to thank me, let me take you out to breakfast after."

He was being so nice it scared her. "Okay. But my treat."

"We can argue about that later."

Deirdre rummaged through the dresser in her room and found a white T-shirt to wear with her leggings. She ran a brush through her hair, and scrawled a note for Henry and her mother in case they got up and found her missing. Carefully she folded the dress around the knife again and tucked them in her messenger bag. At the last minute, she stuffed the folder with her father's manuscript in the bag, too.

When she drove off, it was still dark. It took only ten minutes to drive to the little park that was home to the fountain. She parked around the corner and made her way across the hard-packed dirt path leading to the tiled piazza. The moon was a substantial crescent that hung right over the head of the kneeling Indian on the plinth in the center of the circular fountain. As always, his head was bent and he held his hands out in front of him as if to capture the water playing around him. Or perhaps he was offering thanks to the gods for finding him, among all his compatriots, such a cushy permanent home.

Even at this odd hour the plaza wasn't deserted. A young couple was entwined, necking on one of the benches. Deirdre picked a spot upwind from the fountain's spray, feeling first to be sure the bench was dry. The parade of colored lights in the fountain was still going, but as the sky was starting to lighten, the jets of water looked pale rather than vibrant—powder blue, then seafoam green, then pink, cycling through color after color until the grand finale, all the colors at once. When she was little, her father would occasionally bring her there after getting ice cream at Baskin-Robbins. Even as they faded, the lights still seemed magical.

Traffic was sparse in the usually busy intersection of Santa Monica and Wilshire. Deirdre remembered when there'd been a vast empty field across the street where the Hilton Hotel now stood. Trader Vic's, attached to the hotel's near end, stuck its palm-tree-lined, Tiki-bedecked entrance into the intersection. More and more, Los Angeles and Disneyland were merging into a single entity with reality at a far remove.

Tyler loped across the plaza in jeans and a black T-shirt that showed off a muscular chest and powerful shoulders and upper arms. "Hey, sorry. I got held up," he said. He held a black backpack with white letters stenciled on: ARSON.

"It's been ages since I was down here when the lights were going," Deirdre said. "I forgot how cool it is."

"Me too. I feel personally responsible for that," Tyler said, pointing to a sign that read NO SKATEBOARDING ALLOWED. "We used to come down here when they were doing repairs and the fountain was empty. We'd race around in circles inside the fountain. Jump in and out. Popped more than a few tiles, I'm ashamed to say."

Deirdre said, "My brother claimed he and some friends put a box of Tide in the fountain once. Supposedly the suds spread all the way out onto the street and stopped traffic. He was very proud of that accomplishment."

"Adolescent boys are all idiots." Tyler sat next to her on the bench. Deirdre could smell his aftershave. "So what you want tested is in there?" He indicated the bag in her lap. "Let's have a look, see what you've got."

"It's a dress," Deirdre said, opening the bag. "It's probably nothing." Leaving the knife in the bag, she pulled out the dress and handed it to him.

Tyler turned his back to the fountain and took the dress from her, holding it gingerly away from him. "Like I said, we need to take this somewhere dark enough to see the reaction." Just then the lights in the fountain went out and the fountain's jets turned off. Deirdre looked back at Wilshire. The streetlights had gone off, too.

"We should do this now, before it gets much lighter. Behind there." He pointed to the tall wall that formed the back of a long bench at the rear of the plaza.

Deirdre followed him out and around to where tall bushes lined the back of the wall. It smelled just like it had years and years ago when she'd hunkered down, waiting for Henry to find her. Pee and rotten eggs.

Tyler turned on a penlight, crouched in the shadow between the bushes, and crept in closer to the wall. Taking shallow breaths and steadying herself with her hands, Deirdre followed him, frog walking in close to the base of the wall where it was darkest.

Tyler waited until she was right there in position, too. Then he opened his pack and pulled out a plastic spray bottle. "Okay. You ready?"

"Ready." She hoped she really was.

"Let's see what we have here." Tyler turned off the flashlight and waited. In moments, Deirdre's eyes adjusted to the dark. Tyler held the dress in front of them and gave her the spray bottle. "Just give it a spritz or two." Deirdre aimed the nozzle and gave it two squeezes. An instant later, bluish-green puddles of light glowed on the under-skirt and the netting lit up like a star-sprinkled fisherman's net.

"Probably blood," Tyler said.

CHAPTER 33

After the blue glow faded, Deirdre returned with Tyler to the park. The air felt laden with moisture even though the fountain was off. The sky had turned pale gray and traffic was coming to life.

"Why *probably* blood?" Deirdre asked.

"It's called a presumptive test. Luminol occasionally gives a false positive."

"It glows like that when it hits something other than blood?"

"Like bleach. That's why people use bleach to clean up a blood spill. It camouflages the stains. Animal blood would luminesce, too. And horseradish. I know, more than you need to know."

Horseradish? How weird was that? Because the cocktail sauce that she'd gorged on at the party and then thrown up all over herself had been spicy. It could have been that. Maybe. But if that's all it was, why would Bunny and then her father have held on to it for all these years?

Deirdre said, "I'm amazed at how bright the reaction is, given how old the stain is."

"The older the stain, the stronger the glow. But like I say, it's not proof positive. If you want to know for sure if it's human blood, I'd need to take a sample to the lab and run more tests."

Knowing whether the stains were blood wouldn't bring her any closer to understanding how they'd gotten there or how her father had ended up with the dress. But it would be another piece of information about what happened that night. Eventually, all of it had to fit together.

"Could you?" she said.

"Sure. I'll take a sample."

While he was digging in his backpack, she considered whether to show him the knife and ask him to test it, too. But he'd said luminol glowed when it came in contact with animal blood, and surely the knife had been used to carve meat.

Tyler used scissors to cut a small square of stained fabric from the dress and tucked it into a plastic bag. He gave her back the dress and she stuffed it into her bag.

"Sorry," he said. "Forensics is not an exact science. Sometimes the more you know, the less you're sure of. Do I still get to take you to breakfast?"

A little while later, Deirdre was sitting next to him on a stool at the counter at Canter's on Fairfax, inhaling the aroma of pastrami and garlic pickles. The waitress, wearing a shirtwaist with white trim almost exactly like the one Bunny had dressed Deirdre up in for her visit to City Hall, brought them coffee and took their orders. Even as early as it was, the restaurant hummed with customers.

Deirdre sipped her coffee. When she looked across at the mirrored wall opposite them, she caught Tyler staring at her reflection. "Twenty-year-old bloodstains," he said. "So does this have to do with your car accident?"

Deirdre felt her face flush. She looked away. She was ready to call him for help at five in the morning but not ready to spill her guts.

"Okay, don't tell me," Tyler said. "But I might even be able to help with whatever it is that's got you so stuck."

"I'm not stuck."

"Yeah, you are. You can't even look me in the eye and talk about it."

The waitress brought over their plates and topped off their coffees. Deirdre poked at her egg. Took a bite. The potatoes in the corned beef hash were crisp and the eggs were done exactly right.

"I'm sorry." She shook her head. "These last few days have been a bit much. Between my father and the fire and the mess, it's a lot to deal with."

Tyler tucked into his pancakes. "I can't even imagine. Though I do know cleanup is brutal after a fire, even when you're not grieving. You know, there are companies who will come in and do it for you."

"I need to do it myself. At least a first pass. My father named me executor of his literary estate, and a lot of what should have been preserved was up in his office on the second floor of the garage."

"Have you started? Because water can be just as damaging as fire, especially to paper."

"So far, the only thing I've managed to save is a sleazy photograph."

"A photograph?"

Deirdre found it in the bottom of her bag and showed it to Tyler. "How's this for legacy?"

"Joelen Nichol," Tyler murmured. He took the photo from Deirdre. "You two were always together."

Of course Tyler remembered Joelen—he and the rest of the male population of Beverly Hills.

Tyler raised the photograph to the light. "You think that's your dad?" he asked, pointing to the photographer reflected in the mirror over Joelen's head.

"Isn't it?" she said.

He slipped a key ring from his pocket. Hanging on the ring along with keys was a small magnifying glass. Tyler examined the photograph through it. "Have a close look, why don't you?" He handed Deirdre the magnifier.

Deirdre positioned the lens and looked through it. The photographer's face was hidden behind the camera's viewfinder, the lens accordioned from its box. The man had her father's hair. Same general build. Same stance. But that wasn't what sent a shiver down Deirdre's back as she leaned closer to the magnifying glass. On the arm of the photographer's leather jacket was a Harley-Davidson double-winged eagle patch.

Her father wasn't a biker. Her brother was.

CHAPTER 34

Staring at the Harley eagle patch, Deirdre tried to remember when Henry had gotten into muscle bikes. Seemed like it hadn't been until after he dropped out of college with only a collection of electric guitars and a few demo tapes to show for his dreams of becoming a serious musician.

"What are you thinking?" Tyler asked. He pushed away his empty plate and signaled the waitress to top off their coffees.

"I'm thinking it's a shame that my brother never finished college."

"He was cool. I remember in high school, he had that swagger. And girls—" Tyler whistled.

"Yeah. Girls were all over him. I think he had a great time in high school. Not me. I was so glad when it was over."

"Me too."

They talked for a while longer, comparing notes on what Beverly had been like if you didn't cheerlead or play football or drive a Ferrari. Deirdre could easily have stayed and talked longer, but at half past eight Tyler said he had to get to work. He told her that first thing in the morning was the best time to file a request for the record that the insurance adjuster needed. The Records Office at City Hall opened at nine. Deirdre stopped on her way home, pulled the number 12 from the number dispenser, and was out of there twenty minutes later.

As she drove home, she thought about Henry. He'd tacitly deflected the blame to Arthur for photographs that he'd taken. He'd also let her father take the blame for the car accident that left her crippled. Which reminded her of something Arthur had mentioned in his memoir—Bunny's comment that Arthur was as much to blame for what had happened as she was.

When Deirdre got home, she would question her mother and Henry, both of them. Together. She wanted to know exactly what each of them knew about what happened that night. No more sidestepping, shading the truth, or lying to protect anyone, including herself.

But when she neared her father's house, she realized a dark sedan was parked in front. She pulled over to watch from a distance as a pair of uniformed police officers got out of the car and started up the front walk.

Any plan she'd had of confronting Henry and Gloria evaporated. The police must have obtained another search warrant, as Sy had predicted. If they looked in her bag, she didn't have a good explanation, even for herself, for what was in it.

She drove slowly past the front of the house. Caught a glimpse of the front door opening. Just then, a motorcycle came roaring out of the driveway and sped past her, up the block. Deirdre recognized Henry's red-and-gold helmet. He'd probably seen the police arriving and decided to disappear. She made a quick U-turn and took off after him.

Henry slowed at a stop sign a few blocks later. Deirdre tooted her horn and flashed her lights. But he barely glanced over his shoulder. Just flipped her the bird before peeling out and roaring up the street.

So it's like that, is it? She accelerated, peeling out after him. Thirty miles an hour. Forty. Henry slowed but didn't stop to turn left onto Sunset. Deirdre had to screech to a halt at the corner as a stream of cross traffic held her back. Taking advantage of a minuscule gap between cars, she nipped out onto Sunset, earning herself a horn blast and her second expressive middle finger of the morning. Ahead of her, she could see Henry on his bike slowing. Turning into the driveway of the Nichols' estate. Why was he going there?

Without thinking, Deirdre turned in behind him, making it through the gate just before it closed. By then, Henry and his motorcycle had vanished up the driveway.

Deirdre stopped the car. Now what? Should she drive up to the front door, march up the steps . . . and then what? Throw pebbles at Joelen's window? What Henry was up to was his own business. At least it would have been if he hadn't been lying to her, insisting that he had no ongoing relationship with Joelen Nichol. Maybe she could figure out what was going on without embarrassing him.

She drove slowly up the driveway. When she got to the pool, she backed into the carport that was camouflaged by a bank of bougainvillea, then killed the engine, grabbed her crutch, and started to walk up the drive toward the house. Bunny was obviously not addicted to thirty laps a day. Close up, the pool not only looked gross, it smelled scummy, like sour milk and rotting leaves.

Deirdre continued up the hill, moving as quickly as she could. By the time she rounded the final bend she was out of breath. Henry had parked his bike in front and was crouched behind it, looking at the engine or the tires, she couldn't tell which. His fancy, custom-made helmet hung from one of the handlebars.

The minute he stood, Deirdre realized her mistake. The man by the bike wasn't Henry; it was Jackie Hutchinson. He started walking toward the front door, wobbling a little on the chunky heels of a pair of black cowboy boots that, like his helmet, could have been Henry's.

"Looking for someone?" The voice from behind her startled Deirdre. She whipped around to see Bunny Nichol wearing a pink satin quilted bathrobe, a chiffon scarf wrapped around her head and tied over her forehead. She was in full makeup, of course. "You're here a little early for a visit."

"I thought—" Deirdre started. But before she could come up with a plausible excuse for being there, Bunny hooked her arm and called out, "Jackie!"

Jackie turned around as Bunny propelled Deirdre forward toward the house. "You remember Deirdre?" Bunny said. "She was at the house a few days ago?"

"Sure. You were up there." Jackie pointed vaguely in the direction of Bunny's bedroom. "You look . . . different. I'd never have recognized you."

"I didn't recognize you in that helmet," Deirdre said.

Jackie looked down at the helmet hanging from his hand. "Pretty cool, isn't it?"

"I've only seen one other like it."

"You must know Henry Unger."

"He's my brother."

Jackie narrowed his eyes at Deirdre. "You and Henry? Really. I was just over there. Small world."

Maybe not that small. "You work with him?" Deirdre said.

"Not with him. *For* him. He's an old friend of Bunny's."

"Deirdre," Bunny said, "I know you need to be on your way. I'll walk you back to your car." She started escorting Deirdre down the driveway.

Deirdre didn't mind being given the bum's rush, as her father used to call it. She was as anxious to get out of there as Bunny was to be rid of her. But as they walked away from the house, she picked up her head. Was that the *woop-woop* of a siren?

"Shit," Bunny said under her breath. "You parked at the pool?"

Deirdre nodded.

"You must have triggered the alarm." Bunny gripped Deirdre's arm tighter. "You really should have telephoned first."

As they approached the carport by the pool, the alarm fell silent. A black-and-white car with a row of stars and SECURITY stenciled on the door was parked behind Deirdre's car, blocking it in. A uniformed guard with a brushy salt-and-pepper mustache emerged from under the overhanging bougainvillea. "Der-dra Unger?" he said, mispronouncing Deirdre's name. He had her wallet open in his hand and was holding her messenger bag. "That your Mercedes parked in there?"

"Yes. And that's my bag."

"She's all right, Martin," Bunny said. "False alarm. I'll take those."

Martin the security guard reached into Deirdre's bag and pulled out the knife. "You sure she's all right, ma'am?"

"She's just returning that to me," Bunny said, and held out her hand. Martin gave her the knife, hilt first.

Bunny turned the knife over. The blade flashed in the sun. "Did you know," she said, giving Martin a coy smile, "that I once worked with quite a famous magician? In the early days, of course. Before I became a star." She rotated the knife so she had the blade between her fingertips. "Can you imagine this? I'm dressed"—she poked a bent knee through the opening in her robe—"scantily." She gave Martin a wink. "Strapped to a board. Then Jasper sets me spinning. Backs away. Looks out at the audience as if to say *Dare me*. Pretends he's about to throw the knife but doesn't. Not yet. Suspense builds. Tension thick. You can hear a pin drop." Bunny reared back, holding the knife aloft. "Then suddenly Jasper throws the knife. The audience gasps. The board slowly stops spinning and everyone can see where it's landed, right between my legs." She drew her leg demurely back into the folds of her robe.

Martin exhaled audibly.

"Pure skill," Bunny said. "Not an illusion, as so many magic tricks are." She lowered the knife, moving it to her other hand and grasping it by the handle. "It was simply quite amazing that he could throw as accurately as he could. Frankly, I was terrified. I needed a stiff drink before each performance and kept my eyes shut from the moment he set that board spinning until it stopped."

Bunny's gaze softened, focused in midair. "He also used to make the knife vanish." She blinked. "Now that's a trick I can show you. I store some of our props—mementos, really—in the pool house. Of course, I'm not a master like the Great Jasper, but I've always been a quick study, and I saw him do the trick often enough."

Bunny handed Martin the knife and let herself in through the gate to the pool. Moments later, she emerged holding a painted box. "Here we are." She blew on it, raising a cloud of dust, and rubbed it with her sleeve. "Covered in cobwebs. Like we'll all be ourselves one day." The box was red lacquer, decorated with gold stars and crescent moons.

Magic. It's all about misdirection. That was what Bunny had said when she contemplated how to costume Deirdre so she'd be invisible for her visit to City Hall.

With a practiced gesture, Bunny tapped the surface of the box with delicately tapered nails. "Tricks are so much fun when you don't know their secrets." She rotated the box, then twirled it corner to corner until the stars and moons painted on its shiny enamel surface were a blur. Then she held the box perfectly still. She glanced in Deirdre's direction, then lifted the lid and opened a door in the side. Lowered her hand in through the top. Her fingers waggled, visible through the open side door against a black-and-white-striped interior. "See? Nothing whatsoever inside." She pulled her hand from the box, closed the side door, and held out her hand to Martin. He gave her back the knife. With a flourish, Bunny dropped it into the box. It made a thump when it landed.

Bunny snapped the lid shut. Frowned and looked at the box as if she wasn't sure what to do next. Smiled, like a lightbulb had gone off in her head, then twirled the box again. Once, twice, three times. Waved her hand over it. Murmured, "Magic words, magic words, magic words."

Anyone who'd ever seen a magic act knew that the knife would disappear. Even so, Deirdre gasped when Bunny opened a side panel to reveal that it had. She closed that panel and opened the lid, peered in, and gave a momentary look of surprise. Then she reached in and began pulling out a shiny red silk scarf. Knotted to the end of it was a green scarf. Then a yellow one. Scarf after scarf streamed from the box until there were no more.

"*Et voilà!*" Bunny said with a wave of her arm, sending the string of scarves flying in a zigzag overhead before stuffing them back into the box.

Martin applauded. Deirdre applauded. Bunny tucked the magic box under her arm and took a little bow. "I'm sorry, Martin, that you had to bother coming all the way up here for nothing," she said.

"Not a bother," Martin said. "Never a bother, Miss Nichol. Wouldn't have missed this for anything." He dropped Deirdre's wallet into her messenger bag and transferred it into Bunny's arms. "You're sure there's nothing more I can do?"

"I'm sure. Thank you. Thank you so much," Bunny said. She rose on tiptoe and planted a kiss on his cheek. Martin flushed so red that for a moment the lipstick smear she'd left on his cheek seemed to disappear.

A minute later Deirdre stood alone with Bunny, watching the security car disappear down the driveway.

Bunny turned to face Deirdre, hands on her hips. "So."

Deirdre's first instinct was to apologize, but she was through apologizing. She was tired of being treated like a child who had to be lied to. "I thought you might recognize that knife."

"Should I?" Bunny opened the messenger bag and, to Deirdre's astonishment, pulled the knife from within it. Then she peered into the open bag. Lifting the edge of the yellow dress, she added, "I see you still have this. Where did you find it?"

"Among some things Henry says Dad told him to get rid of. I think that's the same dress and knife that you showed my father the night Tito was killed. You told him you were keeping it for insurance. Insurance against what?"

Bunny's eyes turned watchful. "How do you know that?"

"I . . . he told me."

"He told you?"

Deirdre stared hard at Bunny, determined not to let her gaze drop to the bag Bunny was holding. The manuscript was in it, underneath the yellow dress.

"I asked, how do you know that?" Bunny repeated with a cold, hard look.

"He wrote about it in his memoir," Deirdre said defiantly.

Bunny reared back, clearly shaken. "Where did you find this memoir?"

"Does it matter?"

"Where is it?"

"I gave it to Sy," Deirdre said without missing a beat.

"You gave it to Sy?" Bunny narrowed her eyes and stared into Deirdre's.

"He said he'd take it to his office. He thinks publishers will be all over it, given the content."

"Your father wrote musicals and romantic comedies. He got paid to make things up."

And you get paid to act, Deirdre thought.

"Don't you think it's time people knew the truth?" Deirdre said, the words coming out strong and sharp even as her eyes filled with tears. "My father was here. He helped you move Tito's body from Joelen's bedroom. When he asked you where I was, you said he should be asking where Henry was."

Henry. Bunny mouthed the word as her eyes widened. "What else did he write about Henry?"

Deirdre tried to swallow the lump in her throat. "What I want to know is how did the dress I was wearing that night get like this?" She pulled it from the bag. "And how"—Deirdre waved her crutch—"did I get like this?"

Bunny's look softened. "I understand why you feel you need to know. And I'm sorry you've ended up with so many . . . questions." She gave Deirdre a long look, stripped of artifice. "But I'm telling you, as clearly as I possibly can, that it would be much better all around if you simply stopped asking them." She lifted the dress out of the bag and bundled it around the knife. Then she gave Deirdre back her messenger bag, opened the gate to the pool, and went through it. A moment later Deirdre heard a splash.

When Bunny came back through the gate, her arms were empty.

CHAPTER 35

Deirdre waited until she was off the Nichols' estate to pull over and check that her father's manuscript was still in her bag. It was. In an odd way, it was a relief to be rid of the dress and the knife.

When she got back to her father's house, the police car was gone. Henry's car was gone, too. The dogs greeted her at the door. She gave each of them a desultory pat on the head. One glance past the front hall told her that the place had been thoroughly searched. She made her way through the living room and into the den. Rugs were pushed back. Shelves cleared, with books and videocassettes dumped on the floor.

Deirdre continued to her bedroom. She leaned against the door-jamb and took in the disarray. The mattress had been stripped, the bedding piled on the floor. Her duffel bag had been taken out of the closet, unzipped, and its contents emptied out. The hollow-eyed, kitten-holding orphan was staring from the closet at her. Cardboard boxes that she'd piled in front of the orphan had been pulled out and opened, their contents strewn about. High school yearbooks. Scrapbooks. Spiral notebooks from college classes.

Deirdre wondered what on earth the police were looking for. It would take hours to straighten the mess.

She sank down onto the bare mattress, pulled the pillow off the floor, and hugged it to her chest. She wanted nothing more than to tip over, curl up, and shut down.

"Deirdre? Is that you?" her mother's plaintive voice called.

Deirdre squeezed her eyes shut and pulled the pillow over her head.

"Deirdre?"

Deirdre threw the pillow aside and stood, steadying herself with her crutch. She followed her mother's voice into her father's bedroom. On the way past Henry's room she looked in. His prized electric guitars were piled in a corner instead of lined up against the wall. The contents of his bureau had been dumped on the floor, his closet emptied out too.

Gloria was sitting up in Arthur's bed, her turban askew and her eyes red from crying. Spent tissues were crumpled on the bed covers. This room had also been tossed.

"I see the police came back," Deirdre said.

"Twice."

"Twice?"

"First, two of them showed up and took Henry in for questioning."

"They arrested him?"

"I don't think so. Henry said to call Sy." Gloria's voice rose. "But before I could, another police officer arrived to search the house. I couldn't stop him. He tore through the place while I tried to call Sy. I called his office, and I tried him at home. I tried over and over, but I couldn't reach him."

"Did the police officer say what he was looking for?"

"Looking for?"

"Didn't he show you a warrant?"

Gloria hung her feet off the side of the bed, put her hands on her hips, and worked her thumbs into her back. She looked exhausted. "All he did was show me a badge and tell me to keep out of his way."

"And I'll bet he didn't leave behind a list of what he took, either."

"He didn't leave anything and he didn't take anything, either."

One officer. No warrant. Nothing taken. Sounded like a pretty sketchy police search.

Gloria went on. "Look what a disaster he left the place. The funeral is tomorrow. People will be here." Her voice dropped to a whimper. "It's too much. It's just too much."

"And Henry's still not back? He hasn't called?"

"I haven't heard a word from him." Gloria's face crumpled, and she pulled out another tissue. "I'm so glad you're here, at least."

Deirdre imagined Henry being questioned by Detective Martinez in that little room for hours on end, his words captured on a tape recorder without Sy's reassuring presence to guide him. She tried phoning Sy but, like Gloria, got no answer. She hung up and stared at the phone, willing it to ring. But of course it didn't.

"Come on," she said to Gloria. "At least we can start straightening up."

For the next hour, Deirdre and her mother worked their way from room to room, putting the house back together. They were finishing up in the den when the phone rang. Gloria raced to answer it in the kitchen. Deirdre listened, praying it was Henry.

"Vera?" Deirdre heard her mother say. A long pause. "Oh my God, no!" Deirdre rushed into the kitchen. Gloria was ashen, a trembling hand over her mouth as she listened. "Right. Right." A pause. She shook her head. "How awful."

"What is it?" Deirdre whispered.

"Give me a piece of paper, quick."

Deirdre pulled open one kitchen drawer after another until she found a cash register receipt and a pen.

"Okay. Right." Gloria listened. Then wrote on the back of the receipt. Then listened some more. She just stood there for a few moments, staring at the receiver. At last she found her voice. "That was Vera. It's Sy." She waved the receiver. "He was mugged in the parking garage on his way in to his office this morning. That's why we couldn't reach him. He's in the hospital."

"Is he going to be okay?" Deirdre could barely get the words out.

"All Vera could tell me was that he got robbed and beaten up. They've admitted him." Gloria dabbed at her eyes with a fresh tissue. "Vera's been calling people, canceling his appointments. Meanwhile, Sy is all alone. If it were one of us, he'd be there. Like when you were hurt, he was the first one to show up at the hospital to help your father."

He was? Until that moment, Deirdre hadn't remembered that there'd been someone else there. Now it came back to her. She'd woken up strapped to a gurney. Bright fluorescent lights streamed overhead. Unfamiliar smells. She'd been shivering from what was probably shock, not cold. Her leg throbbing with pain.

If she'd been alone, helpless panic would have overwhelmed her. Only she hadn't been alone. Her father had been there, pale and clearly shaken, and beside him was Sy, a calm, comforting presence. Sy had taken charge, demanding blankets from a passing nurse and piling them over her. Rubbing her hands until she stopped quaking. Asking what she remembered. Explaining to her what had happened, how the car had gone off the road. Staying with her and Arthur until she was rolled into the operating room. Promising not to leave until the doctors were finished putting her back together and she was safely in the recovery room.

Henry had abandoned her, broken on the hillside. Sy had been there with her father at the hospital.

Gloria looked down at the handset she was still holding and hung up the phone. "I'm going over there."

"No. I'll go," Deirdre said. She held out her hand for the notes her mother had written. "You're right. He's been there for me."

"Thank you." Gloria gave her the piece of paper and kissed her on the cheek. "You always were my good girl."

CHAPTER 36

Before Deirdre left the house, she stopped in the bathroom and washed her face and hands. Then she soaked the washcloth in hot water and sat on the toilet seat with the cloth pressed to her face. When it had cooled, she dunked it again, wrung it out, and pressed it to the back of her neck. She was so tired it hurt.

As she made her way out to the car, her messenger bag felt heavy even though all it contained was her wallet, her keys, and her father's manuscript. Gloria had written down *Urgent care - Beverly Medical Center*, and an address on San Vicente in Brentwood. Deirdre had never heard of the place. It wasn't all that far away, just the other side of the San Diego Freeway. But even though it wasn't yet rush hour, traffic and roadwork made the trip slow going.

The medical center was tucked in the back of a half-block-long shopping plaza. A small red-and-white sign directed her to underground parking, where she left the car.

Deirdre leaned on her crutch, hitching her bad leg along behind her, her messenger bag bumping against her hip as she followed the signs to an elevator that deposited her in a bright, plant-filled atrium. The medical center was down a corridor, past a dental office, a law office, and a tae kwon do studio. The door was marked BEVERLY MEDICAL CENTER. Underneath that, in smaller print it said COSMETIC SURGERY, and beneath that in still smaller print it said URGENT CARE. Any other time, the irony of that juxtaposition would have cracked her up.

The waiting area was small, only a half-dozen chairs. One patient was waiting, a woman with a bandage over her nose and her face buried in a *Cosmopolitan*. Deirdre made her way over to a counter topped with a sliding glass window. Behind the glass were desks and a wall lined with a bank of vertical file cabinets with multicolored tabs. A poster of a cocker spaniel with a white bandanna and a stethoscope around its neck hung on the wall.

A woman wearing blue scrubs emerged from a door at the back of the inner office. She slid the window open. "Can I help you?"

"I'm here to see Seymour Sterling," Deirdre said.

"Are you a relative?"

"I'm his daughter," Deirdre said without blinking.

"You are?" The woman looked surprised.

Deirdre started to cry. She couldn't help it. She was worn down from sheer exhaustion. But it also made the lie more convincing.

The woman offered her a tissue. "Let me just check in on him. Make sure he's feeling up to visitors."

She disappeared and a few moments later returned, beckoning Deirdre through a doorway. Deirdre followed her down a corridor lined with examining rooms and through double glass doors. At the threshold of an antiseptic-smelling room, Deirdre stopped for a moment. The smells and the sounds of what looked to be a miniature emergency room were terrifyingly familiar. She had to fight the urge to buck and run.

There were just four hospital beds in the room. The attendant eased past her and disappeared behind curtains that were pulled around one of the beds. When she reappeared, she held the drapes open for Deirdre. "I'll leave you. Don't stay too long. Your father needs his rest."

Deirdre thanked her and turned to Sy. She tried to hide her shock. He looked as pale as the sheets he was lying on. The top of his head was bandaged and black stitches tracked down the side of his face. There was a massive bruise on his forehead, and his right eye was filled with blood. She pulled the folding chair by his bed closer and sat.

"I did not realize that I had a daughter. Lucky me," Sy said with a weak smile.

"Surprised the hell out of me, too." Deirdre took his hand. Her lower lip began to quiver as she stared at the back of Sy's hand, livid around the spot where a needle was taped to a tube that was attached to an IV bag hanging by the bed.

"*Sh, sh, sh,*" Sy said, though Deirdre hadn't spoken. "The only reason I am not home? Doctor is afraid I will have another heart attack. Do not worry. This looks worse than it is." He chuckled. Winced. "Ouch. Cracked rib."

Heart. That explained the tubes attached to suction cups that snaked off his bare chest. A monitor by the bed beeped, a repeating fluorescent green wave pattern tracing out on the screen. Deirdre hated that beeping sound.

"Coming here brings it all back?" Sy said.

"Yeah. The sounds. The smell." Deirdre glanced around the room with its three empty beds. "Why did they bring you here? It's so small." And it was less than a mile from UCLA, with its world-class hospital.

"I am just here for monitoring. Besides, I am not good at waiting in line," Sy said. He coughed and winced again. "Plus my doctor is here in the building. No reason to get stuck in a big emergency room for bumps and bruises."

It looked like a whole lot more than bumps and bruises, but Deirdre didn't push it. "What happened?"

"I got—" Sy licked his lips and pointed to a cup with a straw on the metal table by the bed. Deirdre held it to his mouth while he sipped. Then he settled himself again. "I got out of my car in the parking garage this morning. Guy must have come up behind me while I was walking to the lobby. One minute I am thinking about my appointments for the day. Next thing I know I am on the ground, my head hurts like hell, and a cop and a lot of strangers are staring down at me."

"Did anyone see what happened?"

"No one came forward. No surprise there. The parking lot is quiet by the time I get in. After the morning rush. And like I say, seemed like the guy came out of nowhere."

"It was a man?"

Sy's brows drew together. "You know, I am not sure. But I think so."

"Did he get your wallet?"

"Oddly enough, he did not. Or my Rolex. Or my ring." He raised his hand with the diamond pinkie ring. "And I still had my keys out, so he could have driven off with my car, for Chrissake. All he takes is my old briefcase. I have had that since law school. What did he think was in it?" Sy stared up at the ceiling for a few moments, his eyes squinting into the fluorescent light. "If you ask me, whatever he was hoping to find? He was disappointed."

Hoping to find? It took Deirdre a moment to register what Sy was saying. "You think you were targeted because of something he thought you were carrying? But what?"

"I have been asking myself that very question."

Deirdre swallowed hard as one possible answer occurred to her. "This could be my fault. This morning I told Bunny I'd given you Dad's memoir."

CHAPTER 37

"So Arthur *was* writing a memoir." Sy reached down the side of the bed and pulled a lever. With a hum, the head of the bed raised him to a sitting position. "I accepted as much."

Accepted when he meant *expected*—the occasional slip like that was a reminder that Sy's native language wasn't English. "You didn't know?" Deirdre said. "I thought for sure he'd have talked to you about it. Asked you to read it."

"He did not. I can only assume that he had his reasons."

"Earlier today I told Bunny that I'd found it. That I'd given it to you, and you were going to try to find a publisher."

"Which is what I would have done, if you had given it to me."

Deirdre winced at the tacit rebuke. "I'm sorry. I even told her that you thought it would be an easy sell."

"Did you tell her why I thought that?"

"Because he wrote about the night Tito was killed."

"Did he now?"

Deirdre shifted uncomfortably under his gaze. "He wrote about the party. How Bunny called him late that night and he came back and helped move Tito's body from Joelen's bedroom. That must have been before she called you."

Sy let his head drop back against the pillow. The bruise on his forehead was an angry purple against his ashen skin.

Deirdre went on, "He wrote about Bunny showing him the dress that I'd been wearing and a knife that belonged to us. She warned him that if he wanted to protect me and Henry he'd keep his mouth shut about what happened."

"You and *Henry?*" Sy tilted his head, considering. "Henry was there?"

"That's who you saw driving away from the house. Not Dad. Henry crashed the car."

"I always knew your father was hiding something, but I never guessed that. And Bunny thinks that you have given this manuscript to me? At least this is starting to make sense. You still have it. Some-place secure?"

"For now." It was all Deirdre could do to keep herself from look-ing down at the messenger bag she'd dropped on the floor and where the manuscript was safe, at least for the moment. "Of course, it's un-finished. There are just some notes at the end."

"Notes about what?"

"Stuff he was going to write about, I think." Deirdre tried to re-member those scrawls on the final pages that had seemed like random thoughts. "Something about you and Mom and trust."

"Ah, the trust."

"*The* trust?"

"It is one reason why the estate is as small as it is. Years ago your father had me draw up a trust. Every month he paid a set amount into it. Elenor Nichol was empowered to draw money out. The trust expired a few weeks ago."

Her father had been paying Elenor Nichol? That made no sense. Unless . . . "Starting right after Tito was killed?"

Sy's expression told her she'd guessed right. "Some months after."

"She must have been blackmailing him. He was paying her for her silence." Deirdre looked at Sy but saw no reaction. "Sy, it's got to be connected. My father stops paying into the trust. He starts to write about what he knows, but before he can finish, he's killed. His office is burned to destroy the manuscript, only it's not in his office. Today a fake police search of my father's house fails to find it. Then you get mugged because—"

"What fake police search?"

"Two cops came and took Henry in for questioning, and right after that another one showed and ransacked the place."

Sy's eyebrows raised in surprise, then his brow furrowed. "I suppose it makes sense that the police would come back and also take your brother in for questioning."

"Maybe. But the way they executed the search sounded sketchy. Mom said a single officer got out of an unmarked car, came to the door, flashed a badge, and bulled his way into the house. She just assumed he was legit. After all, he was in uniform, and when someone's in uniform you don't really see him, do you? You told us yourself they're supposed to give you a copy of the search warrant and leave behind a list of what's taken. This guy failed on both counts."

"Not every police search goes by the book. Maybe he left the paperwork but your mother was so upset she—"

"Now I know she can be a little out to lunch, but Mom is not a complete idiot. Whoever she let in to search the house was not operating like a cop. I'm wondering if he's the same person who mugged you because I told Bunny I'd given you the manuscript."

"But—"

"In fact—" Deirdre cut Sy off, talking as fast as she was thinking,

"That police officer who was there in your office building when you came to? Are you sure he arrived *after* you got mugged?"

"I . . . he . . . well of course I assumed after."

"But you didn't see who mugged you, did you?"

It took Sy a moment to get what she was suggesting. "You are saying I got mugged by a pretend cop?"

"Could have been. The first passerby would think the cop was there to help." Deirdre remembered what Bunny Nichol had said about magic. *Make the audience attend to what you want them to see.*

"I guess it is possible," Sy said, "but it seems so unlikely—"

"We should be able to figure it out. If a real officer responded, there will be a record of it, won't there?"

"But how—"

"I know someone who can find out."

"A fake cop." Sy shook his head. "Suppose that's what it turns out he was. Then what? Call the police? Deirdre, are you sure that is what you want? Why, they will ask, would anyone go to all that trouble just to keep an old movie hack's memoir from being published?"

"He wasn't a hack."

"I know. I am just telling you what they will say. Before you know it, you find yourself having to speculate about what your father knew that was so"—he paused, searching for the word—"toxic. Do you want the world to know that you and Henry were there the night Tito was killed? Because you have no idea how quickly things can escalate from there."

Sy was silent for a few moments, his eyes focused on the middle distance between them. "Remember those pictures that ran in the paper the morning after Tito was killed?" He shook his head. "Headlines that ran way beyond the facts? It was horrifying. And who do you think allowed photographers to go up to Bunny Nichol's bedroom? Who gave them entrée and permission to photograph a fifteen-year-old girl, still distraught over what happened that night? Joelen hadn't been charged with a crime." His voice shook with rage. "Shameful. But it happened all the time. If you want to find out whether it still does, go ahead and call in the police. Just don't be surprised at what happens next. You saw what it did to your friend."

That stopped Deirdre. The events of that night had derailed both Joelen's and Deirdre's lives, but at least for Deirdre the aftermath had been a private affair.

"Maybe your father's memoir is publishable. Hell, maybe it has the makings of a bestseller. I would need to read it in order to form an opinion on any of that. But for the moment at least, one thing is clear: that manuscript could get someone killed—"

"Someone already did get killed," Deirdre said. "My dad."

Sy gazed at the machine beside his bed, which was tracing out a regular wave pattern. "I'm not going to disagree with you. But if you have it, or maybe you are carrying it around with you"—she squirmed under his intense gaze, even though there was no way he could know that it was right there in her messenger bag—"you are putting your-self in danger. Hide it in the house and the arsonist might burn the house down next time. Carry it around and you could be the next person who gets mugged. My advice? Before anyone else gets hurt, get rid of it and make it widely known that you have done so. Leave it somewhere safe. The only question is: Where?"

When Deirdre got back into her car, she took out the manuscript. Was this what it was all about? Her father's murder. The garage fire. A fake police search. Now Sy's attack. All because someone desper-ately wanted to keep this from being published?

Deirdre riffled through the pages. What was in it that was so, as Sy put it, toxic? What Arthur had to say about the night of Tito's murder hadn't seemed, to Deirdre at least, to be that much of a game changer. Maybe the murderer was afraid of something Arthur hadn't yet gotten around to putting on the page? But what secret could he reveal about Tito's murder? And if there was something he'd kept secret for all these years, then why had *Arthur* been paying Bunny for her silence? Wouldn't she have been paying him?

Sy was right. Deirdre needed to put it somewhere safe, and then get out the word that she'd done so. After going back and forth with Sy on where, they had agreed on Sy's office. Neither Sy nor Vera would be in there for the next few days, and he had an alarm system that went straight to the police if someone tried to break in.

But looking at the manuscript, a thought occurred to her. What she had in her hands was a carbon copy. Which meant that somewhere out there was the original, and possibly even more carbon copies. Placing the manuscript in Sy's safe only took care of the problem in the short term. On the other hand, announcing where she'd put it might tempt whoever wanted it to reveal himself. Or *herself*. The more she thought about it, the more she liked it.

Deirdre picked up takeout from a Japanese restaurant on the way home. Vegetarian maki rolls for her mother; spicy tuna, yellow fin, and salmon maki for her and Henry. Then she stopped to make a Xerox copy of the manuscript. The first few sheets of onionskin jammed the copier, so she had to feed them in a sheet at a time. That gave her plenty of time to think through exactly what she intended to do. The plan she came up with required the help of a man and a woman. She knew who to ask.

She slipped the Xerox copy into a FedEx envelope, addressed it to herself in San Diego, and left it in the copy store's drop box. Then she bought a ream of paper, got some extra change, and used the pay phone to make two calls before heading home.

Deirdre was relieved to find Henry was back, talking to Gloria in the kitchen when she returned. He looked exhausted and he smelled like he needed a shower.

"How was it—?" Deirdre started, intending to ask Henry how it had gone with the police, when Gloria interrupted with "How's Sy?"

"Concussion and a cracked rib. He's shaken and hurt, but he seemed okay. And he claims the only reason they're keeping him there is to monitor his heart. But he looks ragged. He's going to miss the funeral."

"Miss the . . ." Gloria's face fell. "It won't feel right, burying Arthur without Sy there. And he was going to speak." She reached across for Henry's arm. "Henry, you'll say a few words? Deirdre, maybe you'd like to get up and—"

"No," Deirdre said. "I'm sorry, but no. I couldn't. I'd be too emotional."

"I suppose we do have the film clips. And we can ask people to share their memories," Gloria said as she unwrapped and plated the maki rolls. "That's what they do at a Quaker funeral. Silent meditation and the sharing of memories."

Silent meditation? Good luck with that in a room full of movie people.

"I've got a limousine coming at noon tomorrow to drive us to the chapel," Deirdre said.

"A limo?" Gloria asked. She peeled away the rice paper wrapping and sniffed at a piece of cucumber maki before eating it. "Isn't that a bit extravagant?"

"It's what people do," Deirdre said.

"Did they catch the attacker?" Henry asked. He'd already polished off a piece of spicy tuna roll.

"No. And Sy was hit from behind and knocked out, so he didn't see who it was. For all that, the only thing that got taken was his briefcase."

"That's lucky," Gloria said.

"Maybe it was luck. Or maybe that's what the person was after."

"His briefcase?" Gloria said.

"Sy thinks the person wanted Dad's memoir," Deirdre said, even though she'd been the one who came up with the theory.

"*Our* dad?" Henry said.

"Arthur wrote a memoir?" Gloria said.

"Why would anyone care?" Henry said.

"Sy thinks publishers will care," Deirdre said.

"Really?" Henry gave a dismissive snort.

"Of course they will," Gloria said. She ate another cucumber roll. "Your father was a born storyteller. A true raconteur."

"Right," Henry said. "Now he can tell his stories to people who haven't already heard them a million times. But why would someone mug Sy to get Dad's memoir?"

"Maybe because he wrote about what happened the night Tito Acevedo was killed," Deirdre said, watching Gloria and Henry for their reactions.

Gloria winced. Henry, reaching for the last piece of spicy tuna roll, paused.

"Dad was there." Deirdre leaned close to Henry and stage-whispered to him, "And according to his memoir, you were, too."

Henry's eyes widened and he looked momentarily stunned.

"Henry?" Gloria said.

"That's crazy," Henry said, not very convincingly.

"That's what I thought," Deirdre said. "But hey, why would he write it if it wasn't true?"

"Do you have the manuscript?" Gloria asked.

"I do. Sy wants me to take it over to his office and leave it there on the way to the funeral." With each word, as Deirdre felt as if a burden lightened, Henry looked more and more uncomfortable. He pushed away from the table.

"Do you think that's—" Gloria started.

"So do you want to know what happened with me and the police?" Henry said, interrupting her. He didn't wait for an answer. "I expected it to be a lot worse. He took me—"

"He who?" Deirdre asked.

"Martinez. Took me to a room and asked a lot of questions. Most of them I'd already answered. What happened the night Dad died? Where was I? What did I know about a shovel? Then he started in on the fire in the garage. I told him I don't know anything about that, either, and besides, I was at work."

"Did he seem satisfied?" Gloria asked.

"I couldn't read him. I did my best, but I really wish Sy had been there. Because after that he started asking about you." He looked at Deirdre. "Where you were that night. How you and Dad got along. When I last called you from the house." He paused. "He even wanted to know how your gallery was doing."

"And you said?"

"I said I didn't know."

Of course Henry didn't know. God forbid he'd take the time to pay her a visit and see for himself.

"Which made me think," Henry continued, "I should come down one weekend. See the gallery. Meet your business partner. See your house. Would you have room if I wanted to stay over?"

Shocked, it took Deirdre a moment to come up with an answer. "Of course there's room. I'll make room. You can even bring Baby and Bear."

The dogs, sleeping next to each other in the corner, picked up their heads. They seemed as surprised as Deirdre.

CHAPTER 38

Later that night, Deirdre heard a canned laugh track rumbling from her father's bedroom. Sounded as if her mother, who'd lived for the last ten years without television, was catching up on the latest sitcoms. Deirdre crept out into the hall and knocked lightly on Henry's bedroom door. When there was no answer, she knocked again. "Henry?" she whispered.

"Go away. I'm sleeping."

"Henry," Deirdre said through the closed door, "I was there at the house the night Tito was killed, and I know you were there, too."

No response.

"Are you listening to me? I know you were the one who was driving Daddy's car. You may not want to talk about it, but—"

The door opened. Henry had a pair of earphones loose around his neck. "Shh," he said. He let her into his room and pressed the door shut behind her.

"Don't you think it's time you told me what happened?" Deirdre said.

Henry sat down on the edge of the bed, his shoulders slumped. "I had to get us both out of there. I'm sorry."

I'm sorry? Those were two words she never thought she'd hear coming out of her brother's mouth, and certainly not with the kind of genuine contrition that seemed to fuel them now. "I thought Dad came to get me out of there."

"I had no idea she'd even called him. I found you passed out on the floor in one of the upstairs bathrooms. I had to practically carry you down the back stairs and I was afraid I'd have to carry you all the way home. But when I got outside, Dad's car was right there, with the keys in the ignition. The answer to a prayer. Or that's what I thought at the time." He gave a tired smile and shook his head. "I put you in the car. You were so out of it. I reclined the seat and you curled over on your side."

"You said, 'Night night, sleep tight' and kissed me on the forehead. I thought you were Daddy."

Henry blushed. "What I should have done is belted you in. Believe me, I wish to hell I had. And I wish to hell that I'd stopped long enough to put up the convertible top and calm down. But I was so angry and so—" He broke off, a guarded look crossing his face. "Anyway, I got behind the wheel and started the car."

"Why did you drive up into the canyon?"

"I just drove. I wasn't even thinking about where I was going. Before I knew it, I'd turned onto Mulholland. I was cranking, pushing the car, taking those turns just as fast as I could."

Speed. Deirdre understood how it focused the senses. Obliterated second thoughts.

"I lost control. The car crashed into the guardrail. It was so weird, the car came to a dead stop but the engine just kept screaming. I thought I had my foot on the brake but I was practically standing on the gas pedal. The steering wheel was bent and my chest hurt so badly I could barely breathe. When I looked across to see if you were okay, your seat was empty. I'll never forget that moment."

"Then what? You thought you could just walk away and leave me there?"

"No! God, no. I was frantic. I heard you crying. I crawled through the underbrush and found you. Then I scrambled back and flagged down some bikers. Told them I'd been hitchhiking and witnessed a crash. I begged them to go call for help. All I could think was that you were going to die and it would be my fault. But then, when the ambulance got there, I hid."

"You hid? Why?"

"They'd have—" Henry mumbled something.

"They'd have what?"

"Taken away my driver's license."

"Taken your . . . ? I'm lying there, I could have been dying for all you knew, and you were worried about losing your damned driver's license?"

Henry looked down at the floor and swallowed. The years seemed to fall away and Deirdre could see the vulnerable sixteen-year-old he'd been: tall and charming, goofy and sweet. "I know. I was a coward. I was a jerk." He looked mortified. "You should hate me."

But Deirdre didn't hate him. All she felt at that moment was sadness. "You were a kid. Kids do incredibly stupid things."

"That was beyond stupid and then some. And it wasn't just about losing my license. The truth is, I was afraid they'd find out where I'd been and what I'd been up to." Agitated, Henry got up and crossed the room, then crossed back. He stopped and looked at Deirdre. "Did he write about me and her? Did he?" Before she could answer, he went back to pacing the room. "I knew I should stop seeing her. Tito threatened to kill me if he caught me there again. But she'd whistle and back I'd come. Like some kind of trained puppy. Sit up. Roll over. Sit in my lap. Give us a kiss."

Deirdre tried to put together what Henry was saying. "You came to see her after the party?"

Henry stood still. "I did. She'd told me to meet her at the pool. I rode over on my bicycle. On my *bike*, for Chrissake. At the last minute, I grabbed a knife, thinking I'd flash it at Tito if he showed up. I got to the pool and waited and waited. She never came."

After the party. That was when Deirdre and Joelen were making themselves sick gorging on leftovers, finishing off drinks, and smoking cigarette butts. "She didn't come because we'd gotten smashed. Threw up. Passed out."

"You and Joelen?" Henry blinked. Then he barked a laugh. "You thought I had a thing for Joelen?"

"Didn't you?"

"I . . . I guess I did. Sort of. But not like that."

Not like that? Then she got it. Of course it hadn't been Joelen. A wave of pity and disgust came along with the realization. "You were meeting Bunny Nichol?"

Henry put his hands to his face and closed his eyes. An image of him came back to her. Onstage with his guitar and a microphone in front of him, an ambitious kid swaggering with unearned experience. And Bunny, twenty years older. *Queen of wanton amorous fire*, as her father had described her in his memoir. "What a sleazy—" She couldn't finish.

"I guess that's how it looks now. At the time, it was amazing. I thought I was such a big deal. Supersuave. In charge."

"Oh, Henry. She seduced you. She was glamorous. A famous movie star, for God's sake." Deirdre could only imagine what would have happened if people had found out. Bunny Nichol, involved with a younger man—that might have made a few waves. But that she was sleeping with a sixteen-year-old kid? A tsunami of bad press and ill will, and probably the end of her career. "Did you come up to the house looking for her?"

Henry looked sick. "I did. Even from outside the house I could hear them arguing. She was shouting. Tito bellowing. Then just her, screaming and screaming.

"I ran into the house. I don't know what I thought I was going to do, but I ran inside. I can remember standing at the base of the stairs, looking up. They weren't arguing anymore. Now there was complete silence, so quiet I could hear my own heart pounding.

"Then Bunny was there, like she'd just materialized on the upstairs landing, cold as ice. She came down and took away the knife. I didn't even realize I was holding it. She told me to get the hell out of there, to take you with me, and not to even think about coming back. Ever. So that's what I did. Except the not thinking part. It took me a long time to stop doing that."

Deirdre felt ashamed that for all these years she'd just assumed Henry was Teflon, holding every girlfriend who came along at arm's length emotionally. They came and then they went at his whim, or so it had seemed. This, at least, explained why.

"Did you know why they were fighting? That she'd told him she was pregnant?"

Henry narrowed his eyes. "How do you know that?"

"Sy told me."

"And he knew because . . . ?"

"Bunny told him. He came over later and she had him call the police."

"No. I didn't know that." Henry shook his head.

"But you did know she was pregnant."

"I didn't find out until later, when the baby was born and she came to Dad to negotiate terms and Sy set up the trust. She said the baby was mine. All you have to do is look at Jackie to know that's true."

Of course. She'd seen the resemblance too. She'd felt that frisson of recognition when she first saw Jackie Hutchinson standing on the stairs. There had been something about him. The way he carried himself, his sardonic smile, his hair—all of them echoes of Henry.

"Jackie knows you're his dad?"

"He thinks I'm a friend of the family, and that's what I've tried to be. It's the one good thing that came out of that mess. He's a great kid, even if he is a little lost right now."

That made two lost boys, Deirdre thought as she looked around the room. Henry's prized electric guitars were once again lined up against the wall. Above them on the shelf stood the Battle of the Bands trophies he'd won. Best Band. Best Guitar. He and his buddies had taken top prizes. Henry had had real talent. Looks and charm, too. And he'd been on his way.

But by his senior year of high school, his grades had slipped. He'd stopped playing in the band. Never applied for summer jobs, just hung around, got high, and slept. Gloria and Arthur, distracted by their own unhappiness and Deirdre's surgeries, had barely noticed. After a few months of college, he dropped out and moved home. And he was still there, lost on the way to a real life.

Now Deirdre understood why her father had kept the mysterious baby announcement that she'd found tucked in with his manuscript. Jackie Hutchinson had been the unnamed baby whose arrival was heralded in the card mailed in an envelope postmarked twenty-one years ago. Of course her father had saved it. He was the baby's grandfather.

She also understood one of the notes that her father had jotted on the last page of the manuscript: *Sy trust.* Her father hadn't been paying Bunny hush money. It had been child support. And Arthur had been bound and determined to write about it. He was going to blow the story wide open, and blow away Bunny's reputation in the process.

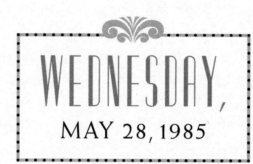

WEDNESDAY,
MAY 28, 1985

CHAPTER 39

The next morning, the dull roar of a vacuum cleaner reached down and hauled Deirdre from a deep sleep. She lay in bed, listening to the nozzle bang against the baseboards in the hallway outside her bedroom. Sounded as if her mother still hated housekeeping and was taking it out on the house.

Deirdre propped herself up on her elbows. It was half past nine already. Rain beat steadily on the window. After her talk with Henry, she'd gone for a drive to clear her head and to find an all-night drugstore where she could buy a disposable camera. Even though she hadn't gotten to sleep until well past midnight, it was the best night's sleep she'd had since she found her father's body floating in the pool.

All these years she'd blamed her father for crippling her when it was Henry who'd been driving. In the end, Henry had been crippled, too, in his own way. The two of them had more in common than she'd ever have imagined.

She got out of bed and took a quick shower. Toweled her hair dry and ran her fingers through it. Her new cut didn't need more than that.

Beyond her trench coat, she hadn't thought about what she had to wear to the funeral service. She couldn't go swanning about the chapel in leggings and a long silk shirt. Her Xeno Art T-shirt was out, too. Ditto her father's chambray shirt. Which left . . . she poked through the old clothes hanging in the closet and pulled out the navy blue, swingy tent dress that she'd worn in college before abandoning dresses for long paisley skirts or hip-hugging bell-bottoms with embroidered peasant blouses.

She slipped the dress on. It was a little tight on top but it would do. She draped her new scarf loosely around her neck and checked herself out in the full-length mirror. Innocuous. Unremarkable. Perhaps even a little retro chic. The skirt length was the only problem—it was ridiculous how short hems had been back then. But she could live with it. Besides, she'd be wearing a coat over it, so it hardly mattered.

She got her crutch and made her way out into the hall. Gloria was dusting the living room. She was wearing a dark straight skirt and matching shell she'd taken from Deirdre's closet. Too small for Deirdre, they fit her mother with room to spare.

"Would you stop!" Deirdre said. "No one's going to expect a perfectly clean house."

Gloria gave Deirdre an appraising look. "We bought that dress at Robinsons. I like it with that scarf, but—" She came over and removed the scarf from around Deirdre's neck, then redraped and tied it. "Better."

Deirdre smiled. There was the shadow of the old Gloria Unger, the woman who had a subscription to *Vogue* and bought her shoes at Delman's.

"Why don't you go wake up your brother," Gloria said.

Henry's bedroom door was closed. Deirdre rapped on it. "Henry? Henry, wake up!"

"Go away." Henry's voice was a barely audible croak.

"The car is coming for us in an hour."

"I'll drive myself over."

"You will not. Now get up!" She waited. Didn't hear anything. "Henry, are you getting up?" She pushed the door open and looked in.

The covers heaved and she heard the bed creak. "All right, all right. I'm up. Now go away."

"I'm not going until you're *up* up."

Henry picked up his head and glared at her. "I'm not getting up until you get out."

By the time a dark limousine pulled up, Henry looked sober and handsome in a dark shirt and tie and pressed jeans. Gloria looked oddly chic, certainly striking. Her growing-in hair framed her face like a dark shadow, and she wore her turban unraveled and tied loosely like a cowl around her neck. A pair of Deirdre's thick, red enameled hoop earrings gave her an exotic, Caribbean look. Her shoes were the only off note—battered black Birkenstock sandals.

Gloria stepped out into the rain, raising the cowl to loosely cover her head as she walked quickly to the car. Henry followed. Deirdre locked the door and carried a large envelope out to the black Cadillac limousine.

The driver in dark livery, the brim of his cap pulled low over a pair of wraparound sunglasses, held the door open for them. The dark interior of the car was cool and smelled of leather and Old Spice. As the car pulled away from the curb, Deirdre leaned forward and gave the driver Sy's office address.

"I see you're going incognito," Henry cracked, a comment on Deirdre's belted trench coat, head scarf, and dark glasses. Deirdre ignored him. Henry ignored her ignoring, instead practicing the informal tribute he planned to give, using notecards and talking about what Arthur had taught him to do. Play guitar, drive a car, mix drinks, pick up girls, and take all the fun out of TV movies by providing a running critique of the dialogue. By the time the limo turned into Westwood Village and pulled up in front of the three-story, pink stucco office building that housed Sy's office, Deirdre was wiping away tears.

"That was perfect," she told Henry. She was glad she'd had a chance to hear his speech.

"I don't know why you have to take care of this right now," Gloria said.

"Sy made me promise I'd leave Dad's manuscript in his office this morning. It'll just take me a minute."

Deirdre got out and speed-walked—as fast as she could with her crutch—out of the rain and in through the arched doorway marked PUBLIC PARKING. The interior, with its gated entry and ramp to upper parking levels, smelled of rubber tires and warm, moist pavement. She wondered if this had been the spot where Sy was attacked.

She pushed through a door to the building's lobby and made her way up a flight of tile-covered stairs, holding on to the wrought-iron railing. Sy's office was halfway along a shadowy, second-floor corridor that was lit by metal sconces with orangey, flame-shaped glass shades. She took off her sunglasses and unlocked the door with the key Sy had given her.

The moment Deirdre pushed open the door and set her crutch in the dark room, an alarm started to beep. She'd known it would, but still the piercing sound rattled her. She turned on the overhead light and hurried over to the wall where Sy told her she'd find the security panel, though with its flashing lights, she'd have easily found it on her own. She punched in the code and the alarm fell silent.

Deirdre turned on the lights and looked around. On a corner table, a copper lamp with a golden mica shade gave off an eerie glow. This outer room where Vera presided—Arthur used to say she was like a lioness guarding the gate—seemed smaller without Vera in it.

On the wall behind Vera's desk were two doors. One connected to Sy's office. The other was a louvered door to a walk-through supply closet. When Deirdre was little, before she started kindergarten even, she often came here with her father. While Sy talked with Arthur, he'd leave both supply closet doors and the connecting office door open so Deirdre could ride her tricycle from Vera's office to Sy's and around through the supply closet on her own miniature speedway.

Deirdre stepped into the supply closet, letting the door click shut behind her. Lines of light shined through between the slats in the door on the opposite side. Through the openings she could see Sy's massive desk, large enough for a pair of law partners to work facing each other. Behind it a pair of casement windows overlooked the street. No coats hung from a coat stand made of deer antlers, the perfect foreground for a large oil painting of a Hollywood western landscape, complete with a cowboy astride a stallion that reared against the sunrise.

At the funeral, Deirdre would let everyone she talked to know exactly where she'd left the memoir. She hoped that the person who'd been looking for it would hear. The closet would be the perfect vantage point from which to watch and see who took the bait. Deirdre slipped the disposable camera that she'd picked up the night before from her pocket, held it up to her face, and aimed the lens through an opening between the louvers. Through the viewfinder she had a perfect view of Sy's desk. She pressed the shutter. *Click. Whirr.* The film wound itself.

Deirdre left the camera within reaching distance on a shelf and pushed her way through the door at the back of the closet into Sy's office. A glass bowl filled with cellophane-wrapped peppermints was on the desk. She put her hand into it and felt around for the desk key. It was there, right where Sy said it would be. Then she unlocked the desk's wide center drawer and placed in it the envelope she'd brought with her. The words, written on the front in dark marker, would be hard to miss: *One Damned Thing After Another by Arthur Unger.*

With that, Deirdre locked the desk, just in case someone got there before she got back. She took the key with her and left, rearming the alarm on her way out. When she got down to the lobby, she put her sunglasses back on and tightened her head scarf. Then she exited through the parking garage and out into the drizzling rain. The limo was waiting at the curb.

The driver got out and opened the door for her. "All set?" he whispered.

Even she wouldn't have recognized Tyler in that uniform and sunglasses.

CHAPTER 40

The cemetery and funeral chapel were just minutes away. The limousine turned in through a driveway between buildings. Hidden behind them was an oasis of green lawn and flowers, a true secret garden that was Westwood Memorial Park. The limo pulled up in front of the path to the chapel. Its sides were lined with benches, tidy flower beds, and shrubs clipped into perfect circles and domes. It struck Deirdre how much effort had gone into controlling the outdoor space—ironic, given that death was so not something that humans could control.

The three of them got out of the car. Deirdre hooked her arm in Henry's, held her crutch in her free hand, and started up the path, through the misty rain, thick with cigarette smoke and crowded with umbrellas.

Arthur would have been pleased by the size of the crowd that overflowed the narrow A-framed chapel. Gloria embraced a man in a dark suit who greeted her and drew her over into a group. Among them, Deirdre recognized Vera, Sy's secretary. Deirdre waved, but she didn't follow. She had a mission, to get out the word that her father had written a memoir, that it had survived the fire, and that it was in Sy Sterling's office even as Sy was in the hospital recovering from being attacked.

It felt awkward at first, approaching people she recognized from the parties her parents had thrown, people who'd come over to dinner. "Yes, it's very sad. And so unexpected," she said, trying her story out first on Milton Breen and his wife, Anne. He'd been a screenwriter, now a director, who had a house with a pool up in the canyon. Arthur and Gloria had taken Deirdre and Henry there to swim before they built a pool of their own. "And then on top of everything else," Deirdre added, "the garage caught fire and we lost all the papers Dad had up in his office. Fortunately we were able to save his memoir. In it, he sets the record straight." She added, even though it sounded a bit lame, "I left the manuscript in Sy's office for safekeeping."

The Breens didn't ask which record got set straight. When she ran the same tape by Lee Golden and a man Lee introduced as another set designer, the reaction was more one of surprise. A little glee, perhaps, at whose secrets might be revealed.

As Deirdre worked her way through the crowd, she noted how each of Arthur's friends reacted to her announcement that Arthur had written a memoir. To one and all, she added that Sy would be handling its publication as soon as he was released from the hospital.

A blond woman Deirdre didn't recognize put her hand on Deirdre's arm and air kissed both her cheeks. Along with the kisses came a familiar blast of rose and jasmine mixed with musk. Probably Joy. "Deirdre darling, I was so sorry to hear about your dad," she said. The voice Deirdre knew: this was once-upon-a-time brunette Marianne Wasserman, her high school's queen bee. "You haven't changed a bit," Marianne added.

Deirdre wondered how Marianne could tell since Deirdre had on

a coat and head scarf and sunglasses. The crutch, probably. "Marianne," she said. "It's so sweet of you to come."

"You remember Nancy Kellogg?" Marianne said, indicating the
woman standing behind her. Deirdre never would have recognized
the once-chunky redhead who was now a blonde, too, and skeletal.

Deirdre slapped down the bitchy voice in her head. It was nice
of the two of them to show up, even if they hadn't known her father
at all and even if they hadn't seen or talked to Deirdre since high
school.

Nancy gave Deirdre's hand a wooden shake. "We thought Joelen
might be here," she said, rising up on her toes and looking around.
We. That made Deirdre smile. Apparently she and Marianne were still
attached at the hip.

"Oh, there's Henry," Marianne said. "Hi!" She waved at Henry,
who was on his way over to join them.

"Joelen Nichol," Deirdre said. As Henry joined the group she
shot him a look that she hoped conveyed *don't contradict me.* "Gosh. I
haven't heard from Joelen in ages. No, I doubt very much that she'll
be here. But you are, so you never know."

"Hello, Henry," Nancy said.

Henry colored slightly. "We should go in," he said. "Come on.
Let's get out of the rain. The service is supposed to start soon."

Henry started to pull Deirdre up the path to the chapel. Deirdre waggled her fingers at Marianne and Nancy and mouthed *See
you,* even though she knew that was unlikely. "Sounds like they know
you," she said to Henry under her breath.

"Knew me. Briefly. Nancy wanted to be in pictures."

"Polaroid pictures?"

Henry chuckled. "I told you, I was an asshole. Where's Mom?"

Turned out Gloria was already inside. She was sitting in the front
row, which was cordoned off for family. Mourners had already filled
about half the chairs in the chapel. Some Deirdre recognized as

family friends. Others anyone would recognize. Gene Kelly. Ernest Borgnine. Ray Bolger. They'd all worked with her dad.

As Henry walked Deirdre down the aisle, simple piano chords accompanied Ella Fitzgerald's sweet, silvery voice on the sound system. "With a Song in My Heart." Deirdre's eyes teared up. She'd helped pick the music.

Henry walked her up to the casket. Deirdre ran her hand lightly over its smooth coffered lid. The words *I'm sorry* echoed in her head. For blaming him all these years. For not accepting him for the complicated human being he was. For not getting down off her high horse, as he'd have put it, and just enjoying their time together. And for what she was about to do: run out on his funeral service. She knew it wasn't respectful, but respect had never been her father's strong suit either. Besides, she was sure he wouldn't have wanted whoever killed him to get away with it.

She sat between Henry and her mother. A movie screen was set up in the front of the chapel. When she turned to look behind her again, the rows had filled and people were standing at the back. Frank Sinatra was on the sound system now, crooning about how he'd done it *my way*. Her father might have argued with that choice— he'd always said Sinatra was a thug and a bully. But the lyrics were perfect for a man who, facing the final curtain, would have thought he'd been king.

A little while later, the lights dimmed in the chapel and the hum of voices went silent. The screen at the front of the room lit up with the words ARTHUR UNGER 1926–1985, white lettering on a royal-blue ground. There was a long pause to allow stragglers to file in, and then the back doors shut and the slides began. First was a stiff, old-world portrait of Arthur as a baby in his bearded father's arms, surrounded by his mother and three older brothers. Then, Arthur sitting on the front stoop of a New York City brownstone with one of his brothers. Arthur, handsome and muscled in bathing trunks at a pool where he'd spent summers as a lifeguard and sometime emcee at a resort in the Poconos. As a bridegroom in a dark suit, Gloria in a tailored suit, too, carrying a bouquet of roses. Both of them looked impossibly young and handsome and—Deirdre tried to find the right word—tentative.

Silence, piano chords, and Nat King Cole's smoky voice began singing. "Unforgettable" . . . Her father would have found the choice entirely too mushy, but it was Deirdre's cue. She made sure that her scarf and sunglasses were secure and leaned over to her mother and then to Henry. "I'll be right back," she told each of them. Without waiting for a response, she grabbed her crutch and made her way to the back of the chapel.

With her sunglasses on and the lights low, the audience was pretty much a sea of indistinct faces. But when Deirdre pushed into the lobby where it was brighter, she recognized the one person still out there: Detective Martinez. She appreciated that he was keeping a respectful distance from the mourners, and fortunately he was preoccupied writing some notes and didn't notice her until she was nearly to the ladies' room.

"Miss Unger?" She heard his voice as the restroom door closed behind her.

The white-and-blue Mexican-tiled room with gleaming brass fixtures was empty. No one stood at the sinks. No feet were visible under the doors to the stalls. Music from the service was muted but still audible.

Deirdre really did need to pee. While she was in the stall, she heard the door to the room creak open. Deirdre raised her feet so they weren't visible. It wouldn't be Detective Martinez. All he had to do was wait for her to reemerge. She hoped it wasn't Marianne Wasserman, concerned as she was about Deirdre's mental status.

Then she heard a woman's voice. "Zelda?"

"Thalia?" Deirdre lowered her feet. "Hang on."

"There you are," Joelen said when Deirdre opened the stall door.

255

"How do I look?" She turned around to show off a tan raincoat over a short black dress. Her hair was done up in a French twist. She turned her toes out and gave the black umbrella she was holding a Charlie Chaplin twirl.

"Perfect," Deirdre said. "But better when you're wearing this." Deirdre took off her coat and gave it to Joelen. Joelen took off hers and they swapped. Deirdre unwound her scarf and tied it around Joelen's head. Dropped her sunglasses into the pocket of the coat that Joelen was now wearing.

"Thanks for sending Tyler over to get me," Joelen said. "He's pretty cute, though I can't say I remember him."

"Well, he remembers you."

Joelen smiled. "Story of my life, but never with a happy ending."

"So far."

Joelen opened up her large black leather handbag and pulled out a blond wig. Deirdre took it from her, shook it out, and started to put it on her head.

"Wait. First you need to put this on." Joelen took out a net cap with banded edges. She snapped it over Deirdre's curls, then tucked in stray strands of hair, just like in a bathing cap.

Bing Crosby and Frank Sinatra were playing on the sound system now, singing a soused duet and proclaiming *What a swell party this is.* That meant the slide show was past its midpoint.

"Hurry up," Deirdre said, "before they send someone in looking for me."

"Don't have a cow. Hold still." Joelen eased the wig over the cap and tugged it a bit sideways, then back the other way. "There. Done." She stood back and assessed.

Deirdre turned to face the mirror and considered her own reflection. Blond bangs and shoulder-length curls framed her face.

"How do you like it?" Joelen said. "Seriously, you should consider going blond."

"I look like me with a wig on."

"That's because you know you." Joelen got out a comb and teased some of the hair on top, then smoothed it all around with her hands. "There. Fabulous."

Deirdre looked into Joelen's reflected eyes. Suddenly she was right back in Joelen's bathroom, sitting on the fluffy pink fur-covered stool and watching Joelen do her hair and makeup for Bunny's party, just hours before both of their worlds imploded.

"What?" Joelen said.

"Why did you confess if you didn't do it?"

Joelen's eyes widened. "I thought you wanted me to hurry and get back in there."

"Was it to protect your mom? Or my brother?"

After a few beats of silence, Joelen gave a tired laugh. "Does it matter at this point?"

"I don't know. It might. What if what happened twenty-two years ago isn't finished playing out? What if my father's murder is connected to what happened to Tito?" Deirdre turned to face Joelen. "So please, did you kill him?"

Joelen shook her head. She put her finger to her lips. "*Shhh*, don't tell anyone." She paused. "Did you?"

"Did I . . . ?" For a moment Deirdre was too shocked to even form a response. "Are you kidding? You're telling me that you don't know who did it?"

"Let's just say I wasn't sorry he got killed and I'm not sorry I confessed." She glanced toward the door and lowered her voice. "I thought I was protecting my mother. It worked out. I only wish that had put an end to it."

Before Deirdre could ask *Put an end to what?*, she heard a familiar piano introduction, then horns, then Louis Armstrong. "Oh, Lawd, I'm on My Way." They'd picked it not for the lyrics but because her father loved it, and because it was so deeply sad and hopeful at the same time, and because if her father had had his druthers, he'd have wanted a jazz funeral procession that stopped traffic and marched right down the middle of Avenue of the Stars in Century City, once a back lot of the studio where he'd done his finest work.

The song was the last in the medley accompanying the slide show and Deirdre's cue to get going. "Here. Take my crutch," Deirdre said, and gave it to Joelen.

Joelen gave Deirdre a pair of oversized white-rimmed sunglasses and a black umbrella. Deirdre put on the glasses and gripped the umbrella handle—flat instead of a hook. She took a few tentative steps, using it like a cane. The tip, with its corklike rubber fitting, didn't slip on the tile floor.

"Looking good," Joelen said, tightening Deirdre's head scarf around her own head and putting on Deirdre's sunglasses.

"Front row, second seat in on the left," Deirdre said. "Break a leg."

"You break a leg, too," Joelen said, giving Deirdre a hug. "Be careful, okay?" She took Deirdre's crutch and, faking a limp that made her look like Quasimodo, started for the door. "Too much?" she asked over her shoulder.

"Yeah. Dial it back, just a smidge."

CHAPTER 41

Deirdre cracked open the restroom door just in time to catch a glimpse of Detective Martinez following Joelen into the chapel. So far so good. As soon as he was gone, she hurried through the lobby and outside. The umbrella made a surprisingly serviceable substitute for her crutch.

The limousine met her as she reached the end of the walkway. Its front passenger door swung open. She got in. Tyler reached across her and pulled the door shut. "Everything okay?"

Deirdre took off Joelen's sunglasses and dropped them in her coat pocket. "So far so good."

Tyler pulled out into the street and headed back toward Westwood Village. "You were right, by the way. There's no record of a new warrant to search your house. And there's nothing in the West LAPD blotter about any mugging yesterday in or near your lawyer's office building."

"You don't think Detective Martinez was ordered up from Central Casting, too?" Deirdre said hopefully.

"No. He's real. And very competent."

Minutes later, they were double-parked in front of Sy's office. "Your car's up on the second level," Tyler said, offering Deirdre her car keys. "Why won't you tell me what you're doing? Maybe I can help."

"I'm not *doing* anything. I'm just waiting to see who shows up. I'll be invisible."

"Invisible?" He sounded skeptical. "Why do you have to do this alone?"

"I just do." Sure, something could go wrong. She was willing to put herself at risk. She wasn't willing to risk putting yet another person, someone she cared about, in danger. Her thoughtless actions had already harmed Sy. And she wasn't about to go to the police. Not yet, anyway. She was already considered a suspect, and as Sy said, once they had a suspect they did their job and built a case. "Besides, you need to go back for Gloria and Henry, and to rescue Joelen if it turns out she needs rescuing."

"Here." Tyler gave her a slip of paper. "This is the number of the car phone in this rig. Promise you'll call if you need backup. I don't want anything to happen to you."

Deirdre leaned across and kissed Tyler on the cheek. "Thanks." She got out of the car and entered the building, then turned and watched as Tyler pulled the limo away from the curb and drove off. Then she turned back. Centered herself. Reviewed her plan.

First thing she'd do would be to go into Sy's office, unlock the drawer, take out the envelope she'd left in it, and put it on top of the desk in plain sight. Then she'd settle into the closet and wait. She'd photograph, not confront, whoever came. Wait until the person was gone so she could safely emerge from hiding. Develop the snapshots, take her evidence to Sy, and together they'd bring it to the police.

Deirdre started up the stairs. The tip of the umbrella thumped each time it connected with the glazed tile floor. She was halfway down the second-floor hallway when she froze. The door to Sy's law office was ajar. Someone was already there.

She tucked the umbrella under her arm and used the wall for support so she could approach the door silently. The door hadn't been broken in, so whoever it was knew how to pick a lock and disable an alarm. She stood very still, just outside in the hall, listening for sounds. Footsteps. A cough. Anything that would tip her off to whether the person was still there.

She crept closer. Nudged the door open a bit more. It was dark in Vera's outer office. No one was in the room. But the door connecting to Sy's office was open. Creeping even closer, Deirdre heard a thump. The sound of a drawer being slammed shut? She fought the urge to flee. Instead, she forced herself to push the hall door open a bit wider. The hinge squeaked and she pulled back, waiting for someone to emerge. When no one did, she slipped inside, crossed the room, and closed herself in the supply closet.

She waited, her heart banging in her chest, afraid that any moment she'd be discovered. But still, there was silence.

Through the gaps between the louvers in the closet door, Sy's office looked empty, too. But now she heard a shuffling sound. Footsteps? She felt for the camera she'd left on the shelf and took it down.

A black shadow crossed directly in front of her. Deirdre reared back, banging her head against a shelf. The person had been moving fast and was backlit. She'd have to wait—

The phone rang.

Deirdre aimed the camera at the desk where the light on the telephone was blinking. She looked through the viewfinder.

The phone rang again. The figure came back into her field of vision, moving away from her toward the desk. A man.

Click. She took a picture.

The man picked up the phone. After a pause, he said, "I know." *Click.* Deirdre's grip tightened around the camera and she took picture after picture of the man's back, the camera whirring after each click.

He sat in the desk chair. "It's not here," he said. *Eets not hyere.* Deirdre froze. She knew this man's voice. This was no intruder. It was Sy, sitting at his own desk in his own office. He must have been released early from the hospital.

Deirdre didn't want to pop out of the closet and startle him. That was all he needed with his cracked ribs and concussion. So she crept from the closet, through Vera's office, and continued out into the hall. Pretending she'd just arrived, she rapped at the outer office door with the umbrella handle and called out, "Hello?" When Sy didn't answer, she rapped again and started through Vera's office to the open connecting door. "Anybody here?"

She entered Sy's office. He was still at his desk, now talking heatedly into the phone. When he paused, Deirdre came up behind him. "Sy?"

Startled, he swiveled to face her and did a double take. "Deirdre?"

"I didn't expect you to be here," she said, taking off her wig and the cap underneath it and shaking out her hair.

In a quiet voice, Sy said into the receiver, "I have to go." After a brief silence, he added, "I will let you know." He hung up the phone, leaned back in his chair, and gave Deirdre a wry smile.

It took a moment to register. No bandage around Sy's head. No stitches down the side of his face. No blood in his eye. He rubbed his chin, his pinkie ring catching the light. "Tests were all coming back normal. I told them I had enough. All those tubes and wires—too much for bumps and bruises."

Bumps and bruises that had miraculously vanished. Deirdre followed Sy's gaze to the foot of the deer antler coat rack. There sat a bulky briefcase that hadn't been there an hour ago. It was the same one that Sy had brought over to her father's house, the one from which he'd pulled her father's will, the one that had supposedly been stolen when he was attacked.

"The police recovered it," Sy said, answering the question Deirdre hadn't asked.

"Really?" Deirdre wanted to believe him. She wanted to believe that Sy thought he'd been mugged. That he was here in the office because he was a tough guy who'd lost patience with overcautious caregivers. That, throughout her father's life and even after his death, Sy was still her father's best friend, the surrogate uncle who'd always been there for her and Henry and always would be. "Did they catch the guy?"

"No, but they found my briefcase"—and there was just a heartbeat of hesitation, Sy's tell—"just around the corner in a Dumpster."

Sure they did. Deirdre leaned against the desk, feeling sick. Because there beside Sy was the envelope she'd locked in the drawer, the title scrawled across it in black marker. It had been torn open, and the blank sheets of paper that she'd tucked inside were strewn across the desktop.

CHAPTER 42

Sy rocked back in the desk chair and gazed at Deirdre across tented fingers. "I never thought you, of all people, would walk out on your father's funeral."

"I never thought you, of all people, would betray him."

Sy barely blinked as he held her gaze. "Oh, Deirdre. I do wish it had not come to this."

"And what exactly is *this*? You went to a lot of trouble to make us all think you'd been mugged." She knew from his bemused expression that this time she'd gotten it right. There'd been no mugging, and no police officer (phony or otherwise) showing up at the scene. Only a well-connected "victim" who could get himself checked into a tiny private clinic that specialized in cosmetic surgery where, for a fee or perhaps as a favor to one of their regular clients, the staff would pretend to care for "injuries" that had been conjured courtesy of smoke and mirrors, as Bunny would have said, along with a little help from Wardrobe and Makeup.

"I am sorry," Sy said, and he did seem genuinely saddened. "You have been caught up in this from the beginning. We tried to disentangle you. Really we did. And it *was* taken care of. Until your father decided to write a tell-all. I warned him not to. It was not worth it, no matter how much publishers were offering him."

"Publishers were making offers?"

"And a producer was eager to option the rights, according to Arthur at least. No one had actually read it, as far as I can tell. Thank God for that. And of course he hadn't finished writing it. But if there was one thing your father knew how to do, it was pitch."

"So do you really think anyone would have wanted to read it?" Deirdre asked.

"Are you kidding? It has everything. Old Hollywood, glamour, sex, intrigue, and violence. Details about a true crime that captured the imagination of a generation of moviegoers. In other words, a blockbuster. And I'm fine with that. Arthur can have his bestseller. Bunny will have her comeback. I can make all that happen. But the manuscript needs a few tweaks before it can go public. I'm already working on that. And in the meanwhile, I can't have a copy of Arthur's draft floating around."

"Arthur's draft?"

"So where is it?"

"It's in the mail."

"You mean this Xerox copy?" Sy crossed the room to his briefcase, opened it, and pulled out a FedEx envelope. He held it up so Deirdre could see her own handwriting on the mailing label. Deirdre's mouth went dry.

"I had you followed. So where's the original?" He shook the envelope at her.

"The original? Good question," Deirdre's words came out a rasp. "Because as you can see, that's a Xerox of a carbon copy. I've never seen the original. Knowing my father, I'm guessing he gave it to someone to read. Someone whose judgment he respected. Whose integrity he trusted. You."

Sy didn't bother to contradict her.

"And of course, you recognized the potential for disaster. Bunny's audience could forgive her for murdering a murderous boyfriend, but not for seducing a sixteen-year-old boy."

"Yes." Sy rubbed his chin. "It would have been a public relations nightmare. I tried to reason with him. But your father let his ego get in the way. I'm sure you can imagine."

Deirdre could. Serene in his own sense of entitlement, Arthur would have blown off his oldest friend's concerns.

"He was going to reveal details Bunny had been sure he'd never tell," Sy said.

"But he didn't know who killed Tito. He thought it was me or Henry."

"It was."

For a moment Deirdre felt short of breath. "But you told me—"

"I told you it wasn't you. Henry killed Tito."

"Henry killed Tito?" Deirdre parroted the words, but her brain wasn't taking them in. "He didn't."

"He did. He came over late that night after the party. Bunny met him. Tito discovered them together."

"But Henry told me Bunny stood him up."

"Henry lied. He's been lying for so long, I'm not sure he even knows what the truth is."

"Henry?" Deirdre felt the air go out of her. She groped behind her for a chair and sat. "It had to have been self-defense," Deirdre said, her voice sounding wooden.

"Of course it was self-defense. No jury would have found your brother guilty. He was a kid who'd gotten in way over his head. He was ready to confess. But Bunny couldn't let that happen. She'd have been pilloried for having an affair with a teenaged kid. So she called your father and when she saw him driving up, she ordered Henry to take your father's car and drive you home. She promised him that she'd take care of everything. Which she did. She called me.

"Months later, when the news stories had finally died down and

Bunny had given birth, she told Arthur that the baby was his grand-child. They struck a deal. She had me draw up a trust that your father agreed to pay into until Jackie turned twenty-one, and your father agreed he'd never tell a soul that Henry was Jackie's father. In return, Bunny would make sure the police never found out that Henry and you had been in the house at the time of the murder. She'd make sure the police never found these."

Sy rose to his feet and walked over to the coat stand. He bent, picked up his briefcase again, and brought it over to her. Deirdre knew what she'd see even before he got there—the stained yellow dress, looking no more soiled than when Bunny had taken it from her. Lying on top of the dress was the bone-handled knife. The splash Deirdre had heard had been just another of Bunny's tricks, playing to her audience's expectations.

"By the time I got to the house," Sy went on, "she'd switched knives and wiped the one that killed Tito on the dress you'd been wearing earlier that night. Always thinking ahead, you can say that for her. She showed your father the knife and the dress. Promised to give them to him after he had finished paying into the trust. Your father thought he was protecting you and Henry both. These can still be handed over to the police . . . if it becomes useful to do so. You can be sure that will never happen if you just give me the last copy of the manuscript."

"You thought the manuscript was in his office, didn't you?" Deir-dre said. "That's why you set the fire."

"Not me personally. But yes, I hired someone. I had no idea that your mother would be up there looking for the manuscript herself, or that you would come back when you did. The important thing"—Sy grabbed Deirdre's arm and pulled her close to him—"is that you give me the last copy of that manuscript. Now."

Deirdre's shoulder throbbed as Sy's grip tightened. "Is this what you tried with Dad? When persuasion and reasoning and arm-twisting didn't work, you bashed him on the head?"

Sy winced and loosened his grip. "It does not have to be this way. Your father wanted to tell his life story. He wanted to be the star. Give me the manuscript and I will do everything in my power to see that it is finished and well published."

"Too bad it has to be posthumous and filled with lies." Deirdre wrenched free and backed away.

"Not lies. Omissions."

"Henry?"

"Erased."

"Can you explain one thing to me? She could have had anyone in Hollywood. Why Henry?"

Sy seemed taken aback by the question. "He was young." Sy shrugged. "She wasn't." He shook his head. "Bunny wants what she wants, and she is used to getting it. Your father, too, in his way. He thought he was entitled to write whatever he damned well pleased. It was pure, shortsighted hubris on his part. Bunny couldn't let that happen. Too much was at stake."

"Cerulean," Deirdre said, the word sounding like air leaking from a balloon.

"You know about that?"

"Bunny had the art for the ad framed in her dressing room. All very hush-hush, or so she said."

"Selling a dream to a vast and untapped audience: women of a certain age." Sy held up his fingers as if he were framing the slogan. Like her father, he was a pro at pitching an idea. "It's going to be huge. Television ads. Free samples in the Oscar gift bags. International tour. She'll be on Johnny Carson. Barbara Walters. *Good Morning America*. She'll be getting scripts again."

"Arthur's memoir would have soured everything," Deirdre said. "Except for Walters. She'd have wanted her even more. What's more fun than a public shaming?"

"You understand. I tried to convince him of his folly. What she would do if she found out what he was up to."

"And she did find out, didn't she?"

Sy didn't say anything. He didn't need to.

"So what happens now?"

"If I'm writing it, then you give me the last copy of your father's memoir and I fix it."

"And if I don't?"

"Ah. Then Susanna comes forward and challenges your timeline. She tells the police that you left the gallery early and she finished the installation alone. Susanna, not Shoshanna, by the way."

"Susanna? You . . . ?"

"Didn't you think it was just a bit far-fetched that a prominent Israeli artist would want his work shown in a third-rate San Diego art gallery? So desperate, in fact, that he would pay for the privilege? *I yem Avram Sigismund,*" Sy said, affecting a thick accent. "*I yem very well known in Israel, but I hev to show my verk in the United States. . . .* Lucky for me, your partner cannot tell a Russian from an Israeli accent. And you still were not suspicious when, right after that, an arts reporter you never heard of calls and wants to feature your gallery in an article?"

"You bastard."

Sy looked genuinely wounded. He sat back in his chair. "I wasn't trying to hurt you. When your father told me you were going to help him get ready to move, I needed to make sure he would be alone the night Bunny and I came over to reason with him. It was a conversation I could not afford to have interrupted. I had no idea Susanna would get creative and have you paper over the gallery's windows. Or that Bunny would want to come back . . ." Sy's face fell.

"Or that I'd pick up the shovel on my way up the driveway the next morning."

"Yes. I do wish you had not done that. But let's not dwell on missteps."

The scary thing was, the scenario Sy was spinning sounded entirely plausible. Whether Deirdre had gotten to the house in time to kill her father would come down to her word against Susanna's, and her fingerprints on the murder weapon sealed it.

On the other hand, Susanna wasn't real. "How hard do you think it will be for me to discredit someone who's not even a real artist's assistant?"

"She is not. She is a rather mediocre actress. A good detective could demolish her story, and a defense attorney worth his salt could poke holes in it. But it will never come to that because after she comes forward and it becomes clear that you will be arrested and charged, you will find a quicker, cleaner way to extricate yourself." Sy paused and thought for a moment, his gaze snagging on the umbrella she was using for a cane. "A car accident, I think."

Deirdre felt as if ice water were trickling down her back. "You'd kill me?" she said, though she could see from his expression that he was dead serious.

"I am very fond of you, and it will make me very sad. So let's not find out. But there is a great deal at stake. Millions this year. More millions for years to come. Not to mention the legacy of a great actress who is far more ruthless than I. Surely we can come up with a better ending."

A better ending. As if her father could spring back to life like TV's Bobby Ewing in *Dallas*. Instead this would be the ending in which someone gets away with her father's murder.

"Step one is not negotiable," Sy said. "You give me the last copy of Arthur's memoir. In return, Susanna backs your story that you left the gallery late. And I do everything that I can to make sure you are not indicted for your father's murder. As you know, I am very good at my job." Sy picked up a chewed-on cigar from the ashtray on his desk and stuck it in the corner of his mouth. "Then we discover your father's memoir among his papers. Finished, of course. And edited slightly. But basically his life with a never-before-revealed, eyewitness account of the events surrounding Tito Acevedo's murder.

"Most of the story will be a familiar to you. The glamorous party.

You were sleeping over. Your father came back to get you. Wonderful stuff, how he comforts Bunny in her distress. She practices the confession she plans to deliver when the police get there. We take out the part where they move Tito's body from Joelen's bedroom. It just makes things more complicated than they need to be."

"Is that where Tito was killed?"

"According to Bunny"—Sy raised his eyebrows—"and on this I take her at her word, Henry burst into her bedroom, yelling at Tito to leave her alone and brandishing a knife. But he did not have the nerve to use it. Tito chased him. Henry hid in Joelen's bedroom, but Tito came after him. It was pure chance that Tito was the one who ended up dead. Pure chance that you were not there. Tito died in the bed you had been sleeping in."

Deirdre closed her eyes and for a moment she was back in Joelen's bedroom, smelling hairspray and feet and ripe pungent sawdust in the cage where Joelen's pet guinea pigs lived. *I thought I was protecting my mother.* That's why Joelen said she'd confessed. In the end, her confession had protected Bunny and Henry both.

"Like I said, we leave all that out," Sy went on. "Before the police arrive, your father drives off with you. Next thing he knows is the morning headlines: Joelen's confession and arrest for murder. We add a third act. The trial. Bunny's triumph in court. Happy ending: Justice is served. In its way."

"And Henry? Is he in the movie?"

"Who's Henry?" Sy chuckled, the sound rumbling deep in his chest.

"What about Jackie?"

"A mere footnote. Bunny will endorse the book. Publishers will be crawling all over one another to get their hands on it. Movie rights will go at auction. You and Henry will cash in. And Bunny will go back to her favorite private clinic, Beverly Medical Center, for more plastic surgery in preparation for her product launch and a starring role in the feature film. Arthur will be dancing in his grave. The changes to his story will seem minor. Believe me, he would not have cared."

"If he didn't care, then why are we here talking about this? Why is he dead?"

"Because he would not bend. Do not make the same mistake, Deirdre." Sy's jaw stiffened. "So, which will it be?" He raised his index finger. "Susanna goes to the police and tells them you had plenty of time to drive to Beverly Hills and kill your father?" He raised another finger. "Or I get the last copy of your father's memoir and turn it into a bestselling book and blockbuster movie. Arthur, played by"—he thought for a moment—"Dustin Hoffman. You? What's her name, the blonde in *Footloose*. Joelen? Maybe they'll cast an unknown. Cameos by famous aging stars, all of them publicity whores."

Deirdre held up three fingers. "Or I go through his papers, the way he asked me to. Sort. Cull. Inventory. Preserve. Certainly his memoir, even if it's unfinished, gets preserved."

"I'm running out of patience," Sy said, reaching into the desk drawer and pulling out a small silver handgun. "Do I get the manu- script or don't I?"

It wasn't the gun that scared Deirdre. It was the cold expression on Sy's face as he looked her squarely in the eye.

CHAPTER 43

I cannot believe you tossed it over the side of the road into the canyon," Sy said from the passenger seat as Deirdre pulled her car out of the parking garage. It was all she could do to keep her sweaty hands anchored on the wheel. "You did not think someone would take it?"

"Not where I left it." After her talk with Henry the night before, she'd driven around for an hour looking for somewhere to hide the manuscript. It had been much harder than she'd thought it would be to find a secure spot. Finally it had come to her: people didn't mess with roadside shrines.

"I have never needed to use this before," Sy said, looking down at the gun in his hand. "I bought it for Elenor but she would not take it."

"Guess it's not her weapon of choice," Deirdre said.

Sy ignored that. He braced himself with his other hand on the door as Deirdre rounded a corner a little too fast.

"I drove all over," Deidre said, "thinking I'd leave it in a backyard, under some bushes, buried in mulch. But these people"—she pointed up one of the driveways, where a gate led to hidden backyards—"have gardeners. Automatic sprinkler systems. Motion sensors and alarm systems."

She heard a clicking sound and glanced across at Sy. He was cocking and uncocking the gun that he held in his lap, pointing at her leg.

The car brushed the curb and Deirdre jerked the wheel. There was a deafening pop. Deirdre screamed and locked her hands on the wheel as the car slew to one side of the road and then to the other. A sulfurous smell. Was she hit? She slammed on the brakes and steered into the skid, narrowly missing a parked car.

At last she got the car under control. She took a quick glance down into her lap. In it were beige plastic shards. Pieces of dashboard.

Her heart pounded like a jackhammer and her fingers ached. That's when she realized Sy was gesticulating at her. Waving his hands, including the one holding the gun. Saying something. Shouting probably. But her ears were ringing.

Finally the ringing abated. She looked across at Sy. He was calm now, staring at the gun, white as a sheet. "Gun is loaded," he said.

No kidding. Deirdre's forehead and the back of her neck were coated with cold sweat, and she felt as if she couldn't breathe. As if there weren't enough oxygen in the car to fill her lungs. She rolled down the window. Took some deep breaths.

She glanced across again at Sy. He looked as terrified as she felt. He had the bluster to threaten, but maybe not the nerve to pull the trigger. Either way, as long as he had that thing in his hands he was dangerous.

Her heart still pounding, she turned north on Beverly Glen. The two-lane residential street, most of its houses hidden by tall bushes, climbed slowly. Deirdre steadied herself. *Keep on talking.*

"So then I thought, maybe I could hide it somewhere in a park," she said as she drove past a small park, barely big enough for a few picnickers to lay out their blankets. "In a public restroom or behind a storage shed or in a trash bin. But I couldn't trust it to remain unnoticed for long. So I thought: How do they do it in the movies? They stash things in lockers in bus or train stations. But do they still have storage lockers? And is there even such a thing as a bus or train station within striking distance of Beverly Hills? Which got me thinking about a locker at a country club."

Her ears popped as they climbed higher and higher. Farther up, the houses were more modest and the road narrowed. Finally she turned onto Mulholland right behind a red Porsche that was moving fast. Deirdre kept on its tail, hoping she was making an impression, that the driver would remember her if anything bad happened.

"Which could have worked except I don't belong to a country club."

Sy held on to the door. He looked like he was about to be carsick. The gun was still in his hand, pointed at her, his finger still on the trigger.

"It's not much farther," Deirdre said. "Would you quit messing with that thing? I know you don't want to shoot me while I'm driving."

"I do not want to shoot you at all."

Deirdre turned tighter than she needed to coming around a bend. Tires screeched and Sy braced himself against the door. But still he held on to the gun. The turnout was just ahead. At least in a few moments they'd be out of the car.

She still hadn't caught her breath when she pulled the car off the road and into the same parking area where she'd spun out, day before yesterday. There were no bikers there today, just a battered, orange-and-white VW bus and an older couple standing at the opposite end of the overlook, taking in the view of the Valley.

Dust settled around Deirdre's car. She started to open the door.

"Not yet." He had the gun steady and pointed directly at her. "First, where is it?"

Deirdre swallowed. "It's over there." She pointed to the tree twenty feet down off the side of the road, its base crowded with mementos of people who'd been injured or lost their lives.

Sy took the keys from the ignition, grabbed Deirdre's umbrella, and got out of the car. He motioned for her to get out, too. She did. He looked around, casting a nervous glance in the direction of the couple. They weren't paying attention to anything but the view.

"Suicide Bend," Sy said, reading the sign and edging closer to the guardrail. He looked over, then gazed up toward the tree branch where the car bumper twisted in the wind. "I guess you are not the only person who got hurt here."

Deirdre limped over to the stretch of guardrail closest to the tree. "I threw it from here."

Sy stared down the steep incline. "Go get it."

"I can't—"

"Then you should not have thrown it." Sy passed her the umbrella she'd been using in place of her crutch.

Deirdre sat on the guardrail. "Or we could just leave it there and it will be our little secret. I'll never tell."

Sy gave her a long, steady look. "You know I cannot risk that. Think of this as part of your role as your father's literary executor."

Deirdre almost laughed. What she was about to do was a gross perversion of the role her father had bestowed upon her. "You're only going to change what he wrote."

"It will still be Arthur Unger's story. Boy from the Bronx makes good. Think about how he would feel if the choice were between dooming it to obscurity or twisting it a bit and making it a smash."

"You must have tried that argument out on him."

"And I think he would have come around. Eventually. But not everyone is as patient as I am."

The worst part was, Deirdre knew Sy was right. She set the tip of the umbrella into the wet soil at the top of the embankment and swung her legs over. Next to the teddy bear and beside a fresh bouquet of flowers, she could see the glint of shiny foil in which she'd wrapped the manuscript. If she gave it to Sy, no one would know that the father of Bunny's son had been a sixteen-year-old kid. Henry could go on pretending to be a friend of the family, taking his son under his wing like a big brother. No one would know that Henry killed Tito.

What would her father have wanted? She knew the answer to that. He'd have wanted to be played by Jack Nicholson.

What mattered to Deirdre? That took her a few moments.

She turned back to Sy. "Will you tell me one thing?"

"Maybe."

"Did you kill my dad?"

"No." Sy's voice was firm. She wasn't sure if it was regret or annoyance that flickered across his face. "But I will say that I did, if it comes to that. I will be very convincing. People who confess to protect people they love can even come to believe the lie."

"Bunny killed him, didn't she?" Deirdre said.

Sy's expression didn't change, but that told her all she needed to know.

Deirdre stood, set the tip of the umbrella in the harder-packed soil farther in from the guardrail. Carefully she began to descend toward the base of the tree.

ALMOST TWO YEARS LATER, WEDNESDAY,
MARCH 11, 1987

CHAPTER 44

Silver-haired Johnny Carson bounced a pencil on his desk and raised a hand in a salute to his audience. "My guest tonight is one of the most glamorous movie stars of all time. When her name was on the marquee, bam, they came. Her new movie is about to open, and it's both a public and a very personal triumph. Would you please join me in welcoming the one, the only"—the camera shifted to a robin's-egg blue curtain that drew aside—"Elenor Nichol."

Orchestral fanfare and long, sustained applause exploded as Bunny, her eyes wide, red lips glistening against white teeth, stood framed by the curtain. She wore a slinky black gown. A diamond brooch sparkled at her slender waist, and diamond chandelier earrings grazed her porcelain shoulders. Her black hair was piled high on her head, with tendrils curling down her back.

"She looks spectacular," Deirdre said, watching the show from the bed she now shared with Tyler in their arts-and-crafts bungalow in Los Feliz Village. Deirdre's share of the income from her father's book and the movie deal had been enough for half the down payment on the house and a year's rent on a storefront on Hollywood Boulevard where she'd soon open her own art gallery. Deirdre and Henry had given a share of their earnings to Gloria, who'd opened a yoga and meditation studio at a hot springs resort between Death Valley and Las Vegas.

On TV, Bunny put her hand over her mouth as the applause continued. She seemed genuinely overwhelmed. Carson got up and offered her his hand, then gave a mock bow all the way down on one knee, like he was waiting to be knighted. Bunny smiled as he stood, offered her his arm, and led her over to the guest chair.

When the applause died down, Carson sat and rested his arms on his desk. "As you can hear, you've been missed."

"Thank you. This means so much to me." Bunny leaned forward as if sharing a confidence, her cleavage swelling. "You're all so kind. You know, I never really meant to leave Hollywood. I just needed time." She shifted in the chair, crossing her leg so that her thigh peeked through a slit in the skirt. "Time to find myself."

"And I trust you have," Carson said, glancing at her leg and giving the audience one of his trademark smirks. Then he smiled graciously at Bunny. "We're glad to have you back. You're a true movie star legend."

"You make me sound like an anachronism." She gave him a sly look. "But I am happy."

"Is it your work or something personal?"

"Probably the work. But who can tell? Regret can be very disabling. It took me a long time to learn to let it go."

He smiled an impish grin. "Screw regret."

Bunny gave a *naughty boy* shake of her head. "Am I being good? Am I being bad? Am I this? Am I that? Who cares? Let it all go. I've learned to live with my past. But I do have a few scars." She widened the slit in her skirt to expose her knee. "Can you see my boo-boos?"

"You want to show them to us?"

The audience howled.

Bunny smiled. Blushed.

Carson spread his arms, like he couldn't help himself. "Might there be a new man in your life? Because behind every great woman is a great behind."

The audience laughed, and Bunny turned to them. "Now you all have to stop egging him on."

As the audience response faded, Johnny's look turned serious. "Okay, so you've let it go. You've . . . um . . ." He bounced a pencil on the desk.

"Finished my *film*." Bunny turned to the audience, spread her hands, and was rewarded with applause.

"You want to talk about your film? What's it called?"

"You know what it's called."

"*Notorio*," Carson said, and music swelled, violins in a syncopated tango with flourishes from a snare drum. A movie poster came up. There was Bunny in the same long black dress, waves of long black hair framing her face, wrapped in a dance embrace with her Latin lover. Deirdre could hear Tito's voice whispering in her ear. Yes, it was about the connection.

"*Notorio*," Bunny said. "With Tito Altavista."

"Tito?"

"Just a coincidence."

"In Hollywood, there's no such thing as coincidence."

"He's a young Fernando Lamas."

"Fernando Lamas."

"It was a great experience."

"With Tito Altavista?"

She looked toward the audience. "Yes."

"Have you ever worked with Fernando Lamas?"

Bunny ignored that. "The movie opens in Los Angeles tomorrow."

"And are you having fun with this new movie?"

"I never do anything I don't enjoy," Bunny said without a hint of irony. "Not anymore."

Johnny raised his eyebrows. "I can certainly relate to that."

Bunny tucked her knee demurely back into her skirt.

On the screen now was the cover of Arthur's book. Johnny said, "I understand the movie is based on a book written by an old friend of yours."

True to Sy's word, as soon as Deirdre had given him the manuscript, Shoshanna/Susanna had showed up to confirm Deirdre's story. Shortly after that, the shovel mysteriously disappeared from police evidence, and a few months later, Arthur's death was ruled *by misadventure*. Six months later, Arthur's memoir, *One Damned Thing After Another*, was published. The movie's publicity rollout had pushed it onto the *New York Times* bestseller list.

"Yes. Arthur Unger is"—Bunny gave her head a sad shake—"*was* a writer. A huge talent. One of Hollywood's greats. And one of its most underappreciated. Maybe now the Academy will recognize his work."

The book cover faded and was replaced by a head shot of Arthur himself taken back in the early days, the kind of black-and-white publicity still that the studio had taken of all its contract talent. Then the picture of Arthur faded, replaced by a still from the movie, Bunny and Jerry Orbach in Bunny's pink bedroom with the actor Tito Altavista dead on the floor with a knife sticking out of his abdomen.

Jerry Orbach wasn't Jack Nicholson or Dustin Hoffman—not A-list enough to share the limelight on the *Tonight* show with Bunny, which was probably just as well. But he was smart, handsome, and a terrific actor. A Broadway song-and-dance man, too. Arthur would have appreciated that.

On TV, Carson asked Bunny, "I understand you worked with Mr. Unger on his book."

"Yes. We collaborated before his tragic death."

Collaborated? That made Deirdre laugh out loud.

"In fact, we talked about it the very day he died. Ironic, don't you think?" Bunny pursed her lips. That brazen admission took Deirdre's breath away.

"And I understand Arthur Unger was not just a friend of yours," Carson said. "His book gives an inside look at the most tragic event in your life, a murder almost twenty-five years ago that got worldwide headlines. People still haven't forgotten. It's something you have never talked about publicly before."

"And I'm not starting now."

"So if we want to know—"

"Go see the movie. It's always better than real life."

The camera held for a moment on Carson's face, his eyebrows raised in dismay. "You heard what the lady said. See the film. And with that . . ." he said and pointed off camera.

The TV went to commercial, and there was Bunny again, wearing another low-cut, slinky black dress adorned with diamonds. Deirdre had the odd sensation that she was in Bunny Nichol's dressing room again, the mirrored walls reflecting and reflecting back infinite images of the glamorous star. It wouldn't have surprised her if the doorbell rang to reveal yet another Bunny, this one in person. Except Deirdre hadn't seen or spoken to Bunny Nichol, not since Bunny had pretended to toss the bloodied dress and the knife into her pool. Joelen had ended up brokering the sale of Arthur's house for $1.1 million. That someone had died there in mysterious circumstances only increased the interest in the property. It was, after all, Hollywood. Deirdre and Joelen hadn't spoken since the closing.

During the commercial for Cerulean, violins, piano, and finally an accordion swelled to a tango rhythm. A tall, slender man dressed all in black moved slowly away from the camera toward Bunny, took her in his arms, twirled her once, twice, then bent her backward. The scene dissolved to a close-up of Bunny raising a bottle of Cerulean as if in a champagne toast, arching her head back and spraying her neck with the perfume. In smoke, words wrote themselves out on the screen in front of her.

Because

you're a woman

"Cerulean," Bunny's voice whispered as the words dissolved into a skim of mist that took over the screen and slowly dissipated to reveal a bottle of the perfume.

Deirdre turned the television off.

"That woman is a piece of work," Tyler said.

"She is that," Deirdre said.

"And she makes it sound as if the story is all about her."

"It always is."

Deirdre had been invited to a screening of the movie. She and Henry had gone together. The movie echoed *Sunset Boulevard* without the grit and irony, with the screenwriter aging and the Hollywood star young and glamorous. Arthur's life story was relegated to a few meager flashbacks.

In the movie's climactic scene, Tito works himself into a jealous rage. He hits Bunny repeatedly, then grabs the strand of pearls she's wearing around her neck, twists it tight, and starts to strangle her. Bunny's mouth opens in a silent scream, her eyes go wide, and her face turns red. Joelen, played by Winona Ryder, screams at him from the bedroom doorway to stop. Tito drops Bunny and pivots toward Joelen, fingers flexed.

Bunny screams. She sees Joelen has a knife. Tito does not. He lunges for Joelen.

The camera lingers on Tito's face. Stunned. On Joelen's face. Shocked. On Bunny's face. Horrified. Then the camera pans back as Tito drops to the floor, rolls over onto his back, his glazed eyes staring up at the ceiling.

In the movie, there was not a whiff of Deirdre's presence at the house that night. No trace of Henry's role in the tragedy, either. Henry still had no idea how close he'd come to being thrust into the limelight. Charged with murder. Revealed as the father of Bunny's son.

After they sold Arthur's house, Henry quit his job at the motorcycle dealership and used his share of their earnings to buy a one-story fixer-upper on a canal in Venice. In the garage, he'd opened a small recording studio.

Audio of Bunny's testimony before the coroner's jury had played as the movie's final credits rolled. Sy had gotten Arthur a posthumous screenwriting credit, even though he'd never actually touched the screenplay.

"How would your father feel about the way she hijacked his story?" Tyler asked.

Deirdre paused. How would Arthur have felt? He knew writers got no respect. That his job was to put words on the pages of scripts that directors and actors inevitably rewrote, mangled, or ignored. But now he had a bestselling book. A major motion picture. Earnings that could have easily have paid for a bigger swimming pool and a credit that might yet garner an Academy Award nomination. He was still in the game.

"He'd have been thrilled," Deirdre said.

AUTHOR'S NOTE

Like any young girl growing up in Beverly Hills, I was fascinated by the 1958 murder of Johnny Stompanato. I was ten years old, and I can remember poring over the pictures and articles that ran in the newspapers. The house where it happened was just a few blocks from where we lived, and Cheryl Crane, Lana Turner's daughter who confessed to stabbing her mother's gangster boyfriend to death, was just four years older than me.

Readers may recognize the crime as one of the inspirations for this book. But in researching *Night Night, Sleep Tight,* beyond rereading news accounts that ran at the time of the crime, I deliberately avoided learning anything about the people involved in the real crime. Instead I took the murder and its trappings, along with my own visceral response to it years ago, as a jumping-off point for an entirely fictional story with fictional characters I could build from the ground up.

ABOUT THE AUTHOR

HALLIE EPHRON is the bestselling, award-winning author of suspense novels. Her novels have been finalists for the Edgar, Anthony, and Mary Higgins Clark awards. With *Night Night, Sleep Tight*, she takes readers back to early-'60s Beverly Hills, a time and place she knows intimately. She grew up there, the third of four daughters of Hollywood screenwriting duo Henry and Phoebe Ephron, contract writers for Twentieth Century Fox who wrote screenplays for classics like *Carousel* and *Desk Set*. Ms. Ephron's novels have been called "Hitchcockian" by *USA Today*, and "deliciously creepy" by *Publishers Weekly*. Her award-winning bestseller *Never Tell a Lie* was made into a movie for the Lifetime Movie Network. Her essays have been broadcast on NPR and appeared in magazines including *More*, *Writer's Digest*, and *O: The Oprah Magazine* ("Growing Up Ephron"). She writes a regular crime fiction book review column for the *Boston Globe*. Ms. Ephron lives near Boston with her husband.